P9-CEC-594

Injury & Trauma Sourcebook

Learning Disabilities Sourcebook, 4th Edition

Leukemia Sourcebook

Liver Disorders Sourcebook

Medical Tests Sourcebook, 4th Edition

Men's Health Concerns Sourcebook, 4th Edition

Mental Health Disorders Sourcebook, 5th Edition

Mental Retardation Sourcebook

Movement Disorders Sourcebook, 2nd Edition

Multiple Sclerosis Sourcebook

Muscular Dystrophy Sourcebook

Obesity Sourcebook

Osteoporosis Sourcebook

Pain Sourcebook, 4th Edition

Pediatric Cancer Sourcebook

Physical & Mental Issues in Aging Sourcebook

Podiatry Sourcebook, 2nd Edition

Pregnancy & Birth Sourcebook, 3rd Edition

Prostate & Urological Disorders Sourcebook

Prostate Cancer Sourcebook

Rehabilitation Sourcebook

Respiratory Disorders Sourcebook, 3rd Edition

Sexually Transmitted Diseases Sourcebook,
5th Edition

Sleep Disorders Sourcebook, 3rd Edition

Smoking Concerns Sourcebook

Sports Injuries Sourcebook, 4th Edition

Stress-Related Disorders Sourcebook, 3rd Edition

Stroke Sourcebook, 3rd Edition

Surgery Sourcebook, 3rd Edition

Thyroid Disorders Sourcebook

Transplantation Sourcebook

Traveler's Health Sourcebook

Urinary Tract & Kidney Diseases & Disorders
Sourcebook, 2nd Edition

Vegetarian Sourcebook

Women's Health Concerns Sourcebook, 4th Edition

Workplace Health & Safety Sourcebook

Worldwide Health Sourcebook

Teen Health Series

Abuse & Violence Information for Teens

Accident & Safety Information for Teens

Alcohol Information for Teens,
3rd Edition

Allergy Information for Teens,
2nd Edition

Asthma Information for Teens,
2nd Edition

Body Information for Teens

Cancer Information for Teens,
3rd Edition

Complementary & Alternative
Medicine Information for Teens,
2nd Edition

Diabetes Information for Teens,
2nd Edition

Diet Information for Teens, 3rd Edition

Drug Information for Teens, 3rd Edition

Eating Disorders Information for Teens,
3rd Edition

Fitness Information for Teens,
3rd Edition

Learning Disabilities Information for
Teens

Mental Health Information for Teens,
4th Edition

Pregnancy Information for Teens,
2nd Edition

Sexual Health Information for Teens,
3rd Edition

Skin Health Information for Teens,
3rd Edition

Sleep Information for Teens

Sports Injuries Information for Teens,
3rd Edition

Stress Information for Teens,
2nd Edition

Suicide Information for Teens,
2nd Edition

Tobacco Information for Teens,
2nd Edition

Child Abuse

SOURCEBOOK

Third Edition

Health Reference Series

Third Edition

Child Abuse

SOURCEBOOK

Basic Consumer Health Information about Child Neglect and the Physical, Sexual, and Emotional Abuse of Children, Including Abusive Head Trauma, Bullying, Munchausen by Proxy Syndrome, Statutory Rape, Incest, Educational Neglect, Exploitation, and the Long-Term Consequences of Child Maltreatment, Featuring Facts about Risk Factors, Prevention Initiatives, Reporting Requirements, Legal Interventions, Child Protective Services, and Therapy Options

Along with Information for Parents, Foster Parents, and Adult Survivors of Child Abuse, a Glossary of Related Terms, and Directories of Additional Resources

Edited by
Valarie R. Juntunen, RN

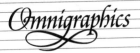

155 W. Congress, Suite 200, Detroit, MI 48226

Bibliographic Note

Because this page cannot legibly accommodate all the copyright notices, the Bibliographic Note portion of the Preface constitutes an extension of the copyright notice.

Edited by Valarie R. Juntunen, RN

Health Reference Series

Karen Bellenir, *Managing Editor*
David A. Cooke, MD, FACP, *Medical Consultant*
Elizabeth Collins, *Research and Permissions Coordinator*
EdIndex, Services for Publishers, *Indexers*

* * *

Omnigraphics, Inc.

Matthew P. Barbour, *Senior Vice President*
Kevin M. Hayes, *Operations Manager*

* * *

Peter E. Ruffner, *Publisher*

Copyright © 2013 Omnigraphics, Inc.

ISBN 978-0-7808-1277-2

E-ISBN 978-0-7808-1278-9

Library of Congress Cataloging-in-Publication Data

Child abuse sourcebook : basic consumer health information about child neglect and the physical, sexual, and emotional abuse of children, including abusive head trauma, bullying, Munchausen by proxy syndrome, statutory rape, incest, educational neglect, exploitation, and the long-term consequences of child maltreatment, featuring facts about risk factors, prevention initiatives, reporting requirements, legal interventions, child protective services, and therapy options, along with information for parents, foster parents, and adult survivors of child abuse, a glossary of related terms, and directories of additional resources / edited by Valarie R. Juntunen.
    pages cm. -- (Health reference series)
  Includes bibliographical references and index.
  Summary: "Provides basic consumer health information about abuse and neglect of children and adolescents, along with facts about prevention and intervention strategies and treatment for survivors of abuse. Includes index, glossary of related terms, and other resources"--Provided by publisher.
  ISBN 978-0-7808-1277-2 (hardcover : alk. paper) 1. Child abuse--United States. 2. Child abuse--United States--Prevention. 3. Abused children--United States. I. Juntunen, Valarie R.
  HV6626.52.C557 2013
  362.76--dc23
                                                                    2013001120

Table of Contents

Visit www.healthreferenceseries.com to view *A Contents Guide to the Health Reference Series*, a listing of more than 16,000 topics and the volumes in which they are covered.

Part IV: Adult Survivors of Child Abuse

Preface

About This Book

According to the U.S. Department of Health and Human Services, state and local child protective services in the United States annually receive more than three million reports of child abuse or neglect. Child maltreatment can create visible welts, bruises, and broken bones, or it can be invisible, producing deep emotional scars and life-long mental health challenges. Children who have been the victims of abuse or neglect can experience alterations in brain chemistry, difficulty with social interaction, physical injuries, and even death.

Child Abuse Sourcebook, Third Edition provides updated information about child neglect and the physical, emotional, and sexual abuse of children, including facts about severe punishment, abusive head trauma, Munchausen by proxy syndrome, rape, incest, exploitation, medical neglect, educational neglect, bullying, and aggression through technology. The book explains the differences between situations that require legal intervention and those considered to be parental choices, even when controversial. Facts about child protective services and interventions by the court system are also included. Parenting issues that may relate to child abuse risks, including domestic violence, postpartum depression, military service, substance abuse, and disciplinary strategies, are addressed, and information for adult survivors of child abuse is provided. The volume concludes with a glossary, a state-by-state list of contact information for reporting suspected child maltreatment, and a directory of resources for finding additional help and information.

How to Use This Book

This book is divided into parts and chapters. Parts focus on broad areas of interest. Chapters are devoted to single topics within a part.

Part I: Child Maltreatment explains the types of intentional actions that U.S. state laws typically recognize as forms of abuse. These include physical abuse, sexual abuse and exploitation, emotional abuse, neglect, and abandonment. Related issues, including bullying and exposure to violence, are also explored. The part concludes with a discussion regarding the physical, psychological, behavioral, and societal consequences of child maltreatment.

Part II: Physical and Sexual Abuse of Children concerns itself with modes of maltreatment that result from physical actions, including family violence, harsh corporal punishment, abusive head trauma (shaken baby syndrome), and Munchausen by proxy syndrome. It also reports on the physical and behavioral indicators of sexual abuse and provides facts about incest and abuse in dating relationships, and it discusses statutory rape laws.

Part III: Child Neglect and Emotional Abuse provides information about forms of abuse that are generally less visible than physical abuse. These can result from the failure of a parent or guardian to take appropriate action on a child's behalf—such as refusing to seek medical care or education—or from other behaviors that negatively impact a child's mental development or psychological wellbeing.

Part IV: Adult Survivors of Child Abuse explains the long-term consequences of experiencing maltreatment during childhood, and it discusses the outcomes that may emerge in adulthood. Mental health issues related to the vestiges of child abuse are also addressed, and the link between child abuse and adult suicide risk is explored.

Part V: Child Abuse Preventions, Interventions, and Treatments reports on various strategies, laws, and regulations intended to reduce the incidence of child abuse. It explains how child protective services can intervene in suspected abuse cases, and it describes therapy options for children and adults who have been impacted by abuse.

Part VI: Parenting Issues and Child Abuse Risks describes some of the most common family challenges that place children in dangerous situations, including domestic violence, mental health issues, parental substance abuse, and inappropriate forms of discipline. It provides tips for improving parenting skills and also offers suggestions for foster and adoptive parents.

Part VII: Additional Help and Information includes a glossary of terms related to child abuse and child protective services, a state-by-state list of contact information for reporting suspected child maltreatment, and a directory of organizations involved in efforts to end child abuse and heal its effects.

Bibliographic Note

This volume contains documents and excerpts from publications issued by the following U.S. government agencies: Administration for Children and Families; Center for Sex Offender Management; Centers for Disease Control and Prevention; Child Welfare Information Gateway; Children's Bureau; Federal Trade Commission; Office on Women's Health; Substance Abuse and Mental Health Services Administration; U.S. Department of Health and Human Services; U.S. Department of Justice; and the U.S. Department of Veterans Affairs.

In addition, this volume contains copyrighted documents from the following organizations, publications, and individuals: Adults Surviving Child Abuse; American Psychological Association; Association for Play Therapy; Australian Institute of Family Studies, Commonwealth of Australia; BioMed Central, Ltd.; *BMC Psychiatry*; Coalition for Children; Court Appointed Special Advocates for Children; Crime Victims' Institute; Education Development Center, Inc.; Future of Children; Helpguide.org; International Initiative to End Child Labor; Dori L. Johnson; Liberty House Center; Massachusetts Children's Trust Fund; McGill Publications; National Center on Shaken Baby Syndrome; National Court Appointed Special Advocates (CASA) Association; Nemours Foundation; North Texas State Hospital; Northern Rocky Mountain Educational Research Association; Ontario Consultants on Religious Tolerance; Prevent Child Abuse America; Rape, Abuse, and Incest National Network; Safe 4Athletes; Sage Publications; Stacey L. Shipley; Stop It Now; University of Michigan Health System; Vanderbilt University, Maternal Infant Health Outreach Worker Program; Virginia Cooperative Extension, Virginia Polytechnic Institute and State University; Witness Justice; and the Woodrow Wilson School of Public and International Affairs at Princeton University.

Full citation information is provided on the first page of each chapter or section. Every effort has been made to secure all necessary rights to reprint the copyrighted material. If any omissions have been made, please contact Omnigraphics to make corrections for future editions.

Acknowledgements

Thanks go to the many organizations, agencies, and individuals who have contributed materials for this *Sourcebook* and to medical consultant Dr. David Cooke and prepress services provider WhimsyInk. Special thanks go to managing editor Karen Bellenir and permissions coordinator Liz Collins for their help and support.

About the Health Reference Series

The *Health Reference Series* is designed to provide basic medical information for patients, families, caregivers, and the general public. Each volume takes a particular topic and provides comprehensive coverage. This is especially important for people who may be dealing with a newly diagnosed disease or a chronic disorder in themselves or in a family member. People looking for preventive guidance, information about disease warning signs, medical statistics, and risk factors for health problems will also find answers to their questions in the *Health Reference Series*. The *Series*, however, is not intended to serve as a tool for diagnosing illness, in prescribing treatments, or as a substitute for the physician/patient relationship. All people concerned about medical symptoms or the possibility of disease are encouraged to seek professional care from an appropriate healthcare provider.

A Note about Spelling and Style

Health Reference Series editors use *Stedman's Medical Dictionary* as an authority for questions related to the spelling of medical terms and the *Chicago Manual of Style* for questions related to grammatical structures, punctuation, and other editorial concerns. Consistent adherence is not always possible, however, because the individual volumes within the *Series* include many documents from a wide variety of different producers and copyright holders, and the editor's primary goal is to present material from each source as accurately as is possible following the terms specified by each document's producer. This sometimes means that information in different chapters or sections may follow other guidelines and alternate spelling authorities. For example, occasionally a copyright holder may require that eponymous terms be shown in possessive forms (Crohn's disease *vs.* Crohn disease) or that British spelling norms be retained (leukaemia *vs.* leukemia).

Locating Information within the Health Reference Series

The *Health Reference Series* contains a wealth of information about a wide variety of medical topics. Ensuring easy access to all the fact sheets, research reports, in-depth discussions, and other material contained within the individual books of the series remains one of our highest priorities. As the *Series* continues to grow in size and scope, however, locating the precise information needed by a reader may become more challenging.

A Contents Guide to the Health Reference Series was developed to direct readers to the specific volumes that address their concerns. It presents an extensive list of diseases, treatments, and other topics of general interest compiled from the Tables of Contents and major index headings. To access *A Contents Guide to the Health Reference Series*, visit www.healthreferenceseries.com.

Medical Consultant

Medical consultation services are provided to the *Health Reference Series* editors by David A. Cooke, MD, FACP. Dr. Cooke is a graduate of Brandeis University, and he received his M.D. degree from the University of Michigan. He completed residency training at the University of Wisconsin Hospital and Clinics. He is board-certified in Internal Medicine. Dr. Cooke currently works as part of the University of Michigan Health System and practices in Ann Arbor, MI. In his free time, he enjoys writing, science fiction, and spending time with his family.

Our Advisory Board

We would like to thank the following board members for providing guidance to the development of this series:

Dr. Lynda Baker, Associate Professor of Library and Information Science, Wayne State University, Detroit, MI

Nancy Bulgarelli, William Beaumont Hospital Library, Royal Oak, MI

Karen Imarisio, Bloomfield Township Public Library, Bloomfield Township, MI

Karen Morgan, Mardigian Library, University of Michigan-Dearborn, Dearborn, MI

Rosemary Orlando, St. Clair Shores Public Library, St. Clair Shores, MI

Health Reference Series *Update Policy*

The inaugural book in the *Health Reference Series* was the first edition of *Cancer Sourcebook* published in 1989. Since then, the *Series* has been enthusiastically received by librarians and in the medical community. In order to maintain the standard of providing high-quality health information for the layperson the editorial staff at Omnigraphics felt it was necessary to implement a policy of updating volumes when warranted.

Medical researchers have been making tremendous strides, and it is the purpose of the *Health Reference Series* to stay current with the most recent advances. Each decision to update a volume is made on an individual basis. Some of the considerations include how much new information is available and the feedback we receive from people who use the books. If there is a topic you would like to see added to the update list, or an area of medical concern you feel has not been adequately addressed, please write to:

Editor
Health Reference Series
Omnigraphics, Inc.
155 W. Congress, Suite 200
Detroit, MI 48226
E-mail: editorial@omnigraphics.com

Part One

Child Maltreatment

Chapter 1

Defining Child Maltreatment

Chapter Contents

Section 1.1

Understanding Child Abuse and Neglect

Recognizing and Preventing Child Abuse

Child abuse is more than bruises and broken bones. While physical abuse might be the most visible, other types of abuse, such as emotional abuse and neglect, also leave deep, lasting scars. The earlier abused children get help, the greater chance they have to heal and break the cycle—rather than perpetuating it. By learning about common signs of abuse and what you can do to intervene, you can make a huge difference in a child's life.

Child Abuse Hotlines

- US or Canada: 1-800-422-4453 (Childhelp)
- UK: 0800 1111 (NSPCC Childline)
- Australia: 1800 688 009 (CAPS)
- New Zealand: 0800-543-754 (Kidsline)
- Other international helplines: ChiWorld.org

Understanding Child Abuse and Neglect

Child abuse is more than bruises or broken bones. While physical abuse is shocking due to the scars it leaves, not all child abuse is as obvious. Ignoring children's needs, putting them in unsupervised, dangerous situations, or making a child feel worthless or stupid are also child abuse. Regardless of the type of child abuse, the result is serious emotional harm.

Myths and Facts about Child Abuse and Neglect

MYTH #1: It's only abuse if it's violent. Fact: Physical abuse is just one type of child abuse. Neglect and emotional abuse can be just as damaging, and since they are more subtle, others are less likely to intervene.

MYTH #2: Only bad people abuse their children. Fact: While it's easy to say that only "bad people" abuse their children, it's not always so black and white. Not all abusers are intentionally harming their children. Many have been victims of abuse themselves, and don't know any other way to parent. Others may be struggling with mental health issues or a substance abuse problem.

MYTH #3: Child abuse doesn't happen in "good" families. Fact: Child abuse doesn't only happen in poor families or bad neighborhoods. It crosses all racial, economic, and cultural lines. Sometimes, families who seem to have it all from the outside are hiding a different story behind closed doors.

MYTH #4: Most child abusers are strangers. Fact: While abuse by strangers does happen, most abusers are family members or others close to the family.

MYTH #5: Abused children always grow up to be abusers. Fact: It is true that abused children are more likely to repeat the cycle as adults, unconsciously repeating what they experienced as children. On the other hand, many adult survivors of child abuse have a strong motivation to protect their children against what they went through and become excellent parents.

Effects of Child Abuse and Neglect

All types of child abuse and neglect leave lasting scars. Some of these scars might be physical, but emotional scarring has long lasting effects throughout life, damaging a child's sense of self, ability to have healthy relationships, and ability to function at home, at work and at school. Some effects include:

- **Lack of trust and relationship difficulties:** If you can't trust your parents, who can you trust? Abuse by a primary caregiver damages the most fundamental relationship as a child—that you will safely, reliably get your physical and emotional needs met by the person who is responsible for your care. Without this base, it is very difficult to learn to trust people or know who is

5

trustworthy. This can lead to difficulty maintaining relationships due to fear of being controlled or abused. It can also lead to unhealthy relationships because the adult doesn't know what a good relationship is.

- **Core feelings of being "worthless" or "damaged":** If you've been told over and over again as a child that you are stupid or no good, it is very difficult to overcome these core feelings. You may experience them as reality. Adults may not strive for more education, or settle for a job that may not pay enough, because they don't believe they can do it or are worth more. Sexual abuse survivors, with the stigma and shame surrounding the abuse, often especially struggle with a feeling of being damaged.

- **Trouble regulating emotions:** Abused children cannot express emotions safely. As a result, the emotions get stuffed down, coming out in unexpected ways. Adult survivors of child abuse can struggle with unexplained anxiety, depression, or anger. They may turn to alcohol or drugs to numb out the painful feelings.

Types of Child Abuse

There are several types of child abuse, but the core element that ties them together is the emotional effect on the child. Children need predictability, structure, clear boundaries, and the knowledge that their parents are looking out for their safety. Abused children cannot predict how their parents will act. Their world is an unpredictable, frightening place with no rules. Whether the abuse is a slap, a harsh comment, stony silence, or not knowing if there will be dinner on the table tonight, the end result is a child that feel unsafe, uncared for, and alone.

Emotional Child Abuse

Sticks and stones may break my bones but words will never hurt me? Contrary to this old saying, emotional abuse can severely damage a child's mental health or social development, leaving lifelong psychological scars. Examples of emotional child abuse include:

- Constant belittling, shaming, and humiliating a child

- Calling names and making negative comparisons to others

- Telling a child he or she is "no good," "worthless," "bad," or "a mistake"

- Frequent yelling, threatening, or bullying
- Ignoring or rejecting a child as punishment, giving him or her the silent treatment
- Limited physical contact with the child—no hugs, kisses, or other signs of affection
- Exposing the child to violence or the abuse of others, whether it be the abuse of a parent, a sibling, or even a pet

Child Neglect

Child neglect—a very common type of child abuse—is a pattern of failing to provide for a child's basic needs, whether it be adequate food, clothing, hygiene, or supervision. Child neglect is not always easy to spot. Sometimes, a parent might become physically or mentally unable to care for a child, such as with a serious injury, untreated depression, or anxiety. Other times, alcohol or drug abuse may seriously impair judgment and the ability to keep a child safe.

Older children might not show outward signs of neglect, becoming used to presenting a competent face to the outside world, and even taking on the role of the parent. But at the end of the day, neglected children are not getting their physical and emotional needs met.

Physical Child Abuse

Physical abuse involves physical harm or injury to the child. It may be the result of a deliberate attempt to hurt the child, but not always. It can also result from severe discipline, such as using a belt on a child, or physical punishment that is inappropriate to the child's age or physical condition.

Many physically abusive parents and caregivers insist that their actions are simply forms of discipline—ways to make children learn to behave. But there is a big difference between using physical punishment to discipline and physical abuse. The point of disciplining children is to teach them right from wrong, not to make them live in fear.

Physical Abuse vs. Discipline

In physical abuse, unlike physical forms of discipline, the following elements are present:

- **Unpredictability:** The child never knows what is going to set the parent off. There are no clear boundaries or rules. The child is constantly walking on eggshells, never sure what behavior will trigger a physical assault.

- **Lashing out in anger:** Physically abusive parents act out of anger and the desire to assert control, not the motivation to lovingly teach the child. The angrier the parent, the more intense the abuse.

- **Using fear to control behavior:** Parents who are physically abusive may believe that their children need to fear them in order to behave, so they use physical abuse to "keep their child in line." However, what children are really learning is how to avoid being hit, not how to behave or grow as individuals.

Child Sexual Abuse: A Hidden Type of Abuse

Help for child sexual abuse:

- 1-888-PREVENT (1-888-773-8368): Stop It Now

- 1-800-656-HOPE: Rape, Abuse and Incest National Network (RAINN)

- Or visit ChiWorld.org for a list of other international child helplines

Child sexual abuse is an especially complicated form of abuse because of its layers of guilt and shame. It's important to recognize that sexual abuse doesn't always involve body contact. Exposing a child to sexual situations or material is sexually abusive, whether or not touching is involved.

While news stories of sexual predators are scary, what is even more frightening is that sexual abuse usually occurs at the hands of someone the child knows and should be able to trust—most often close relatives. And contrary to what many believe, it's not just girls who are at risk. Boys and girls both suffer from sexual abuse. In fact, sexual abuse of boys may be underreported due to shame and stigma.

The Problem of Shame and Guilt in Child Sexual Abuse

Aside from the physical damage that sexual abuse can cause, the emotional component is powerful and far-reaching. Sexually abused children are tormented by shame and guilt. They may feel that they are responsible for the abuse or somehow brought it upon themselves. This can lead to self-loathing and sexual problems as they grow older—often either excessive promiscuity or an inability to have intimate relations.

The shame of sexual abuse makes it very difficult for children to come forward. They may worry that others won't believe them, will be angry with them, or that it will split their family apart. Because of these difficulties, false accusations of sexual abuse are not common, so if a child confides in you, take him or her seriously. Don't turn a blind eye!

Warning Signs of Child Abuse and Neglect

The earlier child abuse is caught, the better the chance of recovery and appropriate treatment for the child. Child abuse is not always obvious. By learning some of the common warning signs of child abuse and neglect, you can catch the problem as early as possible and get both the child and the abuser the help that they need.

Of course, just because you see a warning sign doesn't automatically mean a child is being abused. It's important to dig deeper, looking for a pattern of abusive behavior and warning signs, if you notice something off.

Warning Signs of Emotional Abuse in Children

- Excessively withdrawn, fearful, or anxious about doing something wrong

- Shows extremes in behavior (extremely compliant or extremely demanding; extremely passive or extremely aggressive)

- Doesn't seem to be attached to the parent or caregiver

- Acts either inappropriately adult (taking care of other children) or inappropriately infantile (rocking, thumb-sucking, throwing tantrums)

Warning Signs of Physical Abuse in Children

- Frequent injuries or unexplained bruises, welts, or cuts

- Is always watchful and "on alert," as if waiting for something bad to happen

- Injuries appear to have a pattern such as marks from a hand or belt

- Shies away from touch, flinches at sudden movements, or seems afraid to go home

- Wears inappropriate clothing to cover up injuries, such as long-sleeved shirts on hot days

Warning Signs of Neglect in Children

- Clothes are ill-fitting, filthy, or inappropriate for the weather
- Hygiene is consistently bad (unbathed, matted and unwashed hair, noticeable body odor)
- Untreated illnesses and physical injuries
- Is frequently unsupervised or left alone or allowed to play in unsafe situations and environments
- Is frequently late or missing from school

Warning Signs of Sexual Abuse in Children

- Trouble walking or sitting
- Displays knowledge or interest in sexual acts inappropriate to his or her age, or even seductive behavior
- Makes strong efforts to avoid a specific person, without an obvious reason
- Doesn't want to change clothes in front of others or participate in physical activities
- An STD or pregnancy, especially under the age of 14
- Runs away from home

Child Abuse and Reactive Attachment Disorder

Severe abuse early in life can lead to reactive attachment disorder. Children with this disorder are so disrupted that they have extreme difficulty establishing normal relationships and attaining normal developmental milestones. They need special treatment and support.

Risk Factors for Child Abuse and Neglect

While child abuse and neglect occurs in all types of families—even in those that look happy from the outside—children are at a much greater risk in certain situations.

Domestic violence: Witnessing domestic violence is terrifying to children and emotionally abusive. Even if the mother does her best to protect her children and keeps them from being physically abused, the situation is still extremely damaging. If you or a loved one is in an abusive relationships, getting out is the best thing for protecting the children.

Alcohol and drug abuse: Living with an alcoholic or addict is very difficult for children and can easily lead to abuse and neglect. Parents who are drunk or high are unable to care for their children, make good parenting decisions, and control often-dangerous impulses. Substance abuse also commonly leads to physical abuse.

Untreated mental illness: Parents who suffering from depression, an anxiety disorder, bipolar disorder, or another mental illness have trouble taking care of themselves, much less their children. A mentally ill or traumatized parent may be distant and withdrawn from his or her children, or quick to anger without understanding why. Treatment for the caregiver means better care for the children.

Lack of parenting skills: Some caregivers never learned the skills necessary for good parenting. Teen parents, for example, might have unrealistic expectations about how much care babies and small children need. Or parents who were themselves victims of child abuse may only know how to raise their children the way they were raised. In such cases, parenting classes, therapy, and caregiver support groups are great resources for learning better parenting skills.

Stress and lack of support: Parenting can be a very time-intensive, difficult job, especially if you're raising children without support from family, friends, or the community or you're dealing with relationship problems or financial difficulties. Caring for a child with a disability, special needs, or difficult behaviors is also a challenge. It's important to get the support you need, so you are emotionally and physically able to support your child.

Recognizing Abusive Behavior in Yourself

If you need professional help...

- Do you feel angry and frustrated and don't know where to turn? In the U.S., call 1-800-4-A-CHILD to find support and resources in your community that can help you break the cycle of abuse.

Do you see yourself in some of these descriptions, painful as it may be? Do you feel angry and frustrated and don't know where to turn? Raising children is one of life's greatest challenges and can trigger anger and frustration in the most even tempered. If you grew up in a household where screaming and shouting or violence was the norm, you may not know any other way to raise your kids.

Recognizing that you have a problem is the biggest step to getting help. If you yourself were raised in an abusive situation, that can be extremely difficult. Children experience their world as normal. It may have been normal in your family to be slapped or pushed for little to no reason, or that mother was too drunk to cook dinner. It may have been normal for your parents to call you stupid, clumsy, or worthless. Or it may have been normal to watch your mother get beaten up by your father.

It is only as adults that we have the perspective to step back and take a hard look at what is normal and what is abusive. Read the above sections on the types of abuse and warning signs. Do any of those ring a bell for you now? Or from when you were a child? The following is a list of warning signs that you may be crossing the line into abuse:

How do you know when you've crossed the line?

- **You can't stop the anger:** What starts as a swat on the backside may turn into multiple hits getting harder and harder. You may shake your child harder and harder and finally throw him or her down. You find yourself screaming louder and louder and can't stop yourself.

- **You feel emotionally disconnected from your child:** You may feel so overwhelmed that you don't want anything to do with your child. Day after day, you just want to be left alone and for your child to be quiet.

- **Meeting the daily needs of your child seems impossible:** While everyone struggles with balancing dressing, feeding, and getting kids to school or other activities, if you continually can't manage to do it, it's a sign that something might be wrong.

- **Other people have expressed concern:** It may be easy to bristle at other people expressing concern. However, consider carefully what they have to say. Are the words coming from someone you normally respect and trust? Denial is not an uncommon reaction.

Breaking the Cycle of Child Abuse

If you have a history of child abuse, having your own children can trigger strong memories and feelings that you may have repressed. This may happen when a child is born, or at later ages when you remember specific abuse to you. You may be shocked and overwhelmed by your anger, and feel like you can't control it. But you can learn new ways to manage your emotions and break your old patterns.

Remember, you are the most important person in your child's world. It's worth the effort to make a change, and you don't have to go it alone. Help and support are available.

Tips for Changing Your Reactions

- **Learn what is age appropriate and what is not:** Having realistic expectations of what children can handle at certain ages will help you avoid frustration and anger at normal child behavior. For example, newborns are not going to sleep through the night without a peep, and toddlers are not going to be able to sit quietly for extended periods of time.

- **Develop new parenting skills:** While learning to control your emotions is critical, you also need a game plan of what you are going to do instead. Start by learning appropriate discipline techniques and how to set clear boundaries for your children. Parenting classes, books, and seminars are a way to get this information. You can also turn to other parents for tips and advice.

- **Take care of yourself:** If you are not getting enough rest and support or you're feeling overwhelmed, you are much more likely to succumb to anger. Sleep deprivation, common in parents of young children, adds to moodiness and irritability—exactly what you are trying to avoid.

- **Get professional help:** Breaking the cycle of abuse can be very difficult if the patterns are strongly entrenched. If you can't seem to stop yourself no matter how hard you try, it's time to get help, be it therapy, parenting classes, or other interventions. Your children will thank you for it.

- **Learn how you can get your emotions under control:** The first step to getting your emotions under control is realizing that they are there. If you were abused as a child, you may have an especially difficult time getting in touch with your range of emotions. You may have had to deny or repress them as a child, and now they spill out without your control.

Helping an Abused or Neglected Child

What should you do if you suspect that a child has been abused? How do you approach him or her? Or what if a child comes to you? It's normal to feel a little overwhelmed and confused in this situation. Child abuse is a difficult subject that can be hard to accept and even harder to talk about.

Just remember, you can make a tremendous difference in the life of an abused child, especially if you take steps to stop the abuse early. When talking with an abused child, the best thing you can provide is calm reassurance and unconditional support. Let your actions speak for you if you're having trouble finding the words. Remember that talking about the abuse may be very difficult for the child. It's your job to reassure the child and provide whatever help you can.

Tips for Talking to an Abused Child

- **Avoid denial and remain calm:** A common reaction to news as unpleasant and shocking as child abuse is denial. However, if you display denial to a child, or show shock or disgust at what they are saying, the child may be afraid to continue and will shut down. As hard as it may be, remain as calm and reassuring as you can.

- **Don't interrogate:** Let the child explain to you in his or her own words what happened, but don't interrogate the child or ask leading questions. This may confuse and fluster the child and make it harder for them to continue their story.

- **Reassure the child that they did nothing wrong:** It takes a lot for a child to come forward about abuse. Reassure him or her that you take what is said seriously, and that it is not the child's fault.

- **Safety comes first:** If you feel that your safety or the safety of the child would be threatened if you try to intervene, leave it to the professionals. You may be able to provide more support later after the initial professional intervention.

Reporting Child Abuse and Neglect

If you suspect a child is being abused, it's critical to get them the help he or she needs. Reporting child abuse seems so official. Many people are reluctant to get involved in other families' lives.

Understanding some of the myths behind reporting may help put your mind at ease if you need to report child abuse

- **I don't want to interfere in someone else's family:** The effects of child abuse are lifelong, affecting future relationships, self-esteem, and sadly putting even more children at risk of abuse as the cycle continues. Help break the cycle of child abuse.

- **What if I break up someone's home?** The priority in child protective services is keeping children in the home. A child abuse report does not mean a child is automatically removed from the home—unless the child is clearly in danger. Support such as parenting classes, anger management, or other resources may be offered first to parents if safe for the child.

- **They will know it was me who called:** Reporting is anonymous. In most states, you do not have to give your name when you report child abuse. The child abuser cannot find out who made the report of child abuse.

- **It won't make a difference what I have to say:** If you have a gut feeling that something is wrong, it is better to be safe than sorry. Even if you don't see the whole picture, others may have noticed as well, and a pattern can help identify child abuse that might have otherwise slipped through the cracks.

Next Steps...

- **Reporting child abuse:** As difficult as reporting child abuse or neglect can be, it's important for you to stand up for a child in need. Learn how to communicate effectively in different situations. Read: Child Abuse Reporting Tips [available online at http://beta .helpguide.org/mental/child_abuse_reporting_tips.htm].

Section 1.2

Legal Definitions of Child Abuse and Neglect

From "Definitions of Child Abuse and Neglect," available through the Child Welfare Information Gateway (www.childwelfare.gov), Administration on Children, Youth and Families, Children's Bureau, U.S. Department of Health and Human Services, February 2011. This publication is a product of the State Statutes Series prepared by Child Welfare Information Gateway. While every attempt has been made to be complete, additional information on these topics may be in other sections of a state's code as well as agency regulations, case law, and informal practices and procedures. To find statute information for a particular state, go to www.childwelfare.gov/systemwide/laws_policies/state/index.cfm. To find information on all the states and territories, order a copy of the full-length PDF by calling 800-394-3366, or download it at www.childwelfare.gov/systemwide/laws_policies/statutes/define.pdf.

Child abuse and neglect are defined by federal and state laws. At the state level, child abuse and neglect may be defined in both civil and criminal statutes. This text presents civil definitions that determine the grounds for intervention by state child protective agencies. (States also may define child abuse and neglect in criminal statutes. These definitions provide the grounds for the arrest and prosecution of the offenders. For information on the criminal aspects of child abuse and neglect, visit the National Center for Prosecution of Child Abuse website: www.ndaa.org/ncpca_home.html.)

At the federal level, the Child Abuse Prevention and Treatment Act (CAPTA) defines child abuse and neglect as "Any recent act or failure to act on the part of a parent or caretaker, which results in death, serious physical or emotional harm, sexual abuse, or exploitation, or an act or failure to act which presents an imminent risk of serious harm" (CAPTA Reauthorization Act of 2010 (P.L. 111-320), § 3),

The CAPTA definition of sexual abuse includes these elements [42 U.S.C.A. § 5106g(4) (2010)]:

- The employment, use, persuasion, inducement, enticement, or coercion of any child to engage in, or assist any other person to engage in, any sexually explicit conduct or simulation of such conduct for the purpose of producing a visual depiction of such conduct; or

- The rape, and in cases of caretaker or interfamilial relationships, statutory rape, molestation, prostitution, or other form of sexual exploitation of children, or incest with children

Types of Abuse

Nearly all states, the District of Columbia, American Samoa, Guam, the Northern Mariana Islands, Puerto Rico, and the U.S. Virgin Islands provide civil definitions of child abuse and neglect in statute. (Massachusetts defines child abuse and neglect in regulation.) States recognize the different types of abuse in their definitions, including physical abuse, neglect, sexual abuse, and emotional abuse. Some states also provide definitions in statute for parental substance abuse and/or for abandonment as child abuse.

Physical Abuse

Physical abuse is generally defined as "any nonaccidental physical injury to the child" and can include striking, kicking, burning, or biting the child, or any action that results in a physical impairment of the child. In approximately 38 states and American Samoa, Guam, the Northern Mariana Islands, Puerto Rico, and the Virgin Islands, the definition of abuse also includes acts or circumstances that threaten the child with harm or create a substantial risk of harm to the child's health or welfare. (The word *approximately* is used to stress the fact that the states frequently amend their laws. This information is current through February 2011. The states are Alabama, Alaska, Arkansas, California, Colorado, Florida, Hawaii, Illinois, Indiana, Kansas, Kentucky, Louisiana, Maine, Maryland, Massachusetts, Michigan, Minnesota, Montana, Nebraska, Nevada, New Jersey, New Mexico, New York, North Carolina, Ohio, Oklahoma, Oregon, Pennsylvania, Rhode Island, South Carolina, Tennessee, Texas, Utah, Vermont, Virginia, West Virginia, Wisconsin, and Wyoming.)

Neglect

Neglect is frequently defined as the failure of a parent or other person with responsibility for the child to provide needed food, clothing, shelter, medical care, or supervision to the degree that the child's health, safety, and well-being are threatened with harm. Approximately 24 states, the District of Columbia, American Samoa, Puerto Rico, and the Virgin Islands include failure to educate the child as required by law in their definition of neglect. (The states that define "failure to educate" as neglect include Arkansas, Colorado, Connecticut,

Delaware, Idaho, Indiana, Kentucky, Maine, Minnesota, Mississippi, Missouri, Montana, Nevada, New Hampshire, New Jersey, New Mexico, New York, North Dakota, Ohio, South Carolina, South Dakota, Utah, West Virginia, and Wyoming.)

Seven states (Mississippi, North Dakota, Ohio, Oklahoma, Tennessee, Texas, and West Virginia) specifically define medical neglect as failing to provide any special medical treatment or mental health care needed by the child. In addition, four states define medical neglect as the withholding of medical treatment or nutrition from disabled infants with life-threatening conditions (Indiana, Kansas, Minnesota, and Montana).

Sexual Abuse/Exploitation

All states include sexual abuse in their definitions of child abuse. Some states refer in general terms to sexual abuse, while others specify various acts as sexual abuse. Sexual exploitation is an element of the definition of sexual abuse in most jurisdictions. Sexual exploitation includes allowing the child to engage in prostitution or in the production of child pornography.

Emotional Abuse

Almost all states, the District of Columbia, American Samoa, Guam, the Northern Mariana Islands, Puerto Rico, and the Virgin Islands include emotional maltreatment as part of their definitions of abuse or neglect (all states except Georgia and Washington). Approximately 32 states, the District of Columbia, the Northern Mariana Islands, and Puerto Rico provide specific definitions of emotional abuse or mental injury to a child (Alaska, Arizona, Arkansas, California, Colorado, Delaware, Florida, Hawaii, Idaho, Iowa, Kansas, Kentucky, Maine, Maryland, Massachusetts, Minnesota, Montana, Nevada, New Hampshire, New York, North Carolina, Ohio, Oregon, Pennsylvania, Rhode Island, South Carolina, South Dakota, Tennessee, Texas, Vermont, Wisconsin, and Wyoming). Typical language used in these definitions is "injury to the psychological capacity or emotional stability of the child as evidenced by an observable or substantial change in behavior, emotional response, or cognition" and injury as evidenced by "anxiety, depression, withdrawal, or aggressive behavior."

Parental Substance Abuse

Parental substance abuse is an element of the definition of child abuse or neglect in some states (for summaries of statutes and a more complete discussion of this issue, see Child Welfare Information

Gateway's "Parental Drug Use as Child Abuse," available online at www.childwelfare.gov/systemwide/laws_policies/statutes/drugexposed. cfm). Circumstances that are considered abuse or neglect in some states include:

- Prenatal exposure of a child to harm due to the mother's use of an illegal drug or other substance (Arizona, Arkansas, Colorado, Illinois, Indiana, Iowa, Louisiana, Massachusetts, Minnesota, North Dakota, Oklahoma, Oregon, South Dakota, Wisconsin, and the District of Columbia)

- Manufacture of a controlled substance in the presence of a child or on the premises occupied by a child (Colorado, Indiana, Iowa, Montana, Ohio, Oregon, South Dakota, Tennessee, Virginia, and Washington)

- Allowing a child to be present where the chemicals or equipment for the manufacture of controlled substances are used or stored (Arizona, Arkansas, and Washington)

- Selling, distributing, or giving drugs or alcohol to a child (Arkansas, Florida, Hawaii, Illinois, Minnesota, Ohio, Texas, and Guam)

- Use of a controlled substance by a caregiver that impairs the caregiver's ability to adequately care for the child (California, Delaware, Kentucky, Minnesota, New York, Rhode Island, and Texas)

Abandonment

Approximately 17 states and the District of Columbia include abandonment in their definitions of abuse or neglect, generally as a type of neglect (California, Colorado, Connecticut, Illinois, Kentucky, Louisiana, Minnesota, Nevada, New Jersey, North Carolina, Rhode Island, South Dakota, Utah, Vermont, Virginia, West Virginia, and Wyoming). Approximately 18 states, Guam, Puerto Rico, and the Virgin Islands provide definitions for abandonment that are separate from the definition of neglect (Arizona, Arkansas, Florida, Idaho, Indiana, Kansas, Maine, Massachusetts, Montana, Nebraska, New Hampshire, New Mexico, New York, North Dakota, Ohio, Oklahoma, South Carolina, and Texas). In general, it is considered abandonment of the child when the parent's identity or whereabouts are unknown, the child has been left by the parent in circumstances in which the child suffers serious harm, or the parent has failed to maintain contact with the child or to provide reasonable support for a specified period of time.

19

Standards for Reporting

Generally speaking, a report must be made when an individual knows or has reasonable cause to believe or suspect that a child has been subjected to abuse or neglect. These standards guide mandatory reporters in deciding whether to make a report to child protective services.

Persons Responsible for the Child

In addition to defining acts or omissions that constitute child abuse or neglect, several states' statutes provide specific definitions of persons who can be reported to child protective services as perpetrators of abuse or neglect. These persons have some relationship or regular responsibility for the child. This generally includes parents, guardians, foster parents, relatives, or other caregivers responsible for the child's welfare.

Exceptions

A number of states provide exceptions in their reporting laws that exempt certain acts or omissions from their statutory definitions of child abuse and neglect. For instance, in 12 states and the District of Columbia, financial inability to provide for a child is exempted from the definition of neglect (Arkansas, Florida, Kansas, Louisiana, Massachusetts, New Hampshire, North Dakota, Pennsylvania, Texas, Washington, West Virginia, and Wisconsin). In 16 states, the District of Columbia, American Samoa, and the Northern Mariana Islands, physical discipline of a child, as long as it is reasonable and causes no bodily injury to the child, is an exception to the definition of abuse (Arkansas, California, Colorado, Florida, Georgia, Indiana, Minnesota, Mississippi, Missouri, Ohio, Oklahoma, Oregon, South Carolina, Texas, Utah, and Washington).

CAPTA specifies that nothing in the Act should be construed as establishing a federal requirement that a parent or legal guardian provide any medical service or treatment that is against the religious beliefs of the parent or legal guardian (42 U.S.C. § 5106i). At the state level, 31 states, the District of Columbia, Guam, and Puerto Rico provide in their civil child abuse reporting laws an exception to the definition of child abuse and neglect for parents who choose not to seek medical care for their children due to religious beliefs (Alabama, Alaska, California, Colorado, Delaware, Florida, Georgia, Idaho, Illinois, Indiana, Iowa, Kansas, Kentucky, Louisiana, Maine, Michigan, Minnesota, Mississippi, Missouri, Montana, Nevada, New Hampshire, New

Jersey, New Mexico, Ohio, Oklahoma, Pennsylvania, Utah, Vermont, Virginia, and Wyoming). However, 16 of the 31 states and Puerto Rico authorize the court to order medical treatment for the child when the child's condition warrants intervention (Alabama, Colorado, Florida, Idaho, Indiana, Iowa, Kansas, Kentucky, Louisiana, Michigan, Missouri, Montana, Nevada, Ohio, Oklahoma, and Pennsylvania). Three states (Arizona, Connecticut, and Washington) specifically provide an exception for Christian Science treatment. Five states require mandated reporters to report instances when a child is not receiving medical care so that an investigation can be made (Michigan, Minnesota, Missouri, Ohio, and Oklahoma).

Chapter 2

Infant Maltreatment and Death

Chapter Contents

Section 2.1

Infant Neglect

Excerpted from "Chapter 3: Impact of Neglect," *Child Neglect: A Guide for Prevention, Assessment and Intervention*, by Diane DePanfilis, Office on Child Abuse and Neglect, 2006; available from the Child Welfare Information Gateway (www.childwelfare.gov), a service of the Children's Bureau, Administration for Children and Families. U.S. Department of Health and Human Services. Reviewed by David A. Cooke, MD, FACP, January 2013.

The Impact of Neglect

The impact of neglect on a child may not be apparent at an early stage except in the most extreme cases. However, the effects of neglect are harmful and possibly long-lasting for the victims. Its impact can become more severe as a child grows older and can encompass multiple areas, including health and physical development, intellectual and cognitive development, emotional and psychological development, and social and behavioral development.

Although there are four categories of neglect's effects on an individual, they often are related. For example, if a child experiences neglect that leads to a delayed development of the brain, this may lead to cognitive delays or psychological problems, which may manifest as social and behavioral problems. Because neglected children often experience multiple consequences that may be the result of neglect and related circumstances in their lives, it may be difficult to determine if the impact is related specifically to the neglect, is caused by another factor, or arises from a combination of factors. The impact of neglect can vary based on the child's age; the presence and strength of protective factors; the frequency, duration, and severity of the neglect; and the relationship between the child and caregiver.

The negative impacts of neglect are often associated with the various outcomes children experience in the child welfare system. For example, some of the developmental and health problems linked to neglect are related to higher rates of placement in out-of-home care, a greater number of out-of-home placements, longer out-of-home placements, and a decreased likelihood of children residing with their parents when discharged from foster care.

The Early Years

Research shows that the first few years of children's lives are crucial and sensitive periods for development. During these years, neural synapses are formed at a very high rate. After the age of three, synapses start to be "pruned," and certain pathways that are not used may be discarded. Studies supporting the idea of a sensitive developmental period show that maltreated infants suffer from greater developmental disabilities than those children who were maltreated later in childhood. One example of this is the ability to form attachments with one's primary caregiver. If this process is disrupted early in children's lives, they may have difficulty forming healthy relationships throughout their lives. Although learning can happen throughout life, it often is more difficult for children who were deprived of certain types of early stimulation.

Programs, such as Early Head Start and other infancy and early childhood programs, acknowledge that the first few years of life are extremely significant for development. Child welfare laws and interventions, however, often do not provide or authorize the resources necessary to protect children from neglect during these critical years. Unless children show clear physical signs of neglect, intervention often is unlikely to be mandated. Thus, for many cases of emotional neglect, and especially for young children who cannot tell others about the neglect, interventions may occur too late or not at all. If interventions finally occur, the children may be past critical developmental points and could suffer from deficiencies throughout their lives. Therefore, it is important that professionals working with young children be able to recognize the possible signs of neglect in order to intervene and to keep children from suffering further harm.

Health and Physical Development

Studies show that neglected children can be at risk for many physical problems, including failure to thrive, severe diaper rash and other skin infections, recurrent and persistent minor infections, malnourishment, and impaired brain development. Because neglect includes medical neglect, other health problems can arise from the failure of the parents to obtain necessary medical care for their children. If children do not receive the proper immunizations, prescribed medications, necessary surgeries, or other interventions, there can be serious consequences, such as impaired brain development or poor physical health. The impact of a delay in or lack of treatment might be noticeable immediately or may not be apparent for several weeks, months, or even years. For example, a child who does not receive proper dental care might be all right in the short term, but suffer from tooth decay and gum disease later in life. Children with diabetes may be fine without treatment for a short while, but an extended delay in treatment could have serious consequences and possibly result in death.

Impaired Brain Development

In some cases, child neglect has been associated with a failure of the brain to form properly, which can lead to impaired physical, mental, and emotional development. The brain of a child who has been maltreated may develop in such a way that it is adaptive for the child's negative environment, but is maladaptive for functional or positive environments. A maltreated child's brain may adapt for day-to-day survival, but may not allow the child to develop fully healthy cognitive and social skills. In one study, neglected children had the highest proportion of later diagnoses of mental retardation, which may be due to not getting the necessary care and stimulation for proper brain development. Children who are neglected early in life may remain in a state of "hyper-arousal" in which they are constantly anticipating threats, or they may experience dissociation with a decreased ability to benefit from social, emotional, and cognitive experiences. To be able to learn, a child's brain needs to be in a state of "attentive calm," which is rare for maltreated children. If a child is unable to learn new information, this may cause some areas of the brain to remain inactive, possibly resulting in delayed or stunted brain growth. It also can impair functioning later in life and may lead to the child being anxious, acting overly aggressive, or being withdrawn.

Children who have experienced global neglect, defined as neglect in more than one category, may have significantly smaller brains than the norm. This could be indicative of fewer neuronal pathways available for learning and may lead the children to be at an intellectual disadvantage for their entire lives.

Poor Physical Health

The physical problems associated with neglect may start even before an infant is born, such as when the mother has had little or no prenatal care or smoked during pregnancy. These children may be born prematurely and have complications at birth. Neglected children also can have severe physical injuries, possibly due to the inattention of their parents, such as central nervous system and craniofacial injuries, fractures, and severe burns. They also may be dirty and unhygienic, leading to even more health problems, such as lice or infections. Children also may be exposed to toxins that could cause anemia, cancer, heart disease, poor immune functioning, and asthma. For example, exposure to indoor and outdoor air pollutants, such as ozone, particulate matter, and sulphur dioxide, can cause the development of asthma or increase the frequency or severity of asthma attacks. Additionally, children may have health problems due to a lack of medical attention for injury or illness, including chronic health problems. Neglected children may suffer from dehydration or diarrhea that can lead to more severe problems if unattended.

A medical condition associated with child neglect is "failure to thrive," which can be defined as "children whose growth deviates significantly from the norms for their age and gender." This condition typically occurs in infants and toddlers under the age of two years. Failure to thrive can be manifested as significant growth delays, as well as poor muscle tone; unhappy or minimal facial expressions; decreased vocalizations; and general unresponsiveness.

Failure to thrive can be caused by organic or nonorganic factors, but some doctors may not make such a sharp distinction because physical and behavioral causes often appear together. With organic failure to thrive, the child's delayed growth can be attributed to a physical cause, usually a condition that inhibits the child's ability to take in, digest, or process food. When failure to thrive is a result of the parent's neglectful behavior, it is considered nonorganic.

Treatment for failure to thrive depends on the cause of the delayed growth and development, as well as the child's age, overall health, and medical history. For example, delayed growth due to nutritional factors can be addressed by educating the parents on an appropriate and well-balanced diet for the child. Additionally, parental attitudes and behavior may contribute to a child's problems and need to be examined. In many cases, the child may need to be hospitalized initially to focus on implementation of a comprehensive medical, behavioral, and psychosocial treatment plan. Even with treatment, failure to thrive may have significant long-term consequences for children, such as growth retardation, diminished cognitive ability, mental retardation, socio-emotional deficits, and poor impulse control.

Impact on the Brain of Prenatal Exposure to Alcohol and Drugs

Exposure to alcohol and drugs in utero may cause impaired brain development for the fetus. Studies have shown that prenatal exposure to drugs may alter the development of the cortex, reduce the number of neurons that are created, and alter the way chemical messengers function. This may lead to difficulties with attention, memory, problem

27

solving, and abstract thinking. However, findings are mixed and may depend on what drug is abused. Alcohol abuse has been found to have some of the most detrimental effects on infants, including mental retardation and neurological deficits. One problem with determining the impact of substance abuse on a fetus is isolating whether the negative outcomes are directly associated with the alcohol or drug exposure or with other factors, such as poor prenatal care or nutrition, premature birth, or adverse environmental conditions after birth.

Impact of Malnutrition on Children

Malnutrition, especially early in a child's life, has been shown to lead to stunted brain growth and to slower passage of electrical signals in the brain. Malnutrition also can result in cognitive, social, and behavioral deficits. Iron deficiency, the most common form of malnutrition in the United States, can lead to cognitive and motor delays, anxiety, depression, social problems, and problems with attention.

Intellectual and Cognitive Development

Research shows that neglected children are more likely to have cognitive deficits and severe academic and developmental delays when compared with non-neglected children. When neglected children enter school, they may suffer from both intellectual and social disadvantages that cause them to become frustrated and fall behind. One study found that individuals at 28 years of age who suffered from childhood neglect scored lower on IQ and reading ability tests, when controlling for age, sex, race, and social class, than people who were not neglected as children. Other studies have found that, although both abused and neglected children exhibited language delays or disorders, the problems were more severe for neglected children. Furthermore, neglected children have the greatest delays in expressive and receptive language when compared with abused and nonmaltreated children. When compared to physically abused children, neglected children have academic difficulties that are more serious and show signs of greater cognitive and socio-emotional delays at a younger age. These academic difficulties may lead to more referrals for special education services.

There are also language problems associated with neglect. In order for babies to learn language, they need to hear numerous repetitions of sounds before they can begin making sounds and eventually saying words and sentences. Language development may be delayed if the parent or other caregiver does not provide the necessary verbal interaction with the child.

Impact of Neglect on Academic Performance

Neglect can negatively affect a child's academic performance. Studies have found that:

- Children placed in out-of-home care because of abuse or neglect have below-average levels of cognitive capacity, language development, and academic achievement.

- Neglected children demonstrated a notable decline in academic performance upon entering junior high school.

- Children who were physically neglected were found to have significantly lower IQ scores at 24 and 36 months and the lowest scores on standardized tests of intellectual functioning and academic achievement in kindergarten when compared with children who had experienced either no maltreatment or other forms of maltreatment.

- Neglected children, when compared with nonmaltreated children, scored lower on measures of overall school performance and tests of language, reading, and math skills.

- Neglected boys, but not girls, were found to have lower full-scale IQ scores than physically abused and nonmaltreated children.

Emotional, Psychosocial, and Behavioral Development

Neglect can have a strong impact on, and lead to problems in, a child's emotional, psychosocial, and behavioral development. As with other effects already mentioned, these may be evident immediately after the maltreatment or not manifest themselves until many months or years later.

Neglected children, even when older, may display a variety of emotional, psychosocial, and behavioral problems which may vary depending on the age of the child. Some of these include the following:

- Displaying an inability to control emotions or impulses, usually characterized by frequent outbursts

- Being quiet and submissive

- Having difficulty learning in school and getting along with siblings or classmates

- Experiencing unusual eating or sleeping behaviors

- Attempting to provoke fights or solicit sexual interactions

- Acting socially or emotionally inappropriate for their age
- Being unresponsive to affection
- Displaying apathy
- Being less flexible, persistent, and enthusiastic than non-neglected children
- Demonstrating helplessness under stress
- Having fewer interactions with peers than non-neglected children
- Displaying poor coping skills
- Acting highly dependent
- Acting lethargic and lackluster
- Displaying self-abusive behavior (for example, suicide attempts or cutting themselves)
- Exhibiting panic or dissociative disorders, attention-deficit/hyperactivity disorder, or post-traumatic stress disorder
- Suffering from depression, anxiety, or low self-esteem
- Exhibiting juvenile delinquent behavior or engaging in adult criminal activities
- Engaging in sexual activities leading to teen pregnancy or fatherhood
- Having low academic achievement
- Abusing alcohol or drugs

Emotional and Psychosocial Consequences

All types of neglect, and emotional neglect in particular, can have serious psychosocial and emotional consequences for children. Some of the short-term emotional impacts of neglect, such as fear, isolation, and an inability to trust, can lead to lifelong emotional and psychological problems, such as low self-esteem.

A major component of emotional and psychosocial development is attachment. Children who have experienced neglect have been found to demonstrate higher frequencies of insecure, anxious, and avoidant attachments with their primary caregivers than nonmaltreated children. In fact, studies have demonstrated that 70 to 100 percent of maltreated infants form insecure attachments with their caregivers. Often, emotionally neglected children have learned from their relationships with their primary caregivers that they will not be able to have their needs met by others. This may cause a child not to try to solicit warmth or help from others. This behavior may in turn cause teachers or peers not to offer help or support, thus reinforcing the negative expectations of the neglected child. One mitigating factor, however, may be having an emotionally supportive adult, either within or outside of the family, such as a grandparent or a teacher, available during childhood. Another mitigating factor may be having a loving, accepting spouse or close friend later in life.

Neglected children who are unable to form secure attachments with their primary caregivers may display these characteristics:

- Become more mistrustful of others and may be less willing to learn from adults

- Have difficulty understanding the emotions of others, regulating their own emotions, or forming and maintaining relationships with others

- Have a limited ability to feel remorse or empathy, which may mean that they could hurt others without feeling their actions were wrong

- Demonstrate a lack of confidence or social skills that could hinder them from being successful in school, work, and relationships

- Demonstrate impaired social cognition, which is one's awareness of oneself in relation to others and an awareness of other's emotions. Impaired social cognition can lead a person to view many social interactions as stressful.

Behavioral Consequences

Neglected children may suffer from particular behavioral problems throughout life. Research shows that children who are exposed to poor family management practices are at a greater risk of developing conduct disorders and of participating in delinquent behavior. Neglected children also may be at risk for repeating the neglectful behavior with their own children. Research also shows that neglected children do not necessarily perceive their upbringing to be abnormal or dysfunctional and may model their own parenting behavior on the behavior of their parents. One study estimates that approximately one-third of neglected children will maltreat their own children.

Societal Consequences

Society pays for many of the consequences of neglect. There are large monetary costs for maintaining child welfare systems, judicial systems, law enforcement, special education programs, and physical and mental health systems that are needed to respond to and to treat victims of child neglect and their families. Many indirect societal consequences also exist, such as increased juvenile delinquency, adult criminal activity, mental illness, substance abuse, and domestic violence. There may be a loss of productivity due to unemployment and underemployment associated with neglect. Additionally, supporting children who have developmental delays because of malnutrition often is much more costly than providing adequate nutrition and care to poor women and children.

Early Prevention and Intervention

The incidence of neglect and the harm it does to children can be reduced or mitigated through early prevention and intervention programs. Although the effectiveness of these programs has not been studied adequately, they are most effective when they are comprehensive and long-term. With the effects of neglect being especially damaging during infancy, it also is important to work with families as early as possible—even before the baby is born.

Two promising early prevention and intervention programs are the Olds model and Project STEEP (Steps Toward Effective, Enjoyable Parenting). The Olds model utilizes intensive nurse home visiting during pregnancy and through age two of the child. The program had positive effects on parenting attitudes and behavior and on reports of child maltreatment. Project STEEP includes home visitation and group support and education for expectant mothers and seeks to enhance mother-infant relationships. In the initial implementation of this program, mothers in the experimental group demonstrated a better understanding of child development, better life management skills, fewer depressive symptoms, fewer repeat pregnancies within two years of the birth of their baby, and greater sensitivity to their child's cues and signals.

Section 2.2

Identifying Infant Maltreatment

Infant abuse and neglect leave lasting physical and emotional scars. Abuse and neglect not only lead to trauma and misery, they also can affect the child's future happiness, relationships, and success.

Signs of Abuse

There are many signs that may indicate an infant is being abused/neglected. It's usually a combination of clues and not a single factor that tells the tale of abuse/neglect.

Does the infant:

- have unexplained bruises, burns, welts, fractures, or dislocations?

- show poor physical hygiene, such as severe diaper rash, skins rashes, dirty hair, dirty hands and face, and persistent body odor?

- have poor growth pattern and constant hunger?

- show obvious delays in cognitive or emotional development?

- display frozen watchfulness (excessive staring)?

- appear persistently dull and inactive?

- not physically reach out to parents or caregiver for comfort or attention?

- avoid eye contact?

Parents who were abused as children often become abusers themselves. Poverty, illness, and substance abuse increase the risk. In most cases, parents do not really want to harm their children, but they have a hard time controlling their anger or feel overwhelmed.

There are many signs that may indicate a parent or caregiver is abusing/neglecting an infant.

Does the parent or caregiver:

- refuse to offer or offer farfetched or conflicting explanations about the baby's injuries?

- seem to trust no one?

- seldom touch or look at the infant?

- become unduly tense and irritable when the baby cries or does not respond to baby's cries?

- feel the baby is too demanding?

- express unreal expectations of the infant?

- lack understanding of baby's needs (such as food and supervision)?

- appear to abuse alcohol or drugs?

- appear isolated from normal human relationships with family, friends, neighbors, and community groups?

- make mostly negative comments about the baby?

- behave irrationally or in a bizarre manner?

What You Can Do

Research and Support

- Research child abuse and neglect resources in your community. Know the proper authorities to report suspected abuse and/or neglect to.

- Offer information to families on child development, positive discipline, and stress management during your home visits and through special projects or events.

If you suspect abuse or neglect, it is important not to carry out your own investigation since that can jeopardize the case if it reaches the courts.

Write Down the Facts

- Document as soon as possible what you observe.

- Stick to the facts and leave out your judgements and opinions.

- Write down everything, no matter how trivial it may seem.

Report the Disclosure

[Ed. Note: The following two points address people who are mandatory reporters. For additional information about reporting suspected child abuse, see Chapter 29—Reporting Child Abuse. For more information about mandatory reporters, see Chapter 30—Professionals Who Are Required to Report Child Abuse And Neglect.]

- You are required by law to report child abuse or suspected child abuse to the appropriate state agency. Report your suspicions to your supervisor who will assist you in contacting authorities. If the situation is immediately life threatening, contact 911.

- Discuss with your supervisor ways you can give the mother an opportunity to report the abuse herself, unless it would endanger her or the child to do so.

Section 2.3

Homicides in Children under Age Five

Excerpted from "Homicide Trends in the United States, 1980-2008, Annual Rates for 2009 and 2010," U.S. Department of Justice (www.usdoj.gov), November 2011.

The homicide rate for children under age five has remained stable or declined for all racial groups. The number of homicides of children under age five declined between 1993 and 2006, but increased in 2007 and 2008 (Figure 2.1).

Homicide rates for black children under age five declined 36% between 1993 and 2008, dropping from 11.3 homicides per 100,000 in 1993 to 7.2 homicides per 100,000 in 2008 (Figure 2.2). The homicide rates for black children under age five have remained substantially higher than rates for white children or children of other races.

Homicide rates for white children under age five remained relatively stable between 1980 and 1990, with an average rate of 2.4 homicides per 100,000. The rate rose to 2.8 homicides per 100,000 by 1996, then dropped down to 2.1 homicides per 100,000 in 2006. Since 2006 the rate has risen slightly to 2.3 homicides per 100,000 in 2008.

In general, the younger the child, the greater the risk for being the victim of a homicide (Figure 2.3). Throughout the 28-year period from 1980 to 2008, infants under one year of age had the highest homicide victimization rate of all children under age five.

A parent was the perpetrator in the majority of homicides of children under age 5 (Figure 2.4). These statistics pertain to all children under age five murdered from 1980 through 2008:

- 63% were killed by a parent—33% were killed by their fathers and 30% were killed by their mothers (see Table 2.1)

- 23% were killed by male acquaintances

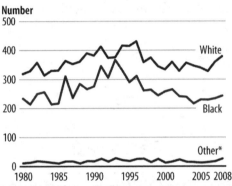

*Other race includes American Indians, Alaska Natives, Asians, Hawaiians, and other Pacific Islanders.

Figure 2.1. *Number of homicides of children under age 5, by race of victim, 1980–2008.*

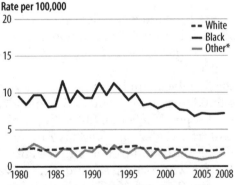

*Other race includes American Indians, Alaska Natives, Asians, Hawaiians, and other Pacific Islanders.

Figure 2.2. *Homicide victimization rates for children under age 5, by race of victim, 1980–2008.*

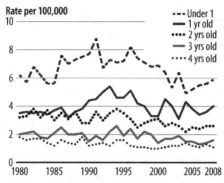

Figure 2.3. Homicides of children under age 5, by age of victim, 1980–2008.

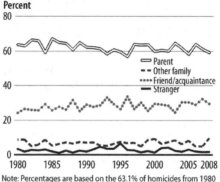

Note: Percentages are based on the 63.1% of homicides from 1980 through 2008 for which the victim/offender relationships were known.

Figure 2.4. Homicides of children under age 5, by relationship with the offender, 1980–2008.

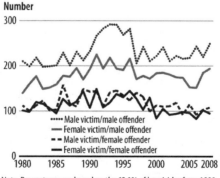

Note: Percentages are based on the 63.1% of homicides from 1980 through 2008 for which the victim/offender relationships were known.

Figure 2.5. Number of homicides of children under age five, by sex of victim and offender, 1980–2008.

- 5% were killed by female acquaintances
- 7% were killed by other relatives
- 3% were killed by strangers

Of children under age five killed by someone other than their parent, 80% were killed by males.

Most of the victims and offenders of homicides involving children under age five were male. Since 1980, the number of homicides involving male children under age five killed by male offenders increased dramatically in the early 1990s before dropping in 1997 and followed a similar pattern for female victims killed by male offenders, although these changes were less pronounced (Figure 2.5).

Table 2.1. Offender relationship to child victim under age five, 1980–2008

Sex of offender	All relationships	Parent	Other family	Friend/ acquaintance	Stranger
All offenders	100%	63%	7%	28%	3%
Male	63%	33%	4%	23%	3%
Female	38%	30%	3%	5%	0%

Note: Detail may not sum to total due to rounding. Percentages are based on the 63.1% of homicides from 1980 through 2008 for which the victim/offender relationships were known.

Section 2.4

Filicide: When Parents Kill Their Children

Excerpted from "Perpetrators and Victims: Understanding and Treating Maternal Filicide Offenders," by Stacey L. Shipley, Psy.D. and Dori L. Johnson, Psy.D, North Texas State Hospital. Presented at the 2007 Annual Meeting of the National Association of State Mental Health Program Directors Forensic Division. © 2007 Stacey L. Shipley, Psy.D. and Dori L. Johnson, Psy.D. Reprinted with permission. The complete text of this presentation is available at www.nasmhpd.org. Reviewed by David A. Cooke, MD, FACP, January 2013.

Filicide

- It is greatest within the first year.

- Among infants in the first week of life, mothers are almost always the ones who committed the filicide.

- Types of filicide: Neonaticide; Infanticide; Filicide

- The most dangerous period for the victim is the first six months of life. This is the time of maternal postpartum psychoses and depressions.

- Men, as compared to women, who kill their children are more likely to kill older children, are more likely to be unemployed, are more likely to be facing separation from their spouse, and are more likely to abuse alcohol or drugs.

Psychosis and/or Depression in Filicide Offenders

- Only a few of the women in the neonaticide group were psychotic, but psychosis was evident in two-thirds of the maternal filicide group.

- Depression was found in 71% of the maternal filicide groups and in only three of the neonaticide cases.

- Suicide attempts accompanied more than one-third of the filicides, but none occurred among the neonaticide cases.

Classification of Filicide by Apparent Motive

- "Altruistic"/associated with suicide: 38%
- To relieve suffering: 11%
- Acutely psychotic: 21%
- Unwanted child: 14%
- Fatal maltreatment: 12%
- Spouse revenge: 4%
- Total (n=131): 100%

Neonaticide

- Most common motive in neonaticide is due to child not being wanted due to the stigma of pregnancy out of wedlock; ashamed, fearful, denial, psychologically isolated, concealment

- Effects of denial can be so great that some women do not show changes in body contour, such as abdominal girth; some women continue menstrual bleeding during pregnancy.

- One consequence of denial of pregnancy is failure to form a significant affective bond with the fetus. Women who commit neonaticide may simply view their fetus as a foreign body passing through them.

Fatal Maltreatment Filicide

- Parental abuse and neglect rarely involve a major mental disease.
- The parent is more likely to have a personality disorder.
- The acts are conscious, voluntary, and there is no delusional distortion of reality.

Spousal Revenge Filicide

- Although borderline personality and dependent personality disorders are common diagnoses, these do not qualify as diseases for purposes of insanity.

- The motive is rational and not based on psychosis. Almost never "not guilty by reason of insanity" (NGRI)

"Acutely Psychotic" Filicide

- This designation includes parents who killed under the influence of hallucinations, epilepsy, or delirium.
- It does not include all of the psychotic child murders.
- This is the weakest category because it contains those cases in which no comprehensible motive could be ascertained.
- Not likely to attempt to hide crime.

Altruistic Filicide

- Associated with suicide: These mothers see their children as an extension of themselves. They do not want to leave a child motherless in a "cruel" world as seen through their depressed eyes.
- Altruistic filicide to relieve victim suffering: The suffering may be real or imagined. Want to relieve child from unbearable suffering

Section 2.5

Differences between Homicide and Filicide Offenders

Excerpted from Putkonen H, Weizmann-Henelius G, Lindberg N, Eronen M, Häkkänen H. "Differences between homicide and filicide offenders: results of a nationwide register-based case–control study." *BMC Psychiatry*. 2009; 9:27. © 2009 Putkonen, et al; licensee BioMed Central Ltd. The original work has been modified: the text has been excerpted. This is an Open Access article distributed under the terms of the Creative Commons Attribution License (http://creativecommons.org/licenses/by/3.0). The electronic version of this article, which includes references, can be found online at: http://www.biomedcentral.com/1471-244X/9/27.

Background

Filicide is defined as the act of a parent killing her/his child. The killing of a child younger than one year is commonly called infanticide; when committed within the first 24 hours of life it is neonaticide.

Over the years, filicide has been studied at length under a number of different classifications. One of the classic systems is that by Resnick [Resnick PJ: Child murder by parents: a psychiatric review of filicide. *Am J Psychiatry* 1969, 126:325-334] proposing a classification of filicide as 1) altruistic, 2) acutely psychotic, 3) unwanted child, 4) accidental, and 5) spousal revenge. Several reviews on the matter have recently been published.

Fortunately, filicide is not a very frequent crime, rates vary from 0.6 per 100,000 children under 15 to 2.5 per 100,000 children under 18. Yet, as is devastatingly clear, each case is highly disturbing. Moreover, rates of child murder are considered underestimates, due to inaccurate coroner rulings and some bodies never being discovered. Filicide is an extraordinary form of homicide. In fact, it has been noted that rates of infanticide parallel suicide rates more closely rather than murder rates. Indeed, suicide is commonly associated with filicide, both attempted and fulfilled suicide. Contrasting findings disagree as to who commits filicide more often, mothers or fathers. Furthermore, numerous studies indicate an association between filicide and parental psychiatric illness, namely major depression with psychotic features. In addition, personality disorders, particularly borderline personality, have been found frequent in both female and male filicide offenders.

Psychopathy is an important construct in explaining criminal behavior and has especially been linked to violent criminality. Characteristics of psychopathy form a particular pattern of interpersonal, affective, and behavioral symptoms. Egocentricity and impulsivity, lack of empathy and remorse, as well as shallow and labile affects are typical personality traits in psychopathy together with a violation of social norms. The most widely used operational definition of psychopathy has been the Hare Psychopathy Checklist – Revised. Although research on psychopathy is quite extensive, to our knowledge, no previous studies on psychopathy of filicide offenders exist. Yet, some of the psychopathic traits, for example, egocentricity and lack of empathy might underlie the act of killing one's own children.

In spite of active research on filicide, nationwide studies are scarce. Moreover, since we have studied Finnish homicide offenders quite extensively, we have come to the conclusion that even though in Finland most homicide offenders, regardless of gender, are substance abusing and personality disordered, there might be subgroups of homicide offenders with a different history and psychiatric morbidity. We suspected that filicide offenders form such a subgroup. The aim of the present nationwide study was to compare the psychosocial history, index offence, and psychiatric morbidity of filicide offenders with those of other homicide offenders. Furthermore, we wanted to compare the prevalence of psychopathy and the discriminating value of the individual items of psychopathy between these groups.

Methods

In this nationwide register-based case-control study all filicide offenders who were in a forensic psychiatric examination in Finland 1995–2004 were examined and compared with an age- and gender matched control group of homicide offenders. The assessed variables were psychosocial history, index offence, and psychiatric variables as well as psychopathy using the PCL-R (Psychopathy Checklist-Revised, a scale developed by Robert D. Hare to help mental health professionals evaluate a person's psychopathic inclinations).

Results

Filicide offenders were not significantly more often diagnosed with psychotic disorders than the controls but they had attempted suicide at the crime scene significantly more often. Filicide offenders had alcohol abuse/dependence and antisocial personality less often than the controls. Filicide offenders scored significantly lower on psychopathy than the controls. Within the group of filicide offenders, the psychopathy items with relatively higher scores were lack of remorse or guilt, shallow affect, callous/lack of empathy, poor behavioral controls, and failure to accept responsibility.

Conclusion

Contrary to previous conclusions, we did not find that the filicide offenders had significantly more mental illness and more serious psychopathology than the other homicide offenders. Psychopathy was certainly not a risk factor for filicide. However, the filicide offender did exhibit emotional problems which should be noted as risk factors and suicidal behavior at the crime scene might signal distress unlike that of the common homicide offender. The filicide offenders might be incapable of handling even everyday difficulties. We therefore conclude that prevention of filicide cannot remain the task of psychiatry alone, but health care and society at large must work to forestall the danger of filicide. Parents who are severely fatigued or otherwise not able to cope should receive adequate support. However, mental health services cannot relax, and our results should be replicated. In order to

43

find in-depth information on filicide and associated social, emotional, and psychopathological issues and, therefore, to enhance prevention, we urgently need international cooperation to study filicide in a large scale database.

Chapter 3

Child Abuse Statistics

Chapter Contents

Section 3.1

Child Maltreatment Facts at a Glance

"Child Maltreatment Facts at a Glance,"
Centers for Disease Control and Prevention (www.cdc.gov), 2010.

Child Maltreatment

- In 2008, U.S. state and local child protective services (CPS) received 3.3 million reports of children being abused or neglected.[1]

- CPS estimated that 772,000 (10.3 per 1,000) of children were victims of maltreatment. Approximately three-quarters of them had no history of prior victimization.

- Seventy-one percent of the children were classified as victims of child neglect; 16 percent as victims of physical abuse; 9 percent as victims of sexual abuse; and 7 percent as victims of emotional abuse.

- A non-CPS study estimated that one in five U.S. children experience some form of child maltreatment: Approximately 1 percent were victims of sexual assault; 4 percent were victims of child neglect; 9 percent were victims of physical abuse; and 12 percent were victims of emotional abuse.[2]

Note: A child is counted each time she or he is a subject of a report, which means a child may be counted more than once as a victim of child maltreatment.

Gender and Race Disparities among Children

- In 2008, some children had higher rates of victimization:
  - African-American (16.6 per 1,000 children)
  - American Indian or Alaska Native (13.9 per 1,000 children)
  - Multiracial (13.8 per 1,000 children)[1]

- Overall, rates of victimization were slightly higher for girls (10.8 per 1,000 children) than boys (9.7 per 1,000 children).[1]

Characteristics of Perpetrators

- Most children are maltreated by their parents versus other relatives or caregivers.[1]
- Perpetrators are typically less than 39 years of age.[1]
- Female perpetrators, mostly mothers, are typically younger than male perpetrators.[1]

Nonfatal Cases of Child Maltreatment

- In 2008, CPS reported the approximate rates of child maltreatment victims:
  - 21.7 per 1,000 for infants less than 1 year old;
  - 12.9 per 1,000 for 1 year-olds;
  - 12.4 per 1,000 for 2 year-olds;
  - 11.7 per 1,000 for 3 year-olds;
  - 11.0 per 1,000 for 4 to 7 year-olds;
  - 9.2 per 1,000 for 8 to 11 year-olds;
  - 8.4 per 1,000 for 12 to 15 year-olds; and
  - 5.5 per 1,000 for 16 to 17 year-olds.[1]

- Non-CPS studies have reported higher rates of nonfatal child maltreatment cases, ranging from 15 to 43 per 1,000 children.[3,4]

Deaths from Child Maltreatment

- In 2008, an estimated 1,740 children ages 0 to 17 died from abuse and neglect (rate of 2.3 per 100,000 children).[1]
  - 80 percent of deaths occurred among children younger than age 4; 10 percent among 4–7 year-olds; 4 percent among 8–11 year-olds; 4 percent among 12–15 year olds; and 2 percent among 16–17 year-olds.
  - 39% of deaths were non-Hispanic White children.
  - 30% of deaths were African-American children.
  - 16% of deaths were Hispanic children.

Note and References

Note: Some numbers have been rounded.

47

1. U.S. Department of Health and Human Services, Administration on Children, Youth and Families. *Child Maltreatment 2008* (Washington, DC: U.S. Government Printing Office, 2010) available at: http://www.acf.hhs.gov.

2. Finkelhor D, Turner H, Ormond R, Hamby SL. Violence, abuse, and crime exposure in a national sample of children and youth. *Pediatrics* 2009; 124:1411–1423.

3. Theodore AD, Chang JJ, Runyan DK, Hunter WM, Bangdewala SI, Agans R. Epidemiologic features of the physical and sexual maltreatment of children in the Carolinas. *Pediatrics* 2005; 115: e331-e337.

4. Finkelhor D, Ormrod H, Turner H, Hamby S. The victimization of children and youth: a comprehensive national survey. *Child Maltreatment* 2005; 10: 5–25.

Section 3.2

Characteristics of Children Aided by Child Protective Services

Excerpted from "Chapter 3—Children," *Child Maltreatment 2010*, U.S. Department of Health and Human Services, 2011. The complete text of this document can be accessed online at http://archive.acf.hhs.gov/programs/cb/pubs/cm10/cm10.pdf.

About This Information

The Child Abuse Prevention and Treatment Act (CAPTA), (42 U.S.C. §5101), as amended by the CAPTA Reauthorization Act of 2010, retained the existing definition of child abuse and neglect as, at a minimum: "Any recent act or failure to act on the part of a parent or caretaker which results in death, serious physical or emotional harm, sexual abuse or exploitation; or an act or failure to act, which presents an imminent risk of serious harm."

Each state defines the types of child abuse and neglect in state statute and policy. State statutes also establish the level of evidence needed to determine a disposition of substantiated or indicated. The local child protective services (CPS) agencies respond to the safety needs of the children who are the subjects of child maltreatment reports based on these state definitions and requirements for levels of evidence.

Ongoing interest in understanding the outcomes of children and their families—as well as advances in state child welfare information systems—has resulted in the ability to assign a unique identifier, within the state, to each child who receives a CPS response. These newer capabilities enable the below-listed types of analyses to be conducted.

- **Duplicate:** Counting a child each time that he or she was a subject of a report that received a CPS response. This count is also known as a report-child pair. This type of count is useful when one is interested in the specific characteristics of an event that has occurred.

- **Unique:** Counting a child once, regardless of the number of reports that received a CPS response. For example, when discussing the age characteristics of children, the unique count may be considered preferable.

In the National Child Abuse and Neglect Data System (NCANDS), a victim is defined as a child for whom the state determined at least one maltreatment was found to be substantiated or indicated; and a disposition of substantiated, indicated, or alternative response victim was assigned for a child in a specific report. It is important to note that a child may be a victim in one report and a nonvictim in another report.

This text provides information about the characteristics of children who were found to be abused and neglected during federal fiscal year (FFY) 2010. National child maltreatment estimates for FFY 2010 are based on 2009 child populations for the 52 reporting states.

Children Who Were Subjects of a Report

Once a referral is screened-in, the local CPS unit typically conducts an investigation response. The investigation includes an assessment of safety and risk, as well as a determination of service needs. At the conclusion of the investigation, a disposition is made as to whether or not the child was maltreated. In most jurisdictions, a disposition is made with regard to each specific allegation of maltreatment. For example, the allegation of neglect could be substantiated, while an allegation of physical abuse could be unsubstantiated.

Some states also are using an alternative approach. One such response is called alternative response. During an alternative response, safety and risk assessments are conducted, but the focus is on working with the family to address issues, as opposed to gathering evidence to substantiate or not substantiate the alleged maltreatment. If alternative response is an option, it is usually offered to families based on the alleged type of maltreatment and the initial assessment of risk to the child. Typically such responses do not result in a finding for each allegation of maltreatment. Each state that uses alternative response decides how to map its codes for these programs to the NCANDS codes. Throughout this report, the term disposition is used for both investigation responses and alternative responses.

All 52 states submitted data to NCANDS about the dispositions of children who received one or more CPS responses. For FFY 2010, more than 3.6 million (duplicate) children were the subjects of at least one report. One-fifth of these children were found to be victims with dispositions of substantiated (19.5%), indicated (1.0%), and alternative response victim (0.5%). The remaining four-fifths of the children were found to be nonvictims of maltreatment. The nonvictim dispositions with the three highest percentages are unsubstantiated (58.2%), no alleged maltreatment (9.1%), and alternative response nonvictim (8.7%) (see Figure 3.1).

Examining the duplicate and unique counts of children who received a CPS response at the state level reveals the amount of duplication. Using a duplicate count, 3.6 million children received a CPS response at a rate of 47.7 children per 1,000 children in the population. Using a unique count, nearly 3 million children received a CPS

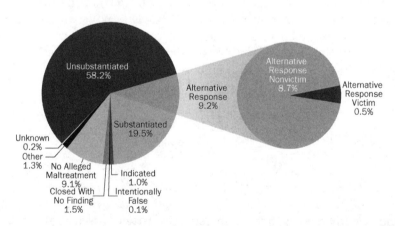

Figure 3.1. Children Who Received a CPS Response by Disposition, 2010 (duplicate count). This pie chart shows the percentages of child dispositions. The alternative response piece is further broken out to show nonvictim and victim. Approximately one-fifth of children were found be victims of maltreatment.

response at a rate of 40.0 children per 1,000 children in the population. The one state that submitted the aggregated data file, the Summary Data Component (SDC), is not included in counting victims uniquely.

As states are increasing their usage of alternative response programs, the numbers and percentages of duplicate children with alternative response dispositions also are increasing. During 2006, 5.9 percent of duplicate children received an alternative response disposition. By 2010, 9.2 percent of duplicate children received such a disposition. The fluctuation in the number of reporting states from 2008 to 2010 is a reflection of one state that piloted and discontinued its alternative response program.

Five-year trend analyses of the child disposition rates reveal slight fluctuations in the rates since 2006, regardless of whether the duplicate or unique analyses are examined. The disposition rate is the rate of all children who received a CPS response.

Number of Child Victims

The duplicate count of child victims counts a child each time he or she was found to be a victim. The unique count of child victims counts a child only once regardless of the number of times he or she was found to be a victim during the reporting year.

One-fifth of children who received an investigation or alternative response were found to have been victims of maltreatment. The FFY

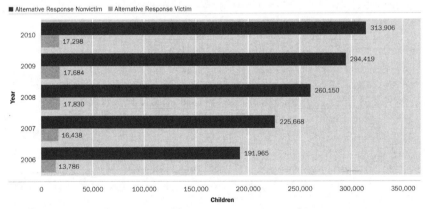

Figure 3.2. Dispositions of Children Who Received an Alternative CPS Response, 2006–2010 (duplicate count). This bar chart displays the number of children who received an alternative child protective services response from federal fiscal years 2006 through 2010. The data are presented in two categories, victim and nonvictim. The purpose is to show how numbers have been increasing.

2010 duplicate victim rate was 10.0 victims per 1,000 children in the population. The unique victim rate was 9.2 victims per 1,000 children in the population.

Analyses of the number and rate of victimization for the past five years show an overall decrease regardless of whether the duplicate or unique analyses are examined. For FFY 2010, an estimated 754,000 duplicate and 695,000 unique children were victims of maltreatment. This year more than one-half of states (29) reported a decreased number of victims when compared to FFY 2009. The decrease may be attributed to several factors, including a decrease in the number of children who received a CPS response and an increase in the number of states with alternative response dispositions. For example, one state had an approximately 30 percent decrease (about 10,000 unique victims) in the number of reported victims due to the implementation of an alternative response program. In another example, one state changed its policy for victim dispositions and this change was reflected in the national victimization decrease for FFY 2007.

First-Time Victims

Three-quarters of unique victims had no history of prior victimization for each year from FFY 2006 through FFY 2010. Information regarding first-time victims is a Federal Performance measure. The Community-Based Child Abuse Prevention Program (CBCAP) reports this measure to the Office of Management and Budget (OMB) each year as an average of all states.

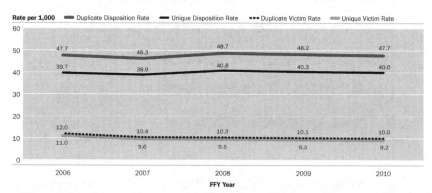

Figure 3.3. Disposition and Victimization Rates, 2006–2010 (duplicate and unique counts). This line chart graphs the rates of duplicate and unique children who received a disposition and were victims of maltreatment. Rates are provided per 1,000 in the population. Analyses of victimization for the past five years show steady decrease.

Perpetrator Relationship

Victim data were analyzed by relationship of duplicate victims to their perpetrators. Four-fifths (81.3%) of victims were maltreated by a parent either acting alone or with someone else. Nearly two-fifths (37.2%) of victims were maltreated by their mother acting alone. One-fifth (19.1%) of victims were maltreated by their father acting alone. One-fifth (18.5%) of victims were maltreated by both parents. Thirteen percent of victims were maltreated by a perpetrator who was not a parent of the child.

Child Victim Demographics

The remaining analyses focus on the demographics of the child victims and were conducted using the unique count of victims. The youngest children are the most vulnerable to maltreatment. More than one-third (34.0%) of all FFY 2010 unique victims were younger than four years. One-fifth (23.4%) of victims were in the age group 4–7 years.

Children younger than one year had the highest rate of victimization at 20.6 per 1,000 children in the population of the same age. Victims with the single-year age of one, two, or three years old had victimization rates of 11.9, 11.4, and 11.0 victims per 1,000 children of those respective ages in the population. In general, the rate and percentage of victimization decreased with age.

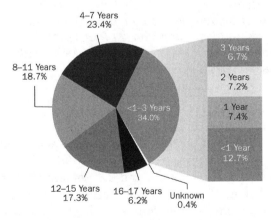

Figure 3.4. *Victims by Age, 2010 (unique count). This pie chart shows the percentage of unique victims by age group. Victims in the group birth–3 years old had highest at 34.0 percent. The youngest group is also broken out to the right.*

Victimization was split between the sexes, with boys accounting for 48.5 percent and girls accounting for 51.2 percent. Fewer than 1 percent of victims had an unknown sex.

Eighty-eight percent of unique victims were comprised of three races or ethnicities—African-American (21.9%), Hispanic (21.4%), and White (44.8%). However, victims of African-American, American Indian or Alaska Native, and multiple racial descent had the highest rates of victimization at 14.6, 11.0, and 12.7 victims, respectively, per 1,000 children in the population of the same race or ethnicity.

The above-mentioned rate and percentage demographics have remained stable for several years, regardless of whether duplicate or unique analyses are examined.

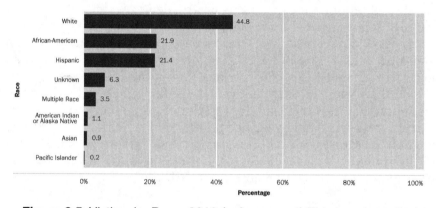

Figure 3.5. *Victims by Race, 2010 (unique count). This bar chart displays the percentages of unique victims by race. The majority comprised three races or ethnicities—African-American (21.9%), Hispanic 21.4%), and White 44.8%). These proportions have remained stable for several years, regardless whether duplicate analyses are examined.*

Maltreatment Types

Four-fifths (78.3%) of unique victims were neglected, 17.6 percent were physically abused, 9.2 percent were sexually abused, 8.1 percent were psychologically maltreated, and 2.4 percent were medically neglected. In addition, 10.3 percent of victims experienced such other types of maltreatment as abandonment, threats of harm to the child, or congenital drug addiction. States may code any maltreatment as *other* if it does not fall into one of the NCANDS categories. These percentages sum to more than 100.0 percent because a child may have suffered more than one type of maltreatment.

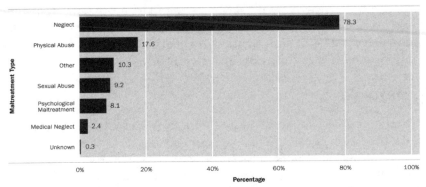

Figure 3.6. *Reported Maltreatment Types of Victims, 2010 (unique count). This bar chart shows the percentages of maltreatment types suffered by unique victims. According to the chart, four-fifths of victims experienced neglect, 17.6 percent physical abuse, and 9.2 sexual abuse. Children could have experienced more than one type, therefore the total is more than 100 percent.*

Risk Factors

Children who were reported with any of the following risk factors were considered as having a disability: mental retardation, emotional disturbance, visual or hearing impairment, learning disability, physical disability, behavioral problems, or another medical problem. Children with risk factors may be undercounted as not every child receives a clinical diagnostic assessment.

Sixteen percent of unique victims were reported as having a disability. Nearly 4 percent (3.9%) of victims were reported as having behavior problems, 3.2 percent of victims were emotionally disturbed, and another 5.2 percent of victims had some other medical condition. A victim could have been reported with more than one type of disability.

The data were examined to determine if the child victims had alcohol abuse, drug abuse, and domestic violence caregiver risk factors. This means that the child was exposed to the risk factor behavior in the home. With respect to domestic violence, the caregiver could have been either the perpetrator or the victim of the domestic violence. For the states that reported on the domestic violence caregiver risk factor, 25.7 percent of victims and 8.1 percent of nonvictims were exposed to this behavior.

Fewer states reported data on the alcohol and drug abuse caregiver risk factors. Eleven percent of victims and 5.7 percent of nonvictims were reported with the alcohol abuse caregiver risk factor, and 18.0 percent of victims and 8.9 percent of nonvictims were reported with the drug abuse caregiver risk factor. It is important to note that some states are not able to differentiate alcohol abuse and drug abuse for some or all children. Those states report both risk factors for the same children in both caregiver risk factor categories.

Recurrence

Through the Child and Family Services Reviews (CFSR), the Children's Bureau has established the current national standard for the absence of maltreatment recurrence as 94.6 percent, defined as: "Of all children who were victims of substantiated or indicated abuse or neglect during the first six months of the reporting year, what percent did not experience another incident of substantiated or indicated abuse or neglect within a six-month period."

The number of states in compliance with this standard has increased from 22 states for FFY 2006 to 27 states for FFY 2010. The percentage of states that met the standard increased from 44.9 percent during FFY 2006 to 52.9 percent for FFY 2010.

Maltreatment in Foster Care

Through the CFSR, the Children's Bureau established a national standard for the absence of maltreatment in foster care as 99.68 percent, defined as: "Of all children in foster care during the reporting period, what percent were not victims of a substantiated or indicated maltreatment by foster parents or facility staff members?"

Counts of children not maltreated in foster care are derived by subtracting the NCANDS count of children maltreated by foster care providers from the Adoption and Foster Care Analysis and Reporting System (AFCARS) count of children placed in foster care. The observation period for this measure is 12 months. The number of states in compliance has increased from 19 states that met this standard for FFY 2006 to 22 states for FFY 2010.

Chapter 4

When Children Are Exposed to Violence

Introductory Message

Children are exposed to violence every day in their homes, schools, and communities. They may be struck by a boyfriend, bullied by a classmate, or abused by an adult. They may witness an assault on a parent or a shooting on the street. Such exposure can cause significant physical, mental, and emotional harm with long-term effects that can last well into adulthood.

Children's Exposure to Violence

This chapter discusses the National Survey of Children's Exposure to Violence (NatSCEV), the most comprehensive nationwide survey of the incidence and prevalence of children's exposure to violence to date, sponsored by the Office of Juvenile Justice and Delinquency Prevention (OJJDP) and supported by the Centers for Disease Control and Prevention (CDC). Conducted between January and May 2008, it measured the past-year and lifetime exposure to violence for children age 17 and younger across several major categories:

Excerpted from "Children's Exposure to Violence: A Comprehensive National Survey," prepared by David Finkelhor, Heather Turner, Richard Ormrod, Sherry Hamby, and Kristen Kracke, Office of Juvenile Justice and Delinquency Programs (OJJDP), U.S. Department of Justice (www.ncjrs.gov), October 2009. The complete text of this document, including references is available online. Access OJJDP publications online at www.ojp.usdoj.gov/ojjdp.

- Conventional crime
- Child maltreatment
- Victimization by peers and siblings
- Sexual victimization
- Witnessing and indirect victimization (including exposure to community violence and family violence)
- School violence and threats
- Internet victimization

This survey is the first comprehensive attempt to measure children's exposure to violence in the home, school, and community across all age groups from birth to age 17, and the first attempt to measure the cumulative exposure to violence over the child's lifetime.

The survey confirms that most of our society's children are exposed to violence in their daily lives. More than 60 percent of the children surveyed were exposed to violence within the past year, either directly or indirectly (that is, as a witness to a violent act; by learning of a violent act against a family member, neighbor, or close friend; or from a threat against their home or school). Nearly one-half of the children and adolescents surveyed (46.3 percent) were assaulted at least once in the past year, and more than one in 10 (10.2 percent) were injured in an assault; one in four (24.6 percent) were victims of robbery, vandalism, or theft; one in 10 (10.2 percent) suffered from child maltreatment (including physical and emotional abuse, neglect, or a family abduction); and one in 16 (6.1 percent) were victimized sexually. More than one in four (25.3 percent) witnessed a violent act and nearly one in 10 (9.8 percent) saw one family member assault another. Multiple victimizations were common: more than one-third (38.7 percent) experienced two or more direct victimizations in the previous year, more than one in 10 (10.9 percent) experienced five or more direct victimizations in the previous year, and more than one in 75 (1.4 percent) experienced 10 or more direct victimizations in the previous year.

Reports of lifetime exposure to violence were generally about one-third to one-half higher than reports of past-year exposure, although the difference tended to be greater for less frequent and more severe types of victimization. (For example, more than three times as many respondents reported being victims of a kidnapping over their lifetimes as did in the past year.) Nearly seven in eight children (86.6 percent) who reported being exposed to violence during their lifetimes also reported being exposed to violence within the past year, which indicated that these children were at ongoing risk of violent victimization. The reports of lifetime exposure also indicate how certain types of exposure change and accumulate as a child grows up; nearly one in five girls ages 14 to 17 (18.7 percent) had been the victim of a sexual assault or attempted sexual assault, and more than one-third of all 14- to 17-year-olds had seen a parent assaulted.

Screening Questions

The survey asked screening questions about 48 types of victimization in the following categories:

- **Conventional crime:** Nine types of victimization, including robbery, theft, destruction of property, attack with an object or weapon, attack without an object or weapon, attempted attack, threatened attack, kidnapping or attempted kidnapping, and hate crime or bias attack (an attack on a child because of the child's or parent's skin color, religion, physical problem, or perceived sexual orientation).

- **Child maltreatment:** Four types of victimization, including being hit, kicked, or beaten by an adult (other than spanking on the bottom); psychological or emotional abuse; neglect; and abduction by a parent or caregiver, also known as custodial interference.

- **Peer and sibling victimization:** Six types of victimization, including being attacked by a group of children; being hit or beaten by another child, including a brother or sister; being hit or kicked in the private parts; being chased, grabbed, or forced to do something; being teased or emotionally bullied; and being a victim of dating violence.

- **Sexual victimization:** Seven types of victimization, including sexual contact or fondling by an adult the child knew, sexual contact or fondling by an adult stranger, sexual contact or fondling by another child or teenager, attempted or completed intercourse, exposure or "flashing," sexual harassment, and consensual sexual conduct with an adult.

- **Witnessing and indirect victimization:** These fall into two general categories, exposure to community violence and exposure to family violence. For exposure to community violence, the survey included 10 types of victimization, including seeing someone attacked with an object or weapon; seeing someone attacked without an object or weapon; having something stolen from the household; having a friend, neighbor, or family member murdered; witnessing a murder; witnessing or hearing a shooting, bombing, or riot; being in a war zone; knowing a family member or close friend who was fondled or forced to have sex; knowing a family member or close friend who was robbed or mugged; and knowing a family member or close friend who was threatened with a gun or knife. For exposure to family violence, eight types of victimization were assessed: seeing a parent assaulted by a spouse, domestic partner, or boyfriend or girlfriend; seeing a brother or sister assaulted by a parent; threat by one parent to assault the other; threat by a parent to damage the other parent's property; one parent pushing the other; one parent hitting or slapping the other; one parent kicking, choking, or beating up the other; and assault by another adult household member against a child or adult in the household.

- **School violence and threat:** Two types of victimization, including a credible bomb threat against the child's school and fire or other property damage to the school.

- **Internet violence and victimization:** Two types of victimization, including internet threats or harassment and unwanted online sexual solicitation.

History of the Current Study

Under the leadership of then Deputy Attorney General Eric Holder in June 1999, OJJDP created the Safe Start Initiative to prevent and reduce the impact of children's exposure to violence. As a part of this initiative and with a growing need to document the full extent of children's exposure to violence, OJJDP launched the National Survey of Children's Exposure to Violence (NatSCEV).

Safe Start's NatSCEV is the first national incidence and prevalence study to examine comprehensively the extent and nature of children's exposure to violence across all ages, settings, and timeframes. It measures their experience of violence in the home, school, and community. It asked children and their adult caregivers about not only the incidents of violence that children suffered and witnessed themselves but also other related crime and threat exposures, such as theft or burglary from a child's household, being in a school that was the target of a credible bomb threat, and being in a war zone or an area where ethnic violence occurred. It includes both the past-year and lifetime exposure to violence of children of all ages up to age 17. The study was developed under the direction of OJJDP, and was designed and conducted by the Crimes against Children Research Center of the University of New Hampshire. It provides comprehensive data on the full extent of violence in the daily lives of children.

The primary purpose of NatSCEV is to document the incidence and prevalence of children's exposure to a broad array of violent experiences across a wide developmental spectrum. The research team asked followup questions about specific events, including where the exposure to violence occurred, whether injury resulted, how often the child was exposed to a specific type of violence, and the child's relationship to the perpetrator and (when the child witnessed violence) the victim. In addition, the study documents differences in exposure to violence across gender, race, socioeconomic status, family structure, region, urban/rural residence, and developmental stage of the child; specifies how different forms of violent victimization cluster or co-occur; identifies individual, family, and community-level predictors of violence exposure among children; examines associations between levels/types of violence exposure and child mental and emotional health; and assesses the extent to which children disclose incidents of violence to various individuals and the nature and source of assistance or treatment provided (if any).

This study began in 2007 with funding from OJJDP's Safe Start Initiative. OJJDP then partnered with CDC to collect additional data on safe, stable, and nurturing relationships—a key focus for CDC's child maltreatment prevention activities. The combined approach by OJJDP and CDC is providing critical national data on levels of violence as well as data on key indicators of protective factors.

Highlights of the Survey Results

NatSCEV estimates both past-year and lifetime exposure to violence across a number of categories, including physical assault, bullying, sexual victimization, child maltreatment, dating violence, and witnessed and indirect victimization. Figure 4.1 illustrates the past-year exposure for all survey respondents to selected categories of violence. Some of the more notable findings are outlined below.

The NatSCEV survey found that children's exposure to violence is common; more than 60 percent of the children surveyed had been exposed to violence in the past year and more than one in 10 reported five or more exposures. This exposure occurs across all age ranges of childhood and for both genders. In general, however, the types of exposure that were most prevalent among younger children were less serious, such as assaults without a weapon or without injury, assaults by a juvenile sibling, or bullying and teasing, all of which were most common among six- to nine-year-olds and declined thereafter. Older adolescents ages 14 to 17 were the most likely to experience more serious forms of violence, including assaults with injury, gang assaults, sexual victimizations, and physical and emotional abuse, and to witness violence in the community. This is not a hard and fast distinction; some serious forms of victimization, including kidnapping and assaults with a weapon, were most common among 10- to 13-year-olds. This age group was also the most likely to witness violence within the home, including domestic violence involving their parents and assaults by other family members.

Developmental Patterns in Exposure to Violence

Victimization in infancy: The most common victimizations during this period are assault by a sibling, assault with no weapon or injury, and witnessing family assault.

Victimization in the toddler years (ages two to five): The most common victimizations during this period are assault by a sibling, assault with no weapon or injury, bullying (physical), and witnessing family assault.

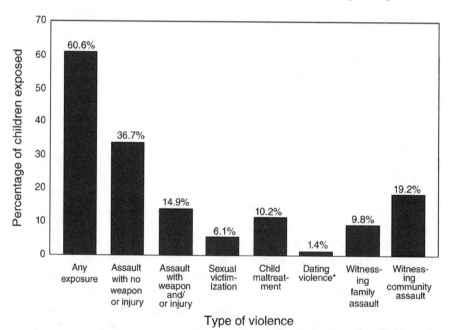

Figure 4.1. Past-Year Exposure to Selected Categories of Violence for All Children Surveyed (*Figures for dating violence are only for children and adolescents age 12 and older.)

Victimization in middle childhood (ages six to nine): This age range represents the peak risk period for assault by a sibling, assault with no weapon or injury, bullying (physical), and emotional bullying/teasing.

Victimization in preteens and early adolescence (ages 10 to 13): This age range represents the peak risk period for assault with weapon, sexual harassment (same rate ages 10 to 17), kidnapping, witnessing family assault, and witnessing intimate partner (interparental) violence.

Victimization in later adolescence (ages 14 to 17): This age range represents the peak risk period for assault with injury, assault by peer (nonsibling), genital assault, dating violence, sexual victimizations of all types, sexual assault, sexual harassment (same rate ages 10 to 17), flashing or sexual exposure, unwanted online sexual solicitation, any maltreatment, physical abuse, psychological or emotional abuse, witnessing community assault, exposure to shooting, and school threat of bomb or attack.

Physical Assault

Nearly one-half (46.3 percent) of all the children surveyed were physically assaulted within the previous year, and more than one-half (56.7 percent) had been assaulted during their lifetime. Physical assaults are extremely common across the entire span of childhood and peak during middle childhood. Assaults by siblings especially show a marked developmental trend, peaking during the middle childhood years (ages six to nine) and then declining. Incidence for the most severe assaults, however, rises steadily with age. Among 14- to 17-year-olds, nearly one in five (18.8 percent) had been injured in the past year in a physical assault. New forms of violence, such as dating violence, also emerge during adolescence, reaching a 5.6-percent past-year incidence rate and an 8.8-percent lifetime rate for the oldest adolescents. The lifetime incidence of assault victimization generally rose steadily as children grew older, with more than seven in ten 14- to 17-year-olds (71.1 percent) reporting that they had been assaulted during their lifetimes.

In general, boys are somewhat more likely than girls to be victims of assault. The past-year incidence of assault is 50.2 percent for boys and 42.1 percent for girls, and the lifetime incidence of assault is 60.3 percent for boys and 52.9 percent for girls. These patterns are consistent with other data on criminal victimization, which typically show that males are the most common targets of physical assault.

Bullying

The survey looked at bullying separately from assault and asked about multiple types of bullying: physical bullying, emotional bullying, and internet harassment. Overall, 13.2 percent of those surveyed reported having been physically bullied within the past year, and more than one in five (21.6 percent) reported having been physically bullied during their lifetimes. The risk of bullying peaks during middle childhood in a pattern similar to that for sibling assault. The highest incidence occurs among six- to nine-year-olds, who had rates of 21.5 percent past-year incidence and 28.0 percent lifetime incidence.

About one in five children (19.7 percent) reported having been teased or emotionally bullied in the previous year and nearly three in 10 reported having been teased or emotionally bullied in their lifetimes. Teasing or emotional bullying followed a similar pattern to physical bullying among age groups, rising to reach a peak among six- to nine-year-olds, nearly one-third of whom (30.4 percent) reported having been teased in the past year and then falling steadily thereafter.

Internet harassment was less common than other forms of bullying. Questions about internet harassment were asked only of youth age 10 and older, who might be most likely to independently use a computer. Unlike other forms of bullying, the peak risk period for internet harassment was ages 14 to 17. In this group, 5.6 percent reported internet harassment within the past year and 7.9 percent during their lifetimes.

Boys were more likely than girls to be physically bullied or threatened, but girls were more likely to be victims of internet harassment. For past-year rates, there were no significant gender differences in emotional bullying; however, for lifetime rates, girls reported more cumulative exposure to emotional bullying than boys.

Sexual Victimization

Overall, 6.1 percent of all children surveyed had been sexually victimized in the past year and nearly one in ten (9.8 percent) over their lifetimes. Sexual victimizations included attempted and completed rape (1.1 percent past year, 2.4 percent lifetime); sexual assault by a known adult (0.3 percent past year, 1.2 percent lifetime), an adult stranger (0.3 percent past year, 0.5 percent lifetime), or a peer (1.3 percent past year, 2.7 percent lifetime); flashing or sexual exposure by an adult (0.4 percent past year, 0.6 percent lifetime) or peer (2.2 percent past year, 3.7 percent lifetime); sexual harassment (2.6 percent past year, 4.2 percent lifetime); and statutory sexual offenses (0.1 percent past year, 0.4 percent lifetime).[1] Adolescents ages 14 to

17 were by far the most likely to be sexually victimized; nearly one in six (16.3 percent) was sexually victimized in the past year, and more than one in four (27.3 percent) had been sexually victimized during their lifetimes. The most common forms of sexual victimization were flashing or exposure by a peer, sexual harassment, and sexual assault.

Girls were more likely than boys to be sexually victimized: 7.4 percent of girls reported a sexual victimization within the past year, and nearly one in eight (12.2 percent) reported being sexually victimized during their lifetimes. Girls ages 14 to 17 had the highest rates of sexual victimization: 7.9 percent were victims of sexual assault in the past year and 18.7 percent during their lifetimes.

Child Maltreatment

Overall, more than one in 10 children surveyed (10.2 percent) suffered some form of maltreatment (including physical abuse other than sexual assault, psychological or emotional abuse, child neglect, and custodial interference) during the past year and nearly one in five (18.6 percent) during their lifetimes. Both the past-year and lifetime rates of exposure to maltreatment rose as children grew older, particularly for children age 10 and older: one in six 14- to 17-year-olds (16.6 percent) suffered maltreatment during the past year and nearly one in three (32.1 percent) during their lifetimes.

Patterns of child maltreatment were similar for girls and boys with the exception of psychological or emotional abuse, the incidence of which was somewhat higher for girls than for boys. Rates of sexual assault by a known adult (not limited to caregivers) were also higher for girls than for boys, in a pattern that was similar to other forms of sexual victimization.

Witnessing and Indirect Exposure to Violence

NatSCEV found that witnessing violence was a common occurrence for children, particularly as they grew older. Overall, more than one-quarter of children surveyed (25.3 percent) had witnessed violence in their homes, schools, and communities during the past year; and more than one-third (37.8 percent) had witnessed violence against another person during their lifetimes. The proportion of children who witnessed violence both within the past year and during their lifetimes rose from one age group to the next.

Of all forms of victimization measured in NatSCEV, witnessing community violence showed the strongest age trends. There was more than a sevenfold increase in rates from toddlers (two- to five-year-olds) to older adolescents (14- to 17-year-olds). More than seven in ten 14- to 17-year-olds had witnessed violence against another person during their lives.

These age trends were due mostly to witnessing violence in the community. The past-year incidence of witnessing assaults in the community rose from 5.8 percent among two- to five-year-olds to 42.2 percent among 14- to 17-year-olds; lifetime incidence rose even more dramatically, from 9.0 percent of two- to five-year-olds to nearly two-thirds (64.2 percent) of 14- to 17-year-olds. Witnessing of shootings also rose sharply in both past-year and lifetime incidence from one age group to the next. Among children younger than two years old, 1.1 percent were exposed to shootings in the past year, whereas more than one in ten 14- to 17-year-olds (10.2 percent) witnessed a shooting in the past year. Similarly, 3.5 percent of two- to five-year-olds had witnessed a shooting during their lifetimes, whereas more than one in five 14- to 17-year-olds (22.2 percent) had witnessed a shooting.[2] As striking as these age trends are, even the lower numbers among young children are cause for great concern.

In contrast to the patterns for witnessing community violence, few age trends in exposure can be seen for witnessing violence within the family. Rates for witnessing family violence were fairly constant across the span of childhood, with all age groups falling in a fairly narrow range of approximately six to 11 percent.

Over the course of their lifetimes, boys overall were slightly more likely than girls to witness violence (40.1 percent of boys and 35.4 percent of girls). Boys were more likely to witness violence in the community, murder, and shootings both in the past year and during their lifetimes. There were no gender differences in witnessing family violence.

Multiple and Cumulative Victimizations

A large proportion of children surveyed (38.7 percent) reported more than one direct victimization (a victimization directed toward the child, as opposed to an incident that the child witnessed, heard, or was otherwise exposed to) within the previous year. Of those who reported any direct victimization, nearly two-thirds (64.5 percent) reported more than one. A significant number of children reported high levels of exposure to violence in the past year: more than one in ten (10.9 percent) reported five or more direct exposures to violence, and 1.4 percent reported 10 or more direct victimizations. (Victimizations that could be counted in more than one category, such as physical abuse by a parent or caregiver that could also be considered an assault, were not included in the counting of multiple victimizations.)

Children who were exposed to one type of violence, both within the past year and over their lifetimes, were at far greater risk of experiencing other types of violence. For example, a child who was physically assaulted in the past year would be five times as likely to also have been sexually victimized and more than four times as likely also to have been maltreated during that period. Similarly, a child who was physically assaulted during his or her lifetime would be more than six times as likely to have been sexually victimized and more than five times as likely to have been maltreated during his or her lifetime.

For Further Information

To learn more about the Safe Start Initiative, visit www.safestartcenter .org. For more information about the National Survey of Children's Exposure to Violence, visit the Crimes against Children Research Center website at www.unh.edu/ccrc.

Endnotes

1. The aggregate figure for any sexual victimization did not include unwanted online sexual solicitation (D. Finkelhor et al., Violence, crime, and exposure in a national sample of children and youth. *Pediatrics* 124[5], November 2009).

2. Previous studies have also noted that low-income and minority youth are many times more likely to have witnessed serious violence in the community. Kracke and Hahn cite studies noting that only one percent of upper-middle-class youth had witnessed a murder and nine percent had witnessed a stabbing, whereas 43 percent of low-income African American school-aged children had witnessed a murder and 56 percent had witnessed a stabbing (Kracke, K., and Hahn, H. 2008. The nature and extent of childhood exposure to violence: What we know, why we don't know more, and why it matters. *Journal of Emotional Abuse* 8(1/2):29–49).

Chapter 5

Child Exploitation

Chapter Contents

Section 5.1

Vulnerable Children and Child Labor

"Child Labor—an Overview," by Lynda Diane Mull. © 2012
International Initiative to End Child Labor (www.endchildlabor.org).
All rights reserved. Reprinted with permission.

Child Labor—An Overview

- "Child labor is the single most important source of child exploitation and child abuse in the world today." —ILO Conference Report, 1996

Children continue to be the most vulnerable in our world's society. While we live in an era of unprecedented global economic integration, competitive pressures feed the need for an ever-cheaper supply of labor, and child labor is the cheapest of all.

Child labor is a socioeconomic problem that encompasses a host of social and economic factors, including the role of children in traditional societies, poverty, and the availability of basic services. The work of children ranges from "work" that does not interfere with the education and development of a child to exhaustive, dangerous, or illegal "labor" that is abusive and exploitative; including child slavery and trafficking, prostitution, soldiering, or hazardous work that places the child's health, safety, or morals at risk.

The problem of child labor has been on the international agenda for a relatively short period of time, most notably since the ratification of the United Nations Convention on the Rights of the Child (CRC) in 1989. Since that time, projects have been designed and implemented throughout the developing world, primarily led by the International Labour Organization (ILO) and the United Nations Children's Fund (UNICEF).

How Many Children Work and What Kind of Work do They Perform?

All around the world 211 million children between the ages of 5 and 14 are working. At least 60 million are working under dangerous

70

or abusive conditions. The majority of working children work in the agricultural industry (70%), but children are working in many other industries as well. Here are some examples of the types of child labor situations that children can be found:

- In West Africa children are exposed to hazards while harvesting cocoa beans.

- In Burma, Burundi, Columbia, the Democratic Republic of Congo and Sudan they serve as soldiers.

- In some parts of the world girls and boys are trafficked into prostitution while others work on agricultural plantations and other industries.

- In Asia, Africa, and Latin America children haul bricks.

Children who work long hours under dangerous conditions are deprived of their rights to an education. The worst forms of child labor place a child's health, safety, and morals at risk and can endanger the child's life.

What Are the Worst Forms of Child Labor and What Is Hazardous Work?

Combating child labor must take into consideration specific cultural and economic contexts. In fact, the World Bank suggests that "the concern of policy makers should be children's welfare, rather than children's work in itself" (World Bank, 2001, page 3). Child work may be a necessary economic or cultural practice; and removing all children from work may not be in the best interest of the child.

To ensure that the work children perform is not hazardous or abusive, activities that a child performs and the conditions under which the child works needs to be examined. While hazardous and exploitive work is often based on the specific situation, the work of children can usually be defined as "acceptable" work or worst forms of "child labor" that need to be immediately confronted.

With less harmful forms of child labor, households can be encouraged to decrease the work load gradually. Wage employment away from the home, on the other hand, has a greater potential for exploitation and abuse. For example, domestic servants are often ill paid, work long hours, and are the subject of physical and sexual abuse. Children working away from homes are also more likely to not attend school (World Bank, 2001). Street or migrant children that have no home are often the most vulnerable. By focusing on the most abusive forms of child labor first, families and service providers can prioritize needs and help those in greatest need.

When examining child labor in a particular country and planning intervention strategies, it is important to understand what job tasks and conditions of work are considered hazardous. Convention 182 on the Elimination of the Worst Forms of Child Labor of the International Labor Organization defines the term of "worst forms of child labor" in Article 3 as:

a) all forms of slavery or practices similar to slavery, such as the sale and trafficking of children, debt bondage, and serfdom and forced or compulsory labor, including forced or compulsory recruitment of children for use in armed conflict;

b) the use, procuring, or offering of a child for prostitution, for the production of pornography or for pornographic performances;

c) the use, procuring, or offering of a child for illicit activities, in particular for the production and trafficking of drugs as defined in the relevant international treaties; and

d) work that, by its nature or the circumstances in which it is carried out, is likely to harm the health, safety, or morals of children.

Within Article 3, sections (a) through (c) are fairly well explained and defined. However, Article 3(d) requires further exploration. Once Convention 182 is ratified by a country and filed with the ILO, defining section (d) is largely left up to the country. The following provides ECACL's [Education to Combat Abusive Child Labor's] interpretation of Article 3(d). The following was developed and discussed with representatives of the ILO and has been used during planning analyses that ECACL has conducted in numerous countries. ECACL recommends that the following tasks be considered when examining work that is "likely to harm the health, safety, or morals of children" under Article 3(d):

a) work that exposes children to physical, psychological, or sexual abuse;

b) work underground, under water, at dangerous heights, or in confined spaces;

c) work with dangerous machinery, equipment and tools, or that involves the manual handling or transport of heavy loads;

d) work in an unhealthy environment that may expose children to (include but not be limited to) hazardous substances, agents or processes, or to temperatures, noise levels, or vibrations damaging to their health; and

e) work under particularly difficult conditions, including but not limited to work for long hours or during the night or work where the child is unreasonably confined to the premises of the employer.

Section 5.2

Sexual Exploitation of Children

Excerpted from "National Strategy for Child Exploitation
Prevention and Interdiction, a Report to Congress," U.S. Department
of Justice (www.justice.gov), August 2010.

- "There can be no keener revelation of a society's soul than the way in which it treats its children."—Nelson Mandela

- "Given the current statistics surrounding child pornography, we are living in a country that is losing its soul."—The Honorable John Adams, Northern District of Ohio, *U.S. v Cunningham*, 1:09-CR-00154-JRA.

The sexual abuse and exploitation of children rob the victims of their childhood, irrevocably interfering with their emotional and psychological development. Ensuring that all children come of age without being disturbed by sexual trauma or exploitation is more than a criminal justice issue, it is a societal issue. Despite efforts to date, the threat of child sexual exploitation remains very real, whether it takes place in the home, on the street, over the internet, or in a foreign land.

Because the sexual abuse and exploitation of children strikes at the very foundation of our society, it will take our entire society to combat this affront to the public welfare. Therefore, this National Strategy lays out a comprehensive response to protect the right of children to be free from sexual abuse and to protect society from the cost imposed by this crime.

In the broadest terms, the goal of this National Strategy is to prevent child sexual exploitation from occurring in the first place, in order to protect every child's opportunity and right to have a childhood that

73

is free from sexual abuse, trauma, and exploitation so that they can become the adults they were meant to be. This Strategy will accomplish that goal by efficiently leveraging assets across the federal government in a coordinated manner. All entities with a stake in the fight against child exploitation—from federal agencies and investigators and prosecutors, to social service providers, educators, medical professionals, academics, non-governmental organizations, and members of industry, as well as parents, caregivers, and the threatened children themselves—are called upon to do their part to prevent these crimes, care for the victims, and rehabilitate the offenders.

Background

In 2008, Congress passed and President Bush signed the Providing Resources, Officers, and Technology to Eradicate Cyber Threats to Our Children Act of 2008 (the "PROTECT Our Children Act" or the "Act"). This Act requires the Department of Justice (the "Department") to formulate and implement a National Strategy to combat child exploitation. The Act also requires the Department to submit a report on the National Strategy (the "National Strategy" or "Report") amount of information, including: (1) an assessment of the magnitude of child exploitation; (2) a review of the Department and other state and federal agencies' efforts to coordinate and combat child exploitation; and (3) a proposed set of goals and priorities for reducing child exploitation. In this inaugural National Strategy report, the Department describes its first-ever threat assessment of the danger that faces the nation's children, its current efforts to combat child exploitation, and posits some goals and plans to fight the threats that are facing our nation's children.

The Threat Assessment

This Report attempts to marshal a massive amount of information about the nature of the child exploitation problem and the significant efforts being undertaken by federal, state, and local agencies to address this epidemic. To evaluate the extent and forms of child exploitation, between approximately February 2009 and February 2010, the National Drug Intelligence Center ("NDIC") prepared a threat assessment (the "Threat Assessment" or "Assessment") that is summarized in this Report. In conducting the Threat Assessment, NDIC interviewed over a hundred prosecutors, investigators, and other experts in the field, conducted interviews to collect information, reviewed thousands of pages of documents from investigations, cases, relevant research, and analyzed data from the National Center for Missing & Exploited Children. In addition to conducting the Threat Assessment, the Department and the Library of Congress have gathered and reviewed an extensive amount of studies and research relevant to the field of child exploitation to help inform the Department and its partners of the most recent information available from academia on this subject.

The Threat Assessment research indicates that the threat to our nation's children of becoming a victim of child exploitation is a very serious one. For example, investigators and prosecutors report dramatic increases in the number, and violent character, of the sexually abusive images of children being trafficked through the internet. They also report the disturbing trend of younger children depicted in these images, even including toddlers and infants. Further, offenders have become proficient at enticing children to engage in risky behavior, like agreeing to meet for sexual activity, or even to display themselves engaging in sexual activity through images or webcams. In addition, the offenders have been able to master internet technologies to better mask their identities.

To address the threat to our nation's children, the National Strategy focuses on the following types of child sexual exploitation: (1) child pornography, often called images of child sexual abuse; (2) online enticement of children for sexual purposes; (3) commercial sexual exploitation of children, and (4) child sex tourism. In short, the threat of sexual exploitation faced by children today is very real.

Child Pornography

The expansion of the internet has led to an explosion in the market for child pornography, making it easier to create, access, and distribute these images of abuse. While "child pornography" is the term commonly used by lawmakers, prosecutors, investigators, and the public to describe this form of sexual exploitation of children, that term largely fails to describe the true horror that is faced by hundreds of thousands of children every year. The child victims are first sexually assaulted in order to produce the vile, and often violent, images. They are then victimized again when these images of their sexual assault are traded over the internet in massive numbers by like-minded people across the globe.

The anonymity afforded by the internet makes the offenders more difficult to locate, and makes them bolder in their actions. Investigations show that offenders often gather in communities over the internet where trading of these images is just one component of a larger relationship that is premised on a shared sexual interest in children.

This has the effect of eroding the shame that typically would accompany this behavior, and desensitizing those involved to the physical and psychological damage caused to the children involved. This self-reinforcing cycle is fueling ever greater demand in the market for these images. In the world of child pornography, this demand drives supply. The individual collector who methodically gathers one image after another has the effect of validating the production of the image, which leads only to more production. Because the internet has blurred traditional notions of jurisdiction and sovereignty, this urgent crime problem is truly global in scope, and requires a coordinated national and international response.

Online Enticement of Children

Child predators often use the internet to identify, and then coerce, their victims to engage in illegal sex acts. These criminals will lurk in chat rooms or on bulletin board websites that are popular with children and teenagers. They will gain the child's confidence and trust, and will then direct the conversation to sexual topics. Sometimes they send the child sexually explicit images of themselves, or they may request that the child send them pornographic images of themselves. Often, the defendants plan a face-to-face [meeting] for the purpose of engaging in sex acts.

The Commercial Sexual Exploitation of Children

Children are being recruited and coerced into the world of prostitution in our own cities. Teen runaways—who are often trying to escape abusive homes—may turn to prostitution as a means of survival. They also frequently fall prey to "pimps" who lure them in with an offer of food, clothes, attention, friendship, love, and a seemingly safe place to sleep. Once the pimps gain this control over the children, they often use acts of violence, intimidation, or psychological manipulation to trap the children in a life of prostitution. Pimps will also cause the children to become addicted to drugs or alcohol (or will increase the severity of a pre-existing addiction) in order to ensure complicity. These children are taught to lie about their age and are given fake ID (identification). They are also trained not to trust law enforcement and to lie to protect their pimps. As a result, these victims are often not recognized as victims, and may be arrested and jailed. The dangers faced by these children—from the pimps, from their associates, and from customers—are severe. These children become hardened by the treacherous street environment in which they must learn to survive. As such, they do not always outwardly present as sympathetic victims. These child victims need specialized services that are not widely available given that they often present with illnesses, drug additions, physical and sexual trauma, lack of viable family and community ties, and total dependence—physical and psychological—on their abusers, the pimps.

Child Sex Tourism

"Child sex tourism" refers to Americans or U.S. resident aliens traveling abroad for the purpose of sexually abusing foreign children (usually in economically disadvantaged countries). Americans, capitalizing on their relative wealth and the lack of effective law enforcement in the destination countries, easily purchase access to young children to engage in illicit sex acts, sometimes for as little as $5. Like child pornography and other internet-facilitated crimes against children, the internet has revolutionized the child sex tourism industry. As a result, a new, emboldened crop of offenders are finding the navigation of travel in developing countries much easier than in the past. Additionally, the internet allows like-minded offenders to gather and exchange information on how and where to find child victims in these foreign locations, making the offenders better informed about where sex tourism is prevalent and where law enforcement is lax. Numerous countries in Southeast Asia are so well-known for child sex tourism that there are entire neighborhoods which are considered brothels, and there are open-air markets where children can be purchased for sex.

A Mother's Story of Child Pornography Victimization

[M]y daughter was abused repeatedly to produce images for the purpose of being traded [and] shared over the internet. Without a market to receive and trade those images, without the encouragement of those who wanted to acquire the images, I truly believe this abuse would not have occurred.

All those who trade these images and thereby create the demand for lurid and violent depictions of children are participants in the exploitation of my daughter. Each traded picture that placed a value on inventiveness, novelty, or cruelty played a role in egging on the abuser to even more vile acts.

The pictures of my daughter were "made for trade"—her abuser adapted to serve his market—whatever his audience was looking to acquire, that's what happened to her...

Producer, distributor, and consumer—everyone who participates in this evil exchange helps create a market, casting a vote for the next abuse. Regardless of whether they directly abused children themselves, reveled in the images of suffering, or persuaded others to abuse children on their behalf (to provide images of the abuse) each participant has a responsibility for the effects...

[A] shadow... comes over her face if a stranger gives her an expected compliment. The pictures are still out there...

Now that she's growing older and realizing the extent of the internet, she's also beginning to grasp the darker side of the story—how many people see those same pictures as something to enjoy rather than abhor.

We have no way of knowing how many pedophiles used the pictures of her being tortured and degraded as an opportunity for personal gratification ...

I can find no words to express the fury I feel at those who participate in this evil, or my scorn for any attempt to minimize responsibility by feeble claims that the crime was "victimless." My daughter is a real person. She was horribly victimized to provide this source of "entertainment." She is exploited anew each and every time an image of her suffering is copied, traded, or sold. While the crime is clearly conscienceless, it is hardly "victimless."

I asked my daughter what she most wanted to ask of the judge. Her request: "Please, don't let them pretend no one's getting hurt."

Chapter 6

Abuse by Other Children

Chapter Contents

Section 6.1

Sibling Abuse

Excerpted from "Sibling Abuse," http://www.med.umich.edu/yourchild/
topics/sibabuse.htm, written and compiled by Kyla Boyse, RN, reviewed
by Brenda Volling, PhD, updated November 2012. Content provided by
the University of Michigan Health System, © 2012. All rights reserved.
Reprinted with permission.

What is sibling abuse?

Sibling abuse is the physical, emotional or sexual abuse of one sibling by another.[1] The physical abuse can range from more mild forms of aggression between siblings, such as pushing and shoving, to very violent behavior such as using weapons.

Often parents don't see the abuse for what it is. As a rule, parents and society expect fights and aggression among siblings. Because of this, parents often don't see sibling abuse as a problem until serious harm occurs.

Besides the direct dangers of sibling abuse, the abuse can cause all kinds of long-term problems on into adulthood.

How common is sibling abuse?

Research shows that violence between siblings is quite common. In fact, it is probably even more common than child abuse (by parents) or spouse abuse.[1] The most violent members of American families are the children.

Experts estimate that three children in 100 are dangerously violent toward a brother or sister.[2,3] A 2005 study puts the number of assaults each year to children by a sibling at about 35 per 100 kids. The same study found the rate to be similar across income levels and racial and ethnic groups.

Likewise, many researchers have estimated sibling incest to be much more common than parent-child incest.

It seems that when abusive acts occur between siblings, family members often don't see it as abuse.[4]

How do I identify abuse? What is the difference between sibling abuse and sibling rivalry?

At times, all siblings squabble and call each other mean names, and some young siblings may "play doctor." But here is the difference between typical sibling behavior and abuse: If one child is always the victim and the other child is always the aggressor, it is an abusive situation. Some possible signs of sibling abuse are:

• One child always avoids their sibling

• A child has changes in behavior, sleep patterns, eating habits, or has nightmares

• A child acts out abuse in play

• A child acts out sexually in inappropriate ways

• The children's roles are rigid: one child is always the aggressor, the other, the victim

• The roughness or violence between siblings is increasing over time

What are some of the risk factors for sibling abuse?

We need more research to find out exactly how and why sibling abuse happens. Experts think there are a number of possible risk factors:

• Parents are not around much at home.

• Parents are not very involved in their children's lives, or are emotionally distant.

• Parents accept sibling rivalry and fights as part of family life, rather than working to minimize them.

• Parents have not taught kids how to handle conflicts in a healthy way from early on.

• Parents do not stop children when they are violent (they may assume it was an accident, part of a two-way fight, or normal horseplay).

• Parents increase competition among children by: playing favorites; comparing children; labeling or type-casting children (even casting kids in positive roles is harmful).

• Parents and children are in denial that there is a problem.

- Children have inappropriate family roles, for example, they are burdened with too much care-taking for a younger sibling.

- Children are exposed to violence: in their family (domestic violence); in the media (for example, in TV shows or video games); among their peers or in their neighborhoods (for example, bullying).

- Parents have not taught children about sexuality and about personal safety.

- Children have been sexually abused or witnessed sexual abuse.

- Children have access to pornography.

How can I prevent abuse from taking place between my children?

- Reduce the rivalries between your children.

- Set ground rules to prevent emotional abuse, and stick to them. For example, make it clear you will not put up with name-calling, teasing, belittling, intimidating, or provoking.

- Don't give your older children too much responsibility for your younger kids. For example, use after-school care programs, rather than leaving older children in charge of younger ones after school.

- Set aside time regularly to talk with your children one-on-one, especially after they've been alone together.

- Know when to intervene in your kids' conflicts, to prevent an escalation to abuse.

- Learn to mediate conflicts.

- Model good conflict-solving skills for your children.

- Model non-violence for your children.

- Teach your children to "own" their own bodies.

- Teach them to say "no" to unwanted physical contact.

- Create a family atmosphere where everyone feels at ease talking about sexual issues and problems.

- Keep an eye on your kids' media choices (TV, video games, and internet surfing), and either join in and then discuss the media messages or ban the poor choices.

- In short, stay actively involved in your kids' lives.

What should I do if there's abuse going on between my kids?

When one sibling hits, bites, or physically tortures a brother or sister, the normal rivalry has become abuse. You can't let this dangerous behavior continue. Here's what to do:

- Whenever violence occurs between children, separate them.

- After a cooling off period, bring all the kids involved into a family meeting.

- Gather information on facts and feelings.

- State the problem as you understand it.

- Help the kids work together to set a positive goal. For example, they will separate themselves and take time to cool off when they start arguing.

- Brainstorm many possible solutions to the problem, and ways to reach the goal.

- Talk together about the list of solutions and pick the ones that are best for everyone.

- Write up a contract together that states the rights and responsibilities of each child. Include a list of expected behavior, and consequences for breaking the code of conduct.

- Make sure you don't ignore, blame, or punish the victim—while at the same time, not playing favorites.

- Make your expectations and the family rules very clear.

- Continue to watch closely your kids' contacts in the future.

- Help your kids learn how to manage their anger.

If problems continue or violent behavior is extreme, your family should get professional help.

Can sibling relationships have lasting effects into adulthood?

In the last few years, more researchers have looked at the lasting effects of early experiences with sisters and brothers. Siblings can have strong, long-lasting effects on one another's emotional development as adults.

Research indicates that the long-term effects of surviving sibling abuse can include:

- Depression, anxiety, and low self-esteem

- Inability to trust; relationship difficulties

- Alcohol and drug addiction

- Learned helplessness

- Eating disorders

Even less extreme sibling rivalry during childhood can create insecurity and poor self-image in adulthood. Sibling conflict does not have to be physically violent to take a long-lasting emotional toll. Emotional abuse, which includes teasing, name-calling, and isolation can also do long-term damage.

The abuser is also at risk—for future violent or abusive relationships, like dating violence and domestic violence.

What are some sources of additional information and support?

- **The National Child Abuse Hotline:** Call 1-800-422-4453 or 1-800-4-A-CHILD . This number provides crisis counseling, child abuse reporting information, and information and referrals for every county in the United States. Referrals include national, state, and local agencies. Mental health professionals staff the hotline 24 hours a day, seven days a week. You can also call your local Department of Social Services. Find those telephone numbers in the phone book in the County Government section.

- *A Parents' Guide to Sibling Sexual Abuse*: This informative guide includes links at the end to age-appropriate booklets to help kids and teens that have gone through abuse (http://www.sasian .org/guide/aguide_en.htm). Also available in French, Spanish, and German.

- **Sibling Abuse Survivors Information and Advocacy Network (SASIAN):** Available online at http://www.sasian.org.

- **Related YourChild resources:** "Sibling Rivalry," "Behavior Problems," "Parenting Resources," "Siblings of Children with Special Needs," and "New Baby Sibling," available online at http://www.med.umich.edu/yourchild/topics/.

What are some good books about sibling abuse?

- *What Parents Need to Know About Sibling Abuse: Breaking the Cycle of Violence*, by Vernon R. Wiehe. A guide just for parents to preventing and addressing verbal and physical sibling abuse.

- *Sibling Abuse: Hidden Physical, Emotional, and Sexual Trauma*, by Vernon R. Wiehe. Written for parents and therapists, a social worker addresses the social problem of the abuse of one sibling by another. He presents testimony from victims, identifies criteria for evaluating sibling interactions, and provides guidelines for prevention and treatment.

- *Sibling Abuse Trauma: Assessment and Intervention Strategies for Children, Families, and Adults*, by John Caffaro and Allison Conn-Caffaro. Written for professionals. Integrating theory, research, and their clinical experiences, the authors address sibling relationship development, and sibling physical, sexual, and psychological abuse. Includes risk factors, case studies, and interviews.

- *Not Child's Play: An Anthology on Brother-Sister Incest*, by Risa Shaw. This anthology of short stories, poetry, prose and art by women survivors of brother-sister sexual abuse brings the issue out in the open in an empowering way. The collection may be useful for survivors (teens and up) and their families, and for counselors/therapists.

- *Sarah's Waterfall*, by Ellery Akers. A fictional story, aimed at girls ages 7–12 (but may appeal to older girls and women, too), about the healing process of a sexual abuse survivor. The story is told in the form of the girl's journal, and includes many useful strategies for coping with abuse. An exceptionally gentle, sensitive tool to aid in the healing process, with lovely illustrations.

What books can help kids with anger management?

- *Hot Stuff to Help Kids Chill Out: The Anger Management Book*, by Jerry Wilde. Speaks directly to children and teens in a language they can easily understand to help them manage their anger rather than be controlled by it. Try reading and discussing it with your children.

References

1. Frazier BH, Hayes KC. Selected Resources on Sibling Abuse: An Annotated Bibliography For Researchers, Educators and

Consumers. SRB 94 – 08 Special Reference Briefs. 1994. Formerly available at URL: http://www.cyfernet.org/research/sibabuse.html. Accessed 23 May 2008.

2. Strauss, MA, Gelles RJ, editors. *Family violence in American families: risk factors and adaptations to violence in 8,145 families*. New Brunswick, NY: Transaction Publishers; 1990.

3. Finkelhor D, Ormrod R, Turner H, Hamby SL. The victimization of children and youth: a comprehensive, national survey. *Child Maltreat*. 2005 Feb;10(1):5–25.

4. American Psychological Association, press release. Childhood sibling abuse common, but most adults don't remember it that way, study finds. No longer available online. Accessed 8 August 2004.

Other Reference

Needleman, R. Sibling rivalry. In: Parker S, Zuckerman B, editors. *Behavioral and developmental pediatrics*. Boston: Little, Brown & Company; 1995. p. 384–386.

Section 6.2

When Children Are Sexually Abused by Other Children

Introduction

Our children are our future. We all have a responsibility to protect them. Take action if you are worried that your child, or a child you know, may be sexually hurting someone. You are not alone. Help is available. Call the Stop It Now! Helpline at 1-888-PREVENT to talk confidentially with professionals who have experience working with individuals and families with similar situations.

As parents and caregivers, we want to do all we can to protect our children, while giving them the freedom they need to develop and become healthy adults. Sometimes, the world can feel full of risks, many of them obvious, and others more confusing. In order to strike the right balance between protection and independence for our children, we adults need the best possible information.

This guide is for everyone involved in bringing up children. It explains that some children do sexually abuse other children, describes how we can recognize the warning signs, and outlines some actions we adults can take to prevent sexual abuse.

Do Children Sexually Abuse Other Children?

"I didn't have the words to tell my parents what was going on. I said I didn't want to be left alone with kids. I wish they had listened to me." —An adolescent with sexual behavior problems

Most people already are aware of the risk of sexual abuse that some adults present to our children. There is growing understanding that the vast majority of children who are sexually abused, are abused by someone they know, and often trust. Unfortunately, very few adults recognize that children and adolescents also can present a risk to other children. In fact, over a third of all sexual abuse of children is committed by someone under the age of 18.

This can be a difficult issue to address, partly because it is often challenging for adults to think of the children or adolescents we know as capable of sexually abusing others. Also, it is not always easy to tell the difference between natural sexual curiosity and potentially abusive behaviors. Children, particularly younger children, may engage in inappropriate interactions without understanding the hurtful impact it has on others. For this reason, it may be more helpful to talk about a child's sexually "harmful" behavior rather than sexually "abusive" behavior.

It is essential that all adults have the information needed to recognize potentially harmful activities at an early stage and to seek help so the behaviors can be stopped. Every adult who cares about children has an opportunity, as both teacher and role model, to show children how to interact without harming others, either while they are still children, or later, as adults. Adults have the added responsibility of ensuring that all children who have been involved in a harmful sexual situation, whatever their role, are given the help they need to live healthy productive lives.

What Is Healthy Sexual Development?

Most adults understand that children pass through different stages of development as they grow. Sometimes, adults have more difficulty acknowledging that, from birth, children are sexual beings. Like other areas of a child's development, it is normal for children's awareness and curiosity about their own sexual feelings to change as they pass from infancy into childhood, and then through puberty to adolescence.

- Each child is an individual and will develop in his or her own way. However, there is a generally accepted range of behaviors linked to children's changing age and developmental stages. These behaviors may include exploration with other children of similar power or stature—by virtue of age, size, ability or social status. Sometimes, it can be difficult to tell the difference between sexual exploration that is appropriate to a developmental stage and interactions that are warning signs of harmful behavior.

- Occasionally, adults may need to set limits when children engage in behaviors we consider inappropriate, even if the children may be unaware of potential harm. This is a chance to talk with them about keeping themselves and others safe, and to let them know that you are someone they can talk to when they have questions. Adults can help children be comfortable with their sexual development and understand appropriate sexual boundaries, for example, adults can model appropriate, respectful behavior.

- Children with disabilities or developmental challenges benefit from special attention to their safety. Depending on the nature of their disability, they may develop at different rates, which can make them more vulnerable to being abused. They may also inadvertently harm another child without understanding the hurtful impact of their actions. For example, children with disabilities sometimes behave sexually in ways that are out of step with their age. Particular care may be needed to help children understand their sexual development and to ensure that these children and their caregivers can communicate effectively about any questions or worries they have.

It is important to recognize that, while people from various backgrounds have different expectations about what is acceptable behavior for children, sexual abuse is present across all ethnic groups, cultures and religious beliefs.

What Is Age-Appropriate or Developmentally Expected Sexual Behavior?

While learning about their bodies and sexuality, children may behave in ways that seem out of sync with their age or developmental stage. Many minor factors—for example, having an older sibling—may increase a child's awareness of knowledge, attitudes and behaviors of an older age group. Usually, unexpected behavior can be redirected with a simple instruction. Of particular concern are behaviors involving another child, in which either child seems unable to control the behavior after being asked to stop.

Preschool (0 to 5 Years)

- **Common:** Sexual language relating to differences in body parts, bathroom talk, pregnancy and birth. Self stimulation at home and in public. Showing and looking at private body parts.

- **Uncommon:** Discussion of specific sexual acts or explicit sexual language. Adult-like sexual contact with other children.

School-Age Children (6 to 12 Years)

May include both pre-pubescent children and children who have already entered puberty, when hormonal changes are likely to trigger an increase in sexual awareness and interest.

Pre-Pubescent Children

- **Common:** Questions about relationships and sexual behavior, menstruation and pregnancy. Experimentation with same-age children, often during games, kissing, touching, exhibitionism and role-playing. Private self stimulation.

- **Uncommon:** Adult-like sexual interactions, discussing specific sexual acts or public self stimulation.

After Puberty Begins

- **Common:** Increased curiosity about sexual materials and information, questions about relationships and sexual behavior, using sexual words and discussing sexual acts, particularly with peers. Increased experimenting including open-mouthed kissing, bodyrubbing, fondling. Masturbating in private.

- **Uncommon:** Consistent adult-like sexual behavior, including oral/genital contact and intercourse. Masturbating in public.

Adolescence (13 to 16)

- **Common:** Questions about decision making, social relationships, and sexual customs. Masturbation in private. Experimenting between adolescents of the same age, including open-mouthed kissing, fondling and body rubbing, oral/genital contact. Also, voyeuristic behaviors are common. Intercourse occurs in approximately on third of this age group.

- **Uncommon:** Masturbating in public and sexual interest directed toward much younger children.

The [list above] shows some examples of common sexual behavior that we might anticipate seeing in our children as they pass through different stages of development from pre-school to adolescence. Remember that each child develops at his or her own pace. Not every child will show all these behaviors at the same stages, or necessarily experience specific behaviors at all.

The chart also describes kinds of behavior that are less common in a given developmental stage, and which may give cause for concern. If you feel uneasy or have any questions or concerns about a child you know, talk to someone you trust, like a friend, family member, your healthcare provider, a counselor, or contact the Stop It Now! Helpline at www.StopItNow.org or 1-888-PREVENT.

For a more complete list or if you have any question or concerns about sexual behaviors of a child in your life, please e-mail or call the Stop It Now! Helpline at www.StopItNow.org or 1-888-PREVENT.

Adapted from Wurtele, S.K. and Miller-Perrin, C.L. *Preventing Sexual Abuse*. University of Nebraska Press. Lincoln, NE. 1992.

What Is Sexually Harmful Behavior?

Sexually harmful behavior by children and young people may range from experimentation that has gone too far to serious sexual assault.

It is important for adults to recognize that many children will engage in some forms of sexual exploration with children of a similar age, size, social status or power. Sometimes a child or young person may engage in sexual play with a much younger or more vulnerable child, or use force, tricks or bribery to involve someone in sexual activity. While such manipulation may be a cause for concern, it is critical to realize that manipulation may not, in itself, indicate a tendency toward sexual aggression. Professional help and advice is needed to determine the best way to support a child in managing any concerning impulses.

Keep in Mind

- Children as young as four or five may unknowingly engage in sexually harmful behavior, although more often those who sexually harm children are adolescents.

- Usually, but not always, the child or young person causing the harm is older than the victim.

- Often the child being harmed is uncomfortable or confused about what is happening, but may feel that he or she is willingly involved or to blame for being in the situation.

- Many times, one or both children do not understand that the behavior is harmful.

What about Sexually Abusive Images of Children— Child Pornography?

Interactions involving both direct contact and non-touching behaviors may cause harm. Examples range from unwelcome repeated touching, to brief touching of genitals to actual intercourse, sexually charged verbal or emotional aggression, photographing a child in sexual poses or exposing a child to sexual acts or images.

There is a growing problem of sexual images of children being available for viewing and downloading on the internet, mobile phones, or other devices. Adults need to supervise children's use of these technologies, provide children with clear information about our expectations and teach them how to make safe choices.

We must educate young people about the risks:

- Viewing abusive images of children may make harmful sexual interactions with children seem normal or acceptable.

- Viewing sexually abusive images of children hurts those children and others by creating a demand for additional images.

- Downloading child pornography is a criminal offense.

- Teens or children who take and share nude images or video of themselves or others can also face criminal charges since these images or video can be considered child pornography.

We adults must also remain aware of the risks of developing technology and of how to access resources when a child does engage in harmful online activities. Social networking sites, text messaging and photocapable cell phones are just a few examples of evolving methods of communication that attract young people, but also can create unanticipated vulnerabilities. For more information and links about safe use of the internet and other technology, visit www.StopItNow.org.

Why Do Some Children Sexually Harm Others?

"The best way to keep your family safe is to educate yourself about child sexual abuse. The earlier we can see what is happening, the earlier we can do something to stop the abuse."
—Mother of an adolescent with sexual behavior problems

The reasons children sexually harm others are complicated, varied and not always obvious. Some of them may have been emotionally, sexually, or physically abused themselves, while others may have witnessed physical or emotional violence at home. Some may have come in contact with sexually explicit movies, video games, or materials that are confusing to them. In some instances, a child or adolescent may act on a passing impulse with no harmful intent, but may still cause harm to themselves or to other children.

Whatever the reason, without help, some sexually abusing youth will go on to abuse children as adults. It is important to seek advice and help promptly whenever there is any concern or question about a child or adolescent.

How Do We Recognize the Warning Signs of Sexually Harmful Behavior?

One of the most difficult discoveries a parent can make is to learn that your child may have sexually harmed or abused another child. Denial, shock, and anger are common reactions. Because a quick and sensitive response can help diminish the harmful effects on the whole family, it is important to get professional advice about what to do as soon as you become aware of warning signs.

The good news is that positive, supportive help for the child or young person and his or her family can make a real difference. Evidence shows that the earlier children get help, the more able they are to learn the skills they need to control their behavior. If you are in this situation, remember that you are not alone. Many other parents who have been through similar experiences found that by taking action the child and family got the help they needed and were able to avoid future abuse. The first step is to recognize the value of talking it over with someone else.

What Are Warning Signs of Sexually Harmful or Abusive Behavior?

Behaviors that may indicate increased risk include:

- Regularly minimizing, justifying, or denying the impact of inappropriate behaviors on others.

- Making others uncomfortable by consistently missing or ignoring social cues about others' personal or sexual limits and boundaries.

- Preferring to spend time with younger children rather than peers.

- Insisting on physical contact with a child even when that child resists.

- Responding sexually to typical gestures of friendliness or affection.

- Reluctance to be alone with a particular child; becoming anxious when a particular child is coming to visit.

- Offering alcohol/drugs, sexual material or inappropriate "privileges" to younger child.

Stronger indicators of risk for abusive behavior include:

- Linking sexuality and aggression in language or behavior; engaging in sexually harassing behavior online or in person; and forcing any sexual interaction.

- Turning to younger or less powerful children rather than peers to explore natural sexual curiosity.

- The inability to control inappropriate sexual behaviors involving another child after being told to stop.

- Taking younger children to "secret" places or hideaways to play "special" undressing or touching games.

While any single behavior may suggest that a child needs help, these behaviors do not, in themselves, indicate that a child is likely to engage in ongoing, sexually harmful behaviors. For more information about concerning behaviors or about resources to get help, please e-mail or contact the Stop It Now! Helpline at www.StopItNow.org or 1-888-PREVENT (1-888-773-8368).

Why Don't Children Tell?

"We couldn't understand at first why he hadn't told us. Now we know how confused he was. He felt that it was his fault, even though he hadn't wanted it to happen." —Parents of teenage boy who was sexually abused by two friends

There are many reasons why children may find it very difficult to tell anyone that they are being abused, whether by an adult or by another child. Most children do not tell anyone about sexual abuse before they become adults themselves. Some common reasons why children do not tell include:

- Children may not understand that the behavior is inappropriate or harmful.

- Sometimes they want to protect the other child or youth, whom they may care about, or they do not want to upset the adults with troubling information.

- Children may feel guilty or that they are to blame for the interaction.

- A child may hope that if he or she is "good enough," the harmful behavior will stop on its own.

- Children may feel obligated to remain silent, having received a combination of gifts, treats, and threats about what will happen if they say "no" or tell someone. Threats may include physical harm to the victim, a relative or a pet, or breakup of the family.

- Children may feel embarrassment about what is happening or fear that they will not be believed.

- Sometimes, a child may be confused by suggestions that they enjoyed the sexual interaction and wanted it to happen.

- The child who is harmed may be confused about his or her feelings and be persuaded that what is happening is "okay" or that "everyone is doing it," particularly if another child or adolescent initiates the sexual behaviors.

- Very young or disabled children may not have the words or means of communication to let people know what is going on.

For these reasons, maintaining open communications—talking with and listening carefully to children—is an important part of preventing child sexual abuse. Because children often find it so hard to tell us in words, it is important to be alert to the behavioral warning signs that they may be being abused, and then act to learn more.

What Are the Signs That a Child or Young Person May Be Being Sexually Abused?

Do you notice some of the following behaviors in a child you know:

- Nightmares, sleep problems, extreme fears without an obvious explanation

- Sudden or unexplained personality changes; seems withdrawn, angry, moody, clingy, "checked-out," or shows significant changes in eating habits

- An older child behaving like a younger child, for example, bedwetting or thumb-sucking

- Develops fear of particular places or resists being alone with particular child or young person for unknown reasons

- Shows resistance to routine bathing, toileting, or removing clothes even in appropriate situations

- Play, writing, drawings, or dreams include sexual or frightening images

- Refuses to talk about a secret he/she has with an adult or older child

- Stomach aches or illness, often with no identifiable reason

- Leaves clues that seem likely to provoke a discussion about sexual issues

- Uses new or adult words for body parts; engages in adult-like sexual activities with toys, objects or other children

- Develops special relationship with older friend that may include unexplained money, gifts or privileges

- Intentionally harming himself or herself; that is, drug/alcohol use, cutting, burning, running away, sexual promiscuity

- Develops physical symptoms; for example, unexplained soreness, pain or bruises around genital or mouth; sexually-transmitted disease; pregnancy

Any of these signs may be caused by other factors and changes in a child's life. If you would like to talk with someone further about concerns, please e-mail or call the Stop It Now! Helpline at www.StopItNow .org or 1-888-PREVENT (1-888-773-8368).

How Can We Protect Our Children?

"I can see now that there was a lot of secrecy in our son's life that we thought was normal, but now we know what he was hiding. If someone had told us that it was OK to talk to our son about these things, or showed us how to do it, maybe this wouldn't have happened." —Mother of an adolescent with sexual behavior problems

There are many things adults can do to prevent the sexual abuse of children: setting clear standards for what is considered appropriate, respectful behavior; staying alert for situations where those expectations are broken; and speaking up promptly to address any concerns are the cornerstones of any effective effort to protect children.

Communication is key. Talking to children about their activities, hopes, and anxieties on a daily basis increases the likelihood that a child, who is worried about his or her own behavior, will be able to tell someone. The sooner adults recognize potentially concerning situations, the better protected children will be.

What Are Some Things That Adults Can Do to Help Prevent Sexually Harmful Behavior Between Children?

1. Set and respect physical boundaries.

Make sure that all members of the family have rights to privacy in dressing, bathing, sleeping, and other personal activities. As adults we are responsible for modeling the boundaries we want our children to honor. Even young children should be respected and their preferences accommodated when possible.

2. Encourage children to also respect themselves and others.

Much of what young people see in the adult world ignores or even ridicules the importance of treating others respectfully and of demanding the same for oneself. Highly sexualized images in advertising, music lyrics, video games, and films can sometimes make it difficult for adolescents—or even young children—to distinguish between innocent experimentation and sexually harmful behaviors.

Teach children to value respectful interactions—including sexual interactions. Create environments at home and in your social groups where children will see that emotionally or sexually aggressive behaviors are not tolerated and that hurtful behaviors are challenged.

3. Demonstrate to children that it is all right to say "no" and that they need to accept "no" from others.

Teach children when it is okay to say "no"—for example when they do not want to play, or be tickled, hugged or kissed. Help them

97

understand what is considered acceptable and unacceptable behavior. Encourage them to always speak up if someone acts in a way that makes them uncomfortable, even if they were unable to object or to say "no" at the time. Teach children that they must listen to and accept others' limits as well.

4. Stay aware of how children are interacting with one another.

Be alert to the warning signs that your child, or another child or young person, may be acting in ways that make it difficult for other children to set a limit, or in ways that are sexually aggressive or abusive. Seek information and help as soon as you feel uncomfortable. Don't keep it a secret.

5. Talk with children, and listen to what they have to say.

Adults and adolescents who sexually abuse children usually rely on secrecy. They often try to silence children and to build trust with adults, counting on them to be silent if they are confused. The first step to breaking through this secrecy is to develop an open and trusting relationship with your children. This means listening carefully to their fears and concerns and letting them know they should not worry about telling you anything. It is important to talk with them about sexuality, offer accurate answers to their questions, and to be comfortable using correct terms for parts of the body.

6. Set clear guidelines and keep a careful eye on children's use of TV, internet, and video games, and other communications technology.

Explain to children the risks associated with using the internet and cell phones. Restrict access to sites that are not age-appropriate, discuss safe use of social networking sites like Facebook, and ask them to tell you if they receive messages or e-mails containing suggestive or sexually explicit material. Keep your computer in a public place so you can easily monitor their use.

Check that TV shows, films, internet content, and videos are age-appropriate. Watch programs with children and use what they see as "teachable moments" to share information and values. Make agreements with other adults that the guidelines of a visiting child's parents or guardians will be respected during play dates or visits.

7. Take sensible precautions about whom you choose to take care of your children.

Be thoughtful about whom you choose to care for your children. Find out as much as you can about baby-sitters and don't leave your child with anyone you have doubts about. If your child is unhappy about spending time with a particular person, talk to the child about his or her concerns.

8. Regularly remind children of other trusted adults whom they can talk to.

Sometimes the child or young person whose behavior concerns us is a close family member or the son or daughter of a friend. In those situations, it may be especially painful for us, as parents and caregivers, to admit what may be happening. It may be even harder for a child to tell that someone the family cares about is harming her or him. An adult outside the immediate family is often in a better position to acknowledge concerns and to take protective actions.

What Can You Do If You Suspect Your Child Is Sexually Harming Another Child or Thinking about Doing So?

It is very disturbing to suspect that your child, or a child you know, may be sexually harming someone. It is so much easier to dismiss such thoughts or to think you're overreacting. You may also be worried about the possible consequences of taking action.

Help is available. It is much better to talk over the situation with someone than to discover later that you were right to be concerned and did nothing.

Remember, you are not alone. Every year thousands of people grapple with situations where someone in their family or circle of friends is suspected of inappropriate sexual behavior. Stop It Now!'s *Parenttalk* newsletter offers insights written by and for parents of children and teens with sexual behavior problems. (www.StopItNow.org/parenttalk).

1. Act quickly. Action is prevention.

If you are worried that your son or daughter may be sexually harming another child, or if you suspect that your child is being abused, act now! Get help from a professional therapist immediately and develop a safety plan addressing the concerning behaviors. Prompt intervention also can get the sexually abusing youth the treatment needed to stop abusing and to grow up as a safe member of our community.

2. Stay steady.

When speaking to children about your concerns, remember to stay calm and ask simple and direct questions. Listen carefully to the responses without suggesting answers. It may be useful to practice with someone else first and get support to help keep your own emotions in check.

Recognize that confusion, guilt, and shame about abuse can make the conversation difficult, both for you and for the child. Acknowledge the child's discomfort and offer praise for his or her courage to talk about a confusing experience. Remember that if it's difficult for you to discuss your concerns, it is likely to be much more difficult for the child.

3. Get support for everyone.

Whatever is revealed, reassure them that you love them and that you are committed to helping them. Children will look to adults for reassurance that they will be all right. Keep reminding yourself that healing for everyone is possible. Children and adolescents frequently respond best to specialized, sex-specific treatment when it is offered early and with the support of trusted adults. Sexual abuse affects all members of a family or group. The entire family, including the adults, is likely to need support.

4. Be prepared to report.

Reporting the abuse to authorities is an upsetting prospect for many families. Yet, filing a report can be a first step to accessing support services. Children who are abused and their families need help to recover from their trauma. Anyone who is harming a child sexually also needs help and support to stop the behavior.

Sometimes, in the most serious cases and depending upon the age of the child or adolescent, reporting may result in legal consequences. Although this can be a difficult process for everyone involved, when combined with specialized treatment, it may be the best way to prevent further harm and even harsher future consequences.

5. Make use of valuable lessons learned.

If you have been involved in helping a child cope with harmful sexual behaviors, your experience and knowledge about abuse and treatment may be extremely valuable to others. The opportunity to prevent sexual abuse does not end with the discovery of abuse. Use the lessons you have learned to educate others about prevention and to support other families facing similar concerns.

Take Action

If you are unsure or worried about the behavior of someone you know (whether they are an adult or a child), we have information that can help you consider your possible next steps. With guidance from our professional Helpline staff, adults can learn about sexual abuse; identify specialized treatment options for themselves or someone they care about; develop a safety plan; find language for an effective conversation when they have concerns, and learn how to report those concerns to authorities when appropriate.

- **Contact:** Stop It Now! Helpline: 1-888-PREVENT
- **E-mail:** helpline@stopitnow.org
- **Visit:** www.StopItNow.org

Chapter 7

Bullying

Chapter Contents

Section 7.1

What Is Bullying?

"Bullying Definition," U.S. Department of
Health and Human Services (www.stopbullying.gov), 2012.

Bullying is unwanted, aggressive behavior among school aged children that involves a real or perceived power imbalance. The behavior is repeated, or has the potential to be repeated, over time. Both kids who are bullied and who bully others may have serious, lasting problems.

In order to be considered bullying, the behavior must be aggressive and include these characteristics:

- **An imbalance of power:** Kids who bully use their power—such as physical strength, access to embarrassing information, or popularity—to control or harm others. Power imbalances can change over time and in different situations, even if they involve the same people.

- **Repetition:** Bullying behaviors happen more than once or have the potential to happen more than once.

Bullying includes actions such as making threats, spreading rumors, attacking someone physically or verbally, and excluding someone from a group on purpose.

Types of Bullying

There are three types of bullying:

- Verbal bullying is saying or writing mean things. Verbal bullying includes tactics such as these:
  - Teasing
  - Name-calling
  - Inappropriate sexual comments
  - Taunting
  - Threatening to cause harm

- Social bullying, sometimes referred to as relational bullying, involves hurting someone's reputation or relationships. Social bullying includes these ploys:
  - Leaving someone out on purpose
  - Telling other children not to be friends with someone
  - Spreading rumors about someone
  - Embarrassing someone in public

- Physical bullying involves hurting a person's body or possessions. Physical bullying includes actions such as the following:
  - Hitting/kicking/pinching
  - Spitting
  - Tripping/pushing
  - Taking or breaking someone's things
  - Making mean or rude hand gestures

Where and When Bullying Happens

Bullying can occur during or after school hours. While most reported bullying happens in the school building, a significant percentage also happens in places like on the playground or the bus. It can also happen travelling to or from school, in the youth's neighborhood, or on the internet.

Frequency of Bullying

There are two sources of federally collected data on youth bullying:

- The 2011 Youth Risk Behavior Surveillance System (Centers for Disease Control and Prevention) indicates that, nationwide, 20% of students in grades 9–12 experienced bullying (see http://www.cdc.gov/HealthyYouth/yrbs/index.htm).

- The 2008–2009 School Crime Supplement (National Center for Education Statistics and Bureau of Justice Statistics) indicates that, nationwide, 28% of students in grades 6–12 experienced bullying (see http://nces.ed.gov/pubs2012/2012314.pdf).

Section 7.2

Bullying Risk Factors and Warning Signs

"Risk Factors," U.S. Department of Health and Human
Services (www.stopbullying.gov), 2012.

No single factor puts a child at risk of being bullied or bullying others. Bullying can happen anywhere—cities, suburbs, or rural towns. Depending on the environment, some groups—such as lesbian, gay, bisexual, or transgendered (LGBT) youth, youth with disabilities, and socially isolated youth—may be at an increased risk of being bullied.

Children at Risk of Being Bullied

Generally, children who are bullied have one or more of the following risk factors:

- Are perceived as different from their peers, such as being overweight or underweight, wearing glasses or different clothing, being new to a school, or being unable to afford what kids consider "cool"

- Are perceived as weak or unable to defend themselves

- Are depressed, anxious, or have low self esteem

- Are less popular than others and have few friends

- Do not get along well with others, seen as annoying or provoking, or antagonize others for attention

However, even if a child has these risk factors, it doesn't mean that they will be bullied.

Children More Likely to Bully Others

There are two types of kids who are more likely to bully others:

- Some are well-connected to their peers, have social power, are overly concerned about their popularity, and like to dominate or be in charge of others.

- Others are more isolated from their peers and may be depressed or anxious, have low self esteem, be less involved in school, be easily pressured by peers, or not identify with the emotions or feelings of others.

Children who have these factors are also more likely to bully others:

- Are aggressive or easily frustrated
- Have less parental involvement or having issues at home
- Think badly of others
- Have difficulty following rules
- View violence in a positive way
- Have friends who bully others

Remember, those who bully others do not need to be stronger or bigger than those they bully. The power imbalance can come from a number of sources—popularity, strength, cognitive ability—and children who bully may have more than one of these characteristics.

Section 7.3

Effects of Bullying

"Effects of Bullying," U.S. Department of
Health and Human Services (www.stopbullying.gov), 2012.

Bullying can affect everyone—those who are bullied, those who bully, and those who witness bullying. Bullying is linked to many negative outcomes including impacts on mental health, substance use, and suicide. It is important to talk to kids to determine whether bullying—or something else—is a concern.

Kids Who Are Bullied

Kids who are bullied can experience negative physical, school, and mental health issues. Kids who are bullied are more likely to experience problems such as the following:

- Depression and anxiety, increased feelings of sadness and loneliness, changes in sleep and eating patterns, and loss of interest in activities they used to enjoy. These issues may persist into adulthood.

- Health complaints

- Decreased academic achievement—GPA and standardized test scores—and school participation. They are more likely to miss, skip, or drop out of school.

A very small number of bullied children might retaliate through extremely violent measures. In 12 of 15 school shooting cases in the 1990s, the shooters had a history of being bullied.

Kids Who Bully Others

Kids who bully others can also engage in violent and other risky behaviors into adulthood. Kids who bully are more likely also to have these traits:

- Abuse alcohol and other drugs in adolescence and as adults

- Get into fights, vandalize property, and drop out of school
- Engage in early sexual activity
- Have criminal convictions and traffic citations as adults
- Be abusive toward their romantic partners, spouses, or children as adults

Bystanders

Kids who witness bullying are more likely to demonstrate these characteristics:

- Have increased use of tobacco, alcohol, or other drugs
- Have increased mental health problems, including depression and anxiety
- Miss or skip school

The Relationship between Bullying and Suicide

Media reports often link bullying with suicide. However, most youth who are bullied do not have thoughts of suicide or engage in suicidal behaviors.

Although kids who are bullied are at risk of suicide, bullying alone is not the cause. Many issues contribute to suicide risk, including depression, problems at home, and trauma history. Additionally, specific groups have an increased risk of suicide, including American Indian and Alaskan Native, Asian American, lesbian, gay, bisexual, and transgender youth. This risk can be increased further when these kids are not supported by parents, peers, and schools. Bullying can make an unsupportive situation worse.

Section 7.4

Preventing and Responding to Bullying

"How to Talk about Bullying," U.S. Department of
Health and Human Services (www.stopbullying.gov), 2012.

Parents, school staff, and other caring adults have a role to play in preventing bullying. They can take these steps:

- Help kids understand bullying. Talk about what bullying is and how to stand up to it safely. Tell kids bullying is unacceptable. Make sure kids know how to get help.

- Keep the lines of communication open. Check in with kids often. Listen to them. Know their friends, ask about school, and understand their concerns.

- Encourage kids to do what they love. Special activities, interests, and hobbies can boost confidence, help kids make friends, and protect them from bullying behavior.

- Model how to treat others with kindness and respect.

Help Kids Understand Bullying

Kids who know what bullying is can better identify it. They can talk about bullying if it happens to them or others. Kids need to know ways to safely stand up to bullying and how to get help.

- Encourage kids to speak to a trusted adult if they are bullied or see others being bullied. The adult can give comfort, support, and advice, even if they can't solve the problem directly. Encourage the child to report bullying if it happens.

- Talk about how to stand up to kids who bully. Give tips, like using humor and saying "stop" directly and confidently. Talk about what to do if those actions don't work, like walking away

- Talk about strategies for staying safe, such as staying near adults or groups of other kids.

- Urge them to help kids who are bullied by showing kindness or getting help.
- Watch the short webisodes available online at http://www.stopbullying.gov/kids/webisodes/index.html and discuss them with kids.

Keep the Lines of Communication Open

Research tells us that children really do look to parents and caregivers for advice and help on tough decisions. Sometimes spending 15 minutes a day talking can reassure kids that they can talk to their parents if they have a problem. Start conversations about daily life and feelings with questions like these:

- What was one good thing that happened today? Any bad things?
- What is lunch time like at your school? Who do you sit with? What do you talk about?
- What is it like to ride the school bus?
- What are you good at? What do you like best about yourself?

Talking about bullying directly is an important step in understanding how the issue might be affecting kids. There are no right or wrong answers to these questions, but it is important to encourage kids to answer them honestly. Assure kids that they are not alone in addressing any problems that arise. Start conversations about bullying with questions like these:

- What does "bullying" mean to you?
- Describe what kids who bully are like. Why do you think people bully?
- Who are the adults you trust most when it comes to things like bullying?
- Have you ever felt scared to go to school because you were afraid of bullying? What ways have you tried to change it?
- What do you think parents can do to help stop bullying?
- Have you or your friends left other kids out on purpose? Do you think that was bullying? Why or why not?
- What do you usually do when you see bullying going on?
- Do you ever see kids at your school being bullied by other kids? How does it make you feel?

111

- Have you ever tried to help someone who is being bullied? What happened? What would you do if it happens again?

Get more ideas for talking with children about life and about bullying. If concerns come up, be sure to respond.

There are simple ways that parents and caregivers can keep up-to-date with kids' lives.

- Read class newsletters and school flyers. Talk about them at home.
- Check the school website
- Go to school events
- Greet the bus driver
- Meet teachers and counselors at "Back to School" night or reach out by e-mail
- Share phone numbers with other kids' parents

Teachers and school staff also have a role to play.

Encourage Kids to Do What They Love

Help kids take part in activities, interests, and hobbies they like. Kids can volunteer, play sports, sing in a chorus, or join a youth group or school club. These activities give kids a chance to have fun and meet others with the same interests. They can build confidence and friendships that help protect kids from bullying.

Model How to Treat Others with Kindness and Respect

Kids learn from adults' actions. By treating others with kindness and respect, adults show the kids in their lives that there is no place for bullying. Even if it seems like they are not paying attention, kids are watching how adults manage stress and conflict, as well as how they treat their friends, colleagues, and families.

Chapter 8

Long-Term Effects and Consequences of Child Abuse and Neglect

Chapter Contents

Section 8.1

Effects of Child Maltreatment on Brain Development

From "Understanding the Effects of Maltreatment on Brain Development,"
U.S. Department of Health and Human Services (HHS), 2009. The complete
text of this document, including references, is available through the Child
Welfare Information Gateway at www.childwelfare.gov.

Babies' brains grow and develop as they interact with their environment and learn how to function within it. When babies' cries bring food or comfort, they are strengthening the neuronal pathways that help them learn how to get their needs met, both physically and emotionally. But babies who do not get responses to their cries, and babies whose cries are met with abuse, learn different lessons. The neuronal pathways that are developed and strengthened under negative conditions prepare children to cope in that negative environment, and their ability to respond to nurturing and kindness may be impaired.

Brief periods of moderate, predictable stress are not problematic; in fact, they prepare a child to cope with the general world. The body's survival actually depends upon the ability to mount a response to stress. Children learn to deal with moderate stress in the context of positive relationships with reliable adult caregivers. Greater amounts of stress may also be tolerable if a child has a reliable adult who can help to buffer the child. But prolonged, severe, or unpredictable stress—including abuse and neglect—during a child's early years is problematic. In fact, the brain's development can literally be altered by this type of toxic stress, resulting in negative impacts on the child's physical, cognitive, emotional, and social growth.

The specific effects of maltreatment may depend on such factors as the age of the baby or child at the time of the abuse or neglect, whether the maltreatment was a one-time incident or chronic, the identity of the abuser (for example, parent or other adult), whether the child had a dependable nurturing individual in his or her life, the type and severity of the abuse, the intervention, and how long the maltreatment lasted.

The sections below give a brief description of abuse and neglect and are followed by descriptions of some of the consequences of maltreatment.

Abuse—Physical, Sexual, and Emotional

Abuse can refer to physical abuse, such as hitting, shaking, burning, or other forms of maltreatment that a parent or other caregiver might inflict. Sexual abuse is a subset of abuse that refers to any type of sexual behavior with a minor, while emotional abuse generally refers to any injury to a child's psychological or emotional stability. Chronic stress may also qualify as emotional abuse. In some states, alcohol or substance abuse or domestic violence that affects the unborn child is considered child abuse.

Physical abuse can cause direct damage to a baby's or child's developing brain. For instance, we now have extensive evidence of the damage that shaking a baby can cause. According to the National Center on Shaken Baby Syndrome, shaking can destroy brain tissue and tear blood vessels. In the short-term, shaking can lead to seizures, loss of consciousness, or even death. In the long-term, shaking can damage the fragile brain so that a child develops a range of sensory impairments, as well as cognitive, learning, and behavioral disabilities.

Babies and children who suffer abuse may also experience trauma that is unrelated to direct physical damage. Exposure to domestic violence, disaster, or other traumatic events can have long-lasting effects. An enormous body of research now exists that provides evidence for the long-term damage of physical, sexual, and emotional abuse on babies and children. We know that children who experience the stress of abuse will focus their brains' resources on survival and responding to threats in their environment. This chronic stimulation of the brain's fear response means that the regions of the brain involved in this response are frequently activated. Other regions of the brain, such as those involved in complex thought and abstract cognition, are less frequently activated, and the child becomes less competent at processing this type of information.

One way that early maltreatment experiences may alter a child's ability to interact positively with others is by altering brain neurochemical balance. Research on children who suffered early emotional abuse or severe deprivation indicates that such maltreatment may permanently alter the brain's ability to use serotonin, which helps produce feelings of well-being and emotional stability.

Altered brain development in children who have been maltreated may be the result of their brains adapting to their negative environment. If a child lives in a threatening, chaotic world, the child's brain may be hyperalert for danger because survival may depend on it. But if this environment persists, and the child's brain is focused on developing and strengthening its strategies for survival, other strategies may not develop as fully. The result may be a child who has difficulty functioning when presented with a world of kindness, nurturing, and stimulation.

Neglect—Lack of Stimulation

While chronic abuse and neglect can result in sensitized fear response patterns, neglect alone also can result in other problems. Malnutrition is a classic example of neglect. Malnutrition, both before and during the first few years after birth, can result in stunted brain growth and slower passage of electrical signals in the brain. This is due, in part, to the negative effect of malnutrition on the myelination process in the developing brain. The most common form of malnutrition in the United States, iron deficiency, can affect the growing brain and result in cognitive and motor delays, anxiety, depression, social problems, and attention problems.

Although neglect often is thought of as a failure to meet a child's physical needs for food, shelter, and safety, neglect also can be a failure to meet a child's cognitive, emotional, or social needs. For children to master developmental tasks in these areas, they need opportunities, encouragement, and acknowledgment from their caregivers. If this stimulation is lacking during children's early years, the weak neuronal pathways that had been developed in expectation of these experiences may wither and die, and the children may not achieve the usual developmental milestones.

For example, babies need to experience face-to-face baby talk and hear countless repetitions of sounds in order to build the brain circuitry that will enable them to start making sounds and eventually say words. If babies' sounds are ignored repeatedly when they begin to babble at around six months, their language may be delayed. In fact, neglected children often do not show the rapid growth that normally occurs in language development at 18–24 months. These types of delays may extend to all types of normal development for neglected children, including their cognitive-behavioral, socio-emotional, and physical development.

Global Neglect

Researchers use the term "global neglect" to refer to deprivations in more than one domain, that is, language, touch, and interaction with others. Children who were adopted from Romanian orphanages in the early 1990s were often considered to be globally neglected; they had little contact with caregivers and little to no stimulation from their environment—little of anything required for healthy development. One study found that these children had significantly smaller brains than the norm, suggesting decreased brain growth.

This type of severe, global neglect can have devastating consequences. The extreme lack of stimulation may result in fewer neuronal pathways available for learning. The lack of opportunity to form an attachment with a nurturing caregiver during infancy may mean that some of these children will always have difficulties forming meaningful relationships with others. But these studies also found that time played a factor—children who were adopted as young infants have shown more recovery than children who were adopted as toddlers.

Emotional and Behavioral Impact

New brain imaging technologies, research with animals, and studies of human growth in optimal and deprived conditions (such as institutions) continue to shed light on the impact of abuse and neglect on brain development. The sections below describe some of the major effects.

Persistent fear response: Chronic stress or repeated traumas can result in a number of biological reactions, including a persistent fear state. Neurochemical systems are affected, which can cause a cascade of changes in attention, impulse control, sleep, and fine motor control. Chronic activation of certain parts of the brain involved in the fear response (such as the hypothalamic-pituitary-adrenal [HPA] axis) can "wear out" other parts of the brain such as the hippocampus, which is involved in cognition and memory. The HPA axis may react to chronic fear or stress by producing excess cortisol—a hormone that may damage or destroy neurons in critical brain areas. Chronic activation of the neuronal pathways involved in the fear response can create permanent memories that shape the child's perception of and response to the environment. While this adaptation may be necessary for survival in a hostile world, it can become a way of life that is difficult to change, even if the environment improves.

Hyperarousal: When children are exposed to chronic, traumatic stress, their brains sensitize the pathways for the fear response and create memories that automatically trigger that response without conscious thought. This is called hyperarousal. These children have an altered baseline for arousal, and they tend to overreact to triggers that other children find nonthreatening. These children may be highly sensitive to nonverbal cues, such as eye contact or a touch on the arm, and they may read these actions as threats. Consumed with a need to monitor nonverbal cues for threats, their brains are less able to interpret and respond to verbal cues, even when they are in a supposedly nonthreatening environment, like a classroom. While these children are often labeled as learning disabled, the reality is that their brains have developed so that they are constantly alert and are unable to achieve the relative calm necessary for learning.

Dissociation: Infants or children who are the victims of repeated abuse may respond to that abuse—and later in life to other unpleasantness—by mentally and emotionally removing themselves from the situation. This coping mechanism of dissociation allows the child to pretend that what is happening is not real. Children who "zone out" or often seem overly detached may be experiencing dissociation. In some cases, it may be a form of self-hypnosis. Dissociation is characterized by first attempting to bring caretakers to help, and if this is unsuccessful, becoming motionless (freezing) and compliant and, eventually, dissociating. Dissociation may be a reaction to childhood sexual abuse, as well as other kinds of active, physical abuse or trauma. Children who suffer from dissociation may retreat to the dissociative state when they encounter other stresses later in life.

This type of response may have implications for the child's memory creation and retention. The brain may use dissociation to smother the memories of a parent's abuse in order to preserve an attachment to the parent, resulting in amnesia for the abuse. However, the implicit memories of the abuse remain, and the child may experience them in response to triggers or as flashbacks or nightmares. In its most extreme form, the child may develop multiple personalities, known as dissociative identity disorder.

Disrupted attachment process: At the foundation of much of our development is the concept of attachment, which refers to the emotional relationships we have with other people. An infant's early attachment to his or her primary caregiver provides the foundation for future emotional relationships. It also provides the base for other learning, because babies and children learn best when they feel safe, calm, protected, and nurtured by their caregivers. If the attachment process is disrupted or never allowed to develop in a healthy manner, as can occur with abusive and neglectful caretakers, the child's brain will be more focused on meeting the child's day-to-day needs for survival rather than building the foundation for future growth.

Disrupted attachment may lead to impairments in three major areas for the developing child:

- Increased susceptibility to stress
- Excessive help-seeking and dependency or excessive social isolation
- Inability to regulate emotions

Young infants depend on positive interactions with caregivers to begin to develop appropriate emotional control and response (affect regulation). For instance, lots of appropriate face-to-face and other contact helps infants recognize and respond to emotional cues. Infants whose caregivers are neglectful or abusive may experience affect dysregulation—meaning that these children are not able to identify and respond appropriately to emotional cues. Ongoing maltreatment may result in insecure or anxious attachment because the child is not able to derive a feeling of security and consistency from the caregiver. Children who have experienced insecure or anxious attachments may have more difficulties regulating their emotions and showing empathy for others' feelings. These children may have difficulties forming attachments later in life as well.

Impact of Abuse and Neglect on Adolescents

Adolescents who are abused or neglected were often maltreated at younger ages, as well. It can be difficult to isolate the effects of abuse and neglect during the adolescent years, because these youth often suffer from the cumulative effects of a lifetime of abuse and neglect.

Most teenagers who have not been victims of abuse or neglect find their teenage years to be exciting and challenging. Normal puberty and adolescence lead to the maturation of a physical body, but the brain lags behind in development, especially in the areas that allow teenagers to reason and think logically. Most teenagers act impulsively at times, using a lower area of their brain—their "gut reaction"—because their frontal lobe is not yet mature. Impulsive behavior, poor decisions, and increased risk-taking are all part of the normal teenage experience.

For teens who have been abused, neglected, or traumatized, this impulsive behavior may be even more apparent. Often, these youth have developed brains that focus on survival, at the expense of the more advanced thinking that happens in the brain's cortex. An underdeveloped cortex can lead to increased impulsive behavior, as well as difficulties with tasks that require higher-level thinking and feeling. These teens

119

may show delays in school and in social skills as well. They may be more drawn to taking risks, and they may have more opportunity to experiment with drugs and crime if they live in environments that put them at increased risk for these behaviors. Teenagers who lack stable relationships with caring adults who can provide guidance and model appropriate behavior may never have the opportunity to develop the relationship skills necessary for healthy adult relationships or for becoming good parents.

Long-Term Effects of Abuse and Neglect

Maltreatment during infancy and early childhood can have enduring repercussions into adolescence and adulthood. As mentioned earlier, the experiences of infancy and early childhood provide the organizing framework for the expression of children's intelligence, emotions, and personalities. When those experiences are primarily negative, children may develop emotional, behavioral, and learning problems that persist throughout their lifetime, especially in the absence of targeted interventions. The Adverse Childhood Experiences (ACE) study is a large-scale, long-term study that has documented the link between childhood abuse and neglect and later adverse experiences, such as physical and mental illness and high-risk behaviors.

Some of the specific long-term effects of abuse and neglect on the developing brain can include the following:

- Diminished growth in the left hemisphere, which may increase the risk for depression

- Irritability in the limbic system, setting the stage for the emergence of panic disorder and posttraumatic stress disorder

- Smaller growth in the hippocampus and limbic abnormalities, which can increase the risk for dissociative disorders and memory impairments

- Impairment in the connection between the two brain hemispheres, which has been linked to symptoms of attention-deficit/ hyperactivity disorder

Section 8.2

Long-Term Consequences of Child Maltreatment

From "Long-Term Consequences of Child Abuse and Neglect," U.S. Department of Health and Human Services (HHS), 2008. The complete text of this document, including references, is available through the Child Welfare Information Gateway at www.childwelfare.gov. Revised by David A. Cooke, MD, FACP, January 2013.

While physical injuries may or may not be immediately visible, abuse and neglect can have consequences for children, families, and society that last lifetimes, if not generations.

The impact of child abuse and neglect is often discussed in terms of physical, psychological, behavioral, and societal consequences. In reality, however, it is impossible to separate them completely. Physical consequences, such as damage to a child's growing brain, can have psychological implications such as cognitive delays or emotional difficulties. Psychological problems often manifest as high-risk behaviors. Depression and anxiety, for example, may make a person more likely to smoke, abuse alcohol or illicit drugs, or overeat. High-risk behaviors, in turn, can lead to long-term physical health problems such as sexually transmitted diseases, cancer, and obesity.

This section provides an overview of some of the most common physical, psychological, behavioral, and societal consequences of child abuse and neglect, while acknowledging that much crossover among categories exists.

Factors Affecting the Consequences of Child Abuse and Neglect

Not all abused and neglected children will experience long-term consequences. Outcomes of individual cases vary widely and are affected by a combination of factors, including the following:

- The child's age and developmental status when the abuse or neglect occurred

- The type of abuse (physical abuse, neglect, sexual abuse, etc.)
- The frequency, duration, and severity of abuse
- The relationship between the victim and his or her abuser

Researchers also have begun to explore why, given similar conditions, some children experience long-term consequences of abuse and neglect while others emerge relatively unscathed. The ability to cope, and even thrive, following a negative experience is sometimes referred to as "resilience." A number of protective and promotive factors may contribute to an abused or neglected child's resilience. These include individual characteristics, such as optimism, self-esteem, intelligence, creativity, humor, and independence, as well as the acceptance of peers and positive individual influences such as teachers, mentors, and role models. Other factors can include the child's social environment and the family's access to social supports. Community well-being, including neighborhood stability and access to safe schools and adequate health care, are other protective and promotive factors.

Physical Health Consequences

The immediate physical effects of abuse or neglect can be relatively minor (bruises or cuts) or severe (broken bones, hemorrhage, or even death). In some cases the physical effects are temporary; however, the pain and suffering they cause a child should not be discounted. Meanwhile, the long-term impact of child abuse and neglect on physical health is just beginning to be explored. According to the National Survey of Child and Adolescent Well-Being (NSCAW), more than one-quarter of children who had been in foster care for longer than 12 months had some lasting or recurring health problem. Below are some outcomes researchers have identified:

Shaken baby syndrome: Shaking a baby is a common form of child abuse. The injuries caused by shaking a baby may not be immediately noticeable and may include bleeding in the eye or brain, damage to the spinal cord and neck, and rib or bone fractures.

Impaired brain development: Child abuse and neglect have been shown, in some cases, to cause important regions of the brain to fail to form or grow properly, resulting in impaired development. These alterations in brain maturation have long-term consequences for cognitive, language, and academic abilities. NSCAW found more than three-quarters of foster children between one and two years of age to be at medium to high risk for problems with brain development, as opposed to less than half of children in a control sample.

Poor physical health: Several studies have shown a relationship between various forms of household dysfunction (including childhood abuse) and poor health. Adults who experienced abuse or neglect during childhood are more likely to suffer from physical ailments such as allergies, arthritis, asthma, bronchitis, high blood pressure, and ulcers.

Psychological Consequences

The immediate emotional effects of abuse and neglect—isolation, fear, and an inability to trust—can translate into lifelong consequences, including low self-esteem, depression, and relationship difficulties. Researchers have identified links between child abuse and neglect and the following:

Difficulties during infancy: Depression and withdrawal symptoms were common among children as young as three who experienced emotional, physical, or environmental neglect.

Poor mental and emotional health: In one long-term study, as many as 80 percent of young adults who had been abused met the diagnostic criteria for at least one psychiatric disorder at age 21. These young adults exhibited many problems, including depression, anxiety, eating disorders, and suicide attempts. Other psychological and emotional conditions associated with abuse and neglect include panic disorder, dissociative disorders, attention-deficit/hyperactivity disorder, depression, anger, posttraumatic stress disorder, and reactive attachment disorder.

Chronic pain disorders: There is increasing recognition that there is a very high prevalence of childhood abuse, particularly sexual abuse, among adults who suffer from severe or disabling chronic pain disorders. While the exact cause and effect relationship is not completely understood, prior abuse appears to be a major risk factor for disability due to chronic low back pain, chronic pelvic pain, fibromyalgia, and a number of other chronic pain conditions.

Cognitive difficulties: NSCAW found that children placed in out-of-home care due to abuse or neglect tended to score lower than the general population on measures of cognitive capacity, language development, and academic achievement. A 1999 LONGSCAN study also found a relationship between substantiated child maltreatment and poor academic performance and classroom functioning for school-age children.

Social difficulties: Children who experience rejection or neglect are more likely to develop antisocial traits as they grow up. Parental neglect is also associated with borderline personality disorders and violent behavior.

Behavioral Consequences

Not all victims of child abuse and neglect will experience behavioral consequences. However, behavioral problems appear to be more likely among this group, even at a young age. An NSCAW survey of children ages three to five in foster care found these children displayed clinical or borderline levels of behavioral problems at a rate of more than twice that of the general population. Later in life, child abuse and neglect appear to make the following more likely:

Difficulties during adolescence: Studies have found abused and neglected children to be at least 25 percent more likely to experience problems such as delinquency, teen pregnancy, low academic achievement, drug use, and mental health problems. Other studies suggest that abused or neglected children are more likely to engage in sexual risk-taking as they reach adolescence, thereby increasing their chances of contracting a sexually transmitted disease.

Juvenile delinquency and adult criminality: According to a National Institute of Justice study, abused and neglected children were 11 times more likely to be arrested for criminal behavior as a juvenile, 2.7 times more likely to be arrested for violent and criminal behavior as an adult, and 3.1 times more likely to be arrested for one of many forms of violent crime (juvenile or adult).

Alcohol and other drug abuse: Research consistently reflects an increased likelihood that abused and neglected children will smoke cigarettes, abuse alcohol, or take illicit drugs during their lifetime. According to a report from the National Institute on Drug Abuse, as many as two-thirds of people in drug treatment programs reported being abused as children.

Abusive behavior: Abusive parents often have experienced abuse during their own childhoods. It is estimated approximately one-third of abused and neglected children will eventually victimize their own children.

Societal Consequences

While child abuse and neglect almost always occur within the family, the impact does not end there. Society as a whole pays a price for child abuse and neglect, in terms of both direct and indirect costs.

Direct costs: Direct costs include those associated with maintaining a child welfare system to investigate and respond to allegations of child abuse and neglect, as well as expenditures by the judicial, law enforcement, health, and mental health systems. A 2001 report by Prevent Child Abuse America estimates these costs at $24 billion per year.

Indirect costs: Indirect costs represent the long-term economic consequences of child abuse and neglect. These include costs associated with juvenile and adult criminal activity, mental illness, substance abuse, and domestic violence. They can also include loss of productivity due to unemployment and underemployment, the cost of special education services, and increased use of the health care system. Prevent Child Abuse America estimated these costs at more than $69 billion per year.

Summary

Much research has been done about the possible consequences of child abuse and neglect. The effects vary depending on the circumstances of the abuse or neglect, personal characteristics of the child, and the child's environment. Consequences may be mild or severe; disappear after a short period or last a lifetime; and affect the child physically, psychologically, behaviorally, or in some combination of all three ways. Ultimately, due to related costs to public entities such as the health care, human services, and educational systems, abuse and neglect impact not just the child and family, but society as a whole.

Part Two

Physical and Sexual Abuse of Children

Chapter 9

Physical Abuse of Children

Chapter Contents

Section 9.1

The Nature and Consequences of Child Physical Abuse

Definition of Child Physical Abuse

Child physical abuse is commonly defined as the non-accidental physical injury to a child by a person responsible for the child's welfare. However, legal definitions of physical abuse vary from state to state. State laws differ in how they define perpetrators of abuse (that is, parents, guardians, relatives) and in how they determine exemptions from such definitions. Religion, cultural practices, and physical punishment are among the most prevalent exemptions.

The most common forms of physical abuse include hitting, kicking, punching, biting, whipping, and burning. Physical abuse can be identified by physical indicators such as welts, human bite marks, bald spots, burns, skeletal and head injuries, lacerations, abrasions, discoloration of skin, and unexplained bruise marks in various stages of healing.

Scope of Child Physical Abuse

In 2008, approximately 122,350 children (16.1 percent of all substantiated cases of child maltreatment) were officially counted as victims of child physical abuse. In 2008, child physical abuse alone was responsible for 308 fatalities (226.9 percent of all CA/N [child abuse/neglect] fatalities).

Nature of Child Physical Abuse

There is no single cause of physical abuse. Instead, there are usually multiple and interacting contributors at the levels of the child, parent, family, community, and society. Examples of contributors include a child with a disability, a parent struggling with depression or substance abuse, intimate partner violence, a father who is not involved in their child's life, a lack of community supports (for example, affordable child care), the burdens associated with poverty, and inadequate policies to support families and parents. These characteristics greatly contribute to the intractability of the problem. Combinations of such problems may impair a parent's ability to ensure his or her child's needs are adequately met.

Consequences of Child Physical Abuse

Child physical abuse is a form of trauma that impacts a child's cognitive, physical, social, and emotional development. Its effects on physical and mental health are far-reaching and often last a lifetime. Children who are physically abused are more likely to have suicidal thoughts, learning impairments, conduct disorder, a poor self-image, abuse drugs or alcohol, act out sexually, and/or show signs of depression.

Adults who were physically abused as children often have problems establishing intimate personal relationships. They are at higher risk for anxiety, depression, substance abuse, medical abuse, medical illness, and problems with school or work. Furthermore, adults abused as children may continue the cycle of abuse by abusing their own children. Research says that approximately one in three adults that were abused as children will subject their children to abuse.

Research conducted by the U.S. Department of Justice indicates that physically abused children were more likely to be arrested for a violent crime than children who suffered from other forms of maltreatment. One in four female prisoners and one in ten male prisoners were physically abused before the age of eighteen.

It is clear that the consequences of physical abuse extend far beyond the affected children and families. Enormous societal costs are involved. Prevent Child Abuse America estimated the economic impact of child abuse and neglect at $104 billion in 2007; and this was likely a conservative estimate. Thus, in addition to the compelling human argument to help optimize children's development, health and safety, there is also a financial impetus to help prevent the neglect of children. The aphorism that "our children are our nation's most valuable resource" should be more than a slogan. Finally, at the heart of child neglect is a concern with their basic rights, their human rights.

The costs associated with the pervasive and long-lasting effects of child abuse and neglect are as undeniable as our obligation to prevent—not just respond to—this problem. In 2007, $33 billion in direct costs for foster care services, hospitalization, mental health treatment, and law enforcement were supplemented by over $70 billion in indirect costs like loss of individual productivity, chronic health problems, special education, and delinquent and criminal justice services.

For more information contact Prevent Child Abuse America at 312-663-3520 or at mailbox@preventchildabuse.org.

Section 9.2

Recognizing Physical Abuse in Children

Nonaccidental physical injury may include severe beatings, burns, biting, strangulation, and scalding with resulting bruises, welts, broken bones, scars, or serious internal injuries (National Committee for the Prevention of Child Abuse). An "abused child," under the law, means a child less than 18 years of age whose parent or other person legally responsible for the child's care inflicts or allows to be inflicted upon the child physical injury by other than accidental means which causes or creates substantial risk of death or serious disfigurement, or impairment of physical health, or loss or impairment of the function of any bodily organ. It is also considered "abuse" if such a caretaker creates or allows to be created situations whereby a child is likely to be in risk of the dangers mentioned above. (see N.Y. Social Services Law, Sec.412;Family Court Act, Sec. 1012).

Please note, any one of these observations in isolation could be indicative of other problems. Part of what we observe in physical abuse is a pattern or series of events. Be particularly aware of frequent occurrences which singularly seem to have a reasonable explanation, but which, as a whole, cause concern.

Physical Indicators

- Bite marks

- Unusual bruises
- Lacerations
- Burns
- High incidence of accidents or frequent injuries
- Fractures in unusual places
- Injuries, swellings to face and extremities
- Discoloration of skin

Behavioral Indicators in Child

- Avoids physical contact with others
- Apprehensive when other children cry
- Wears clothing to purposely conceal injury (for example, long sleeves)
- Refuses to undress for gym or for required physical exams at school
- Gives inconsistent versions about occurrence of injuries, burns, etc.
- Seems frightened by parents
- Often late or absent from school
- Comes early to school, seems reluctant to go home afterwards
- Has difficulty getting along with others
- Little respect for others
- Overly compliant, withdrawn, gives in readily and allows others to do for him/her without protest
- Plays aggressively, often hurting peers
- Complains of pain upon movement or contact
- Has a history of running away from home
- Reports abuse by parents

Family or Parental Indicators

- Many personal and marital problems
- Economic stress

- Parent(s) were abused as children themselves, were raised in homes where excessive punishment was the norm, and use harsh discipline on own children

- Highly moralistic

- History of alcohol or drug abuse

- Are easily upset, have a low tolerance for frustration

- Are antagonistic, suspicious and fearful of other people

- Social isolation, no supporting network of relatives or friends

- See child as bad or evil

- Little or no interest in child's well-being

- Do not respond appropriately to child's pain

- Explanation of injuries to child are evasive and inconsistent

- Blame child for injuries

- Constantly criticize and have inappropriate expectations of child

- Take child to different physicians or hospital for each injury

Section 9.3

Helping First Responders Identify Child Abuse

Excerpted from "Chapter 2: Recognizing Child Maltreatment," *The Role of First Responders in Child Maltreatment Cases: Disaster and Nondisaster Situations,* Child Welfare Information Gateway (www.childwelfare.gov), Children's Bureau, Office on Child Abuse and Neglect, 2010.

First responders have various levels of experience and training regarding the detection of possible child abuse and neglect. While some effects of child maltreatment are easily observable, many require a more in-depth assessment by first responders. The physical, emotional, and behavioral effects of child abuse or neglect are wide-ranging, but many of these also may be caused by something other than maltreatment. First responders should be able to recognize and to assess any possible maltreatment within the context of other problematic situations that may occur in the home, such as domestic violence or substance abuse.

Federal Child Welfare Laws

State laws, sound professional standards for practice, and strong philosophical underpinnings should guide any intervention into family life on behalf of children. The key principles guiding state child protection laws are based largely on federal statutes, primarily the Child Abuse Prevention and Treatment Act (CAPTA), as amended by the Keeping Children and Families Safe Act of 2003 (P.L. 108-36), and the Adoption and Safe Families Act (ASFA) of 1997 (P.L. 105-89). CAPTA provides definitions and guidelines regarding child maltreatment issues, and ASFA promotes three national goals for child protection:

- **Safety:** All children have the right to live in an environment free from abuse and neglect. The safety of children is the paramount concern that must guide child protection efforts.

- **Permanency:** Children need a family and a permanent place to call home. A sense of continuity and connectedness is central to children's healthy development.

135

- **Well-being:** Children deserve nurturing families and environments in which their physical, emotional, educational, and social needs are met. Child protection practices must take into account each child's needs and should promote the healthy development of family relationships.

For additional information on federal and state child welfare laws, visit the Child Welfare Information Gateway website at http://www.childwelfare.gov/systemwide/laws_policies/.

Types of Child Maltreatment

There are four commonly recognized forms of child maltreatment—physical abuse, neglect, psychological abuse, and sexual abuse. The definitions of these types of child maltreatment may vary depending on the state or the locality in which the first responder works. First responders should become familiar with the definitions that apply in their jurisdictions.

Additionally, the signs of child maltreatment listed in this text, such as the behavioral clues listed below, do not indicate absolutely that child maltreatment has occurred. They are meant to act as general guidelines for identifying the possibility of each type of maltreatment. Actual child maltreatment, as well as the perpetrator's identity, can be determined only after a thorough response and investigation.

Behavioral Clues That May Indicate Possible Child Maltreatment

Children who possibly are maltreated may exhibit these behaviors:

- Be aggressive, oppositional, or defiant
- Cower or demonstrate a fear of adults
- Act out, displaying aggressive or disruptive behavior
- Be destructive to self or others
- Come to school too early or not want to leave school, indicating a possible fear of being at home
- Show fearlessness or extreme risk-taking
- Be described as "accident prone"
- Cheat, steal, or lie (may be related to too high expectations at home)

- Be a low achiever

- Be unable to form good peer relationships

- Wear clothing that covers the body and may be inappropriate in warmer months, such as wearing a turtleneck sweater in the summer (Be aware that this may possibly be a cultural issue instead.)

- Show regressive or less mature behavior

- Dislike or shrink away from physical contact (for example, may not tolerate physical praise, such as a pat on the back).

Physical Abuse

The physical abuse of children includes any nonaccidental physical injury caused by the child's caretaker. Physical abuse can vary greatly in frequency and severity. It may include injuries sustained from burning, beating, kicking, or punching. Although the injury is not an accident, neither is it necessarily the intent of the child's caretaker to injure the child. Physical abuse may result from punishment that is inappropriate to the child's age, developmental level, or condition. Additionally, it may be caused by a parent's recurrent lapses in self-control that are brought on by immaturity, stress, or the use of alcohol or illicit drugs. Caretakers may physically abuse children during discipline or as a way to "teach the child a lesson."

These are some signs of possible physical abuse:

- Fractures unexpectedly discovered in the course of an otherwise routine medical examination (for example, discovering a broken rib while listening to the child's heartbeat)

- Injuries that are inconsistent with, or out of proportion to, the history provided by the caretaker or with the child's age or developmental stage (for example, a three-month old burning herself by crawling on top of the stove)

- Multiple fractures, often symmetrical (for example, in both arms or legs), or fractures at different stages of healing

- Fractures in children who are not able to walk

- Skeletal trauma (for example, fractures) combined with other types of injuries, such as burns

- Subdural hematomas, which are hemorrhages between the brain and its outer lining that are caused by ruptured blood vessels

- Burns on the buttocks, around the anogenital region, on the backs of the hands, or on both hands, as well as those that are severe

Some injuries that may have been caused by physical abuse have distinct marks. Some injuries from physical abuse may appear in distinct shapes, especially in cases involving an instrument or burns. Some injuries, however, may not be visible without a complete medical examination. For instance, injuries caused by abuse directed to the abdomen or to the head often are undetected because many of the injuries are internal.

The first response in child physical abuse cases is handled predominately by social service agencies, such as child protective services (CPS). Many jurisdictions across the country have interagency agreements and protocols that define when a joint investigation by law enforcement and CPS will be conducted. Some have put guidelines in place for law enforcement to respond to all physical abuse cases involving young children, as well as to all cases of serious physical abuse. Serious physical abuse cases generally are defined as those requiring medical treatment or hospitalization. A response by law enforcement is also often required in cases involving any blows to the face or the head or the use of a particular instrument (for example, clubs, bats, sticks, chains), which can indicate an attempt to do serious harm.

Physical Abuse vs. Neglect

Neglect involves a caregiver's failure to meet the basic needs of a child, such as food, clothing, shelter, medical care, or supervision. Types of neglect include physical, environmental, emotional, and educational neglect, as well as inadequate supervision.

Caregivers may not provide proper care for a variety of reasons, including a lack of knowledge or understanding about meeting the child's needs, inadequate bonding with the child, or impairment due to substance abuse or to mental illness. Although there are cases of co-occurring maltreatment and poverty, living in poverty, in and of itself, does not mean that a child is being neglected.

Signs of Possible Neglect

Children who possibly are neglected may have these characteristics

- Seem inadequately dressed for the weather (for example, wearing shorts and sandals in freezing weather)

- Appear excessively listless and tired (due to no routine or structure around bedtimes)

- Report caring for younger siblings (when they themselves are underage or are developmentally not ready to do so)

- Demonstrate poor hygiene or smell of urine or feces

- Seem unusually small or thin or have a distended stomach (indicative of malnutrition)

- Have unattended medical or dental problems, such as infected sores or badly decayed or abscessed teeth

- Appear withdrawn

- Crave unusual amounts of attention, even eliciting negative responses in order to obtain it

- Be chronically truant.

Additionally, the first responder should check the home environment for signs of neglect, such as health or safety hazards, no heat, or unsanitary conditions.

Chapter 10

Abusive Head Trauma

Abusive head trauma/inflicted traumatic brain injury—also called shaken baby/shaken impact syndrome (or SBS)—is a form of inflicted head trauma.

Abusive head trauma (AHT) can be caused by direct blows to the head, dropping or throwing a child, or shaking a child. Head trauma is the leading cause of death in child abuse cases in the United States.

How These Injuries Happen

Unlike other forms of inflicted head trauma, abusive head trauma results from injuries caused by someone vigorously shaking a child. Because the anatomy of infants puts them at particular risk for injury from this kind of action, the majority of victims are infants younger than one year old. The average age of victims is between three and eight months, although these injuries can be seen in children up to years old.

The perpetrators in these cases are most often parents or caregivers. Common triggers are frustration or stress when the child is crying. Unfortunately, the shaking may have the desired effect: Although at first the baby cries more, he or she may stop crying as the brain is damaged.

"Abusive Head Trauma (Shaken Baby Syndrome)," January 2011, reprinted with permission from www.kidshealth.org. This information was provided by Kids Health®, one of the largest resources online for medically reviewed health information written for parents, kids, and teens. For more articles like this, visit www.KidsHealth.org, or www.TeensHealth.org. Copyright © 1995–2012 The Nemours Foundation. All rights reserved.

Approximately 60% of identified victims of shaking injury are male, and children of families who live at or below the poverty level are at an increased risk for these injuries as well as any type of child abuse. It is estimated that the perpetrators in 65% to 90% of cases are males— usually either the baby's father or the mother's boyfriend, often someone in his early twenties.

When someone forcefully shakes a baby, the child's head rotates about the neck uncontrollably because infants' neck muscles aren't well developed and provide little support for their heads. This violent movement pitches the infant's brain back and forth within the skull, sometimes rupturing blood vessels and nerves throughout the brain and tearing the brain tissue. The brain may strike the inside of the skull, causing bruising and bleeding to the brain.

The damage can be even greater when a shaking episode ends with an impact (hitting a wall or a crib mattress, for example), because the forces of acceleration and deceleration associated with an impact are so strong. After the shaking, swelling in the brain can cause enormous pressure within the skull, compressing blood vessels and increasing overall injury to its delicate structure.

Normal interaction with a child, like bouncing the baby on a knee, will not cause these injuries. It's important to never shake a baby under any circumstances.

What Are the Effects?

AHT often causes irreversible damage. In the worst cases, children die due to their injuries.

Children who survive may have:

- partial or total blindness

- hearing loss

- seizures

- developmental delays

- impaired intellect

- speech and learning difficulties

- problems with memory and attention

- severe mental retardation

- cerebral palsy

Even in milder cases, in which babies look normal immediately after the shaking, they may eventually develop one or more of these problems. Sometimes the first sign of a problem isn't noticed until the child enters the school system and exhibits behavioral problems or learning difficulties. But by that time, it's more difficult to link these problems to a shaking incident from several years before.

Signs and Symptoms

In any abusive head trauma case, the duration and force of the shaking, the number of episodes, and whether impact is involved all affect the severity of the infant's injuries. In the most violent cases, children may arrive at the emergency room unconscious, suffering seizures, or in shock. But in many cases, infants may never be brought to medical attention if they don't exhibit such severe symptoms.

In less severe cases, a child who has been shaken may experience:

- lethargy
- irritability
- vomiting
- poor sucking or swallowing
- decreased appetite
- lack of smiling or vocalizing
- rigidity
- seizures
- difficulty breathing
- altered consciousness
- unequal pupil size
- an inability to lift the head
- an inability to focus the eyes or track movement

Diagnosis

Many cases of AHT are brought in for medical care as "silent injuries." In other words, parents or caregivers don't often provide a history that the child has had abusive head trauma or a shaking injury, so doctors don't know to look for subtle or physical signs. This can sometimes result in children having injuries that aren't identified in the medical system.

In many cases, babies who don't have severe symptoms may never be brought to a doctor. Many of the less severe symptoms such as vomiting or irritability may resolve and can have many non-abusive causes.

Unfortunately, unless a doctor has reason to suspect child abuse, mild cases (in which the infant seems lethargic, fussy, or perhaps isn't feeding well) are often misdiagnosed as a viral illness or colic. Without a suspicion of child abuse and any resulting intervention with the parents or caregivers, these children may be shaken again, worsening any brain injury or damage.

If shaken baby syndrome is suspected, doctors may look for:

- hemorrhages in the retinas of the eyes
- skull fractures
- swelling of the brain
- subdural hematomas (blood collections pressing on the surface of the brain)
- rib and long bone (bones in the arms and legs) fractures
- bruises around the head, neck, or chest

The Child's Development and Education

What makes AHT so devastating is that it often involves a total brain injury. For example, a child whose vision is severely impaired won't be able to learn through observation, which decreases the child's overall ability to learn.

The development of language, vision, balance, and motor coordination, all of which occur to varying degrees after birth, are particularly likely to be affected in any child who has AHT.

Such impairment can require intensive physical and occupational therapy to help the child acquire skills that would have developed on their own had the brain injury not occurred.

As they get older, kids who were shaken as babies may require special education and continued therapy to help with language development and daily living skills, such as dressing themselves.

Before age three, a child can receive speech or physical therapy through the Department of Public Health/Early Intervention. Federal law requires that each state provide these services for children who have developmental disabilities as a result of being abused.

Some schools are also increasingly providing information and developmental assessments for kids under the age of three. Parents can turn to a variety of rehabilitation and other therapists for early intervention services for children after abusive head trauma. Developmental assessments can assist in improving education outcomes as well as the overall well-being of the child.

After a child who's been diagnosed with abusive head trauma turns three, it's the school district's responsibility to provide any needed additional special educational services.

Preventing AHT

Abusive head trauma is 100% preventable. A key aspect of prevention is increasing awareness of the potential dangers of shaking.

Finding ways to alleviate the parent or caregiver's stress at the critical moments when a baby is crying can significantly reduce the risk to the child. Some hospital-based programs have helped new parents identify and prevent shaking injuries and understand how to respond when infants cry.

The National Center on Shaken Baby Syndrome offers a prevention program, the Period of Purple Crying, which seeks to help parents and other caregivers understand crying in normal infants. By defining and describing the sometimes inconsolable infant crying that can sometimes cause stress, anger, and frustration in parents and caregivers, the program hopes to educate and empower people to prevent AHT.

Another method that may help is author Dr. Harvey Karp's "five S's":

1. **S**hushing (using "white noise" or rhythmic sounds that mimic the constant whir of noise in the womb, with things like vacuum cleaners, hair dryers, clothes dryers, a running tub, or a white noise CD)

2. **S**ide/stomach positioning (placing the baby on the left side—to help digestion—or on the belly while holding him or her, then putting the sleeping baby in the crib or bassinet on his or her back)

3. **S**ucking (letting the baby breastfeed or bottle-feed, or giving the baby a pacifier or finger to suck on)

4. **S**waddling (wrapping the baby up snugly in a blanket to help him or her feel more secure)

5. **S**winging gently (rocking in a chair, using an infant swing, or taking a car ride to help duplicate the constant motion the baby felt in the womb)

If a baby in your care won't stop crying, you can also try the following:

- Make sure the baby's basic needs are met (for example, he or she isn't hungry and doesn't need to be changed).

- Check for signs of illness, like fever or swollen gums.

- Rock or walk with the baby.

- Sing or talk to the baby.

- Offer the baby a pacifier or a noisy toy.

- Take the baby for a ride in a stroller or strapped into a child safety seat in the car.

- Hold the baby close against your body and breathe calmly and slowly.

- Call a friend or relative for support or to take care of the baby while you take a break.

- If nothing else works, put the baby on his or her back in the crib, close the door, and check on the baby in 10 minutes.

- Call your doctor if nothing seems to be helping your infant, in case there is a medical reason for the fussiness.

To prevent potential AHT, parents and caregivers of infants need to learn how to respond to their own stress. It's important to talk to anyone caring for your baby about the dangers of shaking and how it can be prevented.

Chapter 11

Munchausen by Proxy Syndrome

Munchausen by proxy syndrome (MBPS) is a relatively rare form of child abuse that involves the exaggeration or fabrication of illnesses or symptoms by a primary caretaker.

Also known as "medical child abuse," MBPS was named after Baron von Munchausen, an 18th-century German dignitary known for making up stories about his travels and experiences in order to get attention. "By proxy" indicates that a parent or other adult is fabricating or exaggerating symptoms in a child, not in himself or herself.

Munchausen by proxy syndrome is a mental illness and requires treatment.

About MBPS

In MBPS, an individual—usually a parent or caregiver—causes or fabricates symptoms in a child. The adult deliberately misleads others (particularly medical professionals), and may go as far as to actually cause symptoms in the child through poisoning, medication, or even suffocation. In most cases (85%), the mother is responsible for causing the illness or symptoms.

Typically, the cause is a need for attention and sympathy from doctors, nurses, and other professionals. Some experts believe that it isn't just the attention that's gained from the "illness" of the child that drives this behavior, but also the satisfaction in deceiving individuals who they consider to be more important and powerful than themselves.

Because the parent or caregiver appears to be so caring and attentive, often no one suspects any wrongdoing. Diagnosis is made extremely difficult due to the ability of the parent or caregiver to manipulate doctors and induce symptoms in their child.

Often, the perpetrator is familiar with the medical profession and knowledgeable about how to induce illness or impairment in the child. Medical personnel often overlook the possibility of MBPS because it goes against the belief that parents and caregivers would never deliberately hurt their child.

Most victims of MBPS are preschoolers (although there have been cases in kids up to 16 years old), and there are equal numbers of boys and girls.

Diagnosing MBPS

Diagnosis is very difficult, but could involve some of the following:

- A child who has multiple medical problems that don't respond to treatment or that follow a persistent and puzzling course

- Physical or laboratory findings that are highly unusual, don't correspond with the child's medical history, or are physically or clinically impossible

- Short-term symptoms that tend to stop or improve when the victim is not with the perpetrator (for example, when hospitalized)

- A parent or caregiver who isn't reassured by "good news" when test results find no medical problems, but continues to believe that the child is ill and may "doctor shop" to find a professional who believes them

- A parent or caregiver who appears to be medically knowledgeable or fascinated with medical details or seems to enjoy the hospital environment and attention the sick child receives

- A parent or caregiver who's overly supportive and encouraging of the doctor, or one who is angry and demands further intervention, more procedures, second opinions, or transfers to more sophisticated facilities

If you have any concerns about a child you know, it is important to speak to someone at your local child protective services agency—even if you prefer to call in anonymously.

Causes of MBPS

MBPS is a psychiatric condition. In some cases, the perpetrators were themselves abused, physically and/or and sexually, as children. They may have come from families in which being sick was a way to get love.

The parent's or caregiver's own personal needs overcome his or her ability to see the child as a person with feelings and rights, possibly because the parent or caregiver may have grown up being treated like he or she wasn't a person with rights or feelings.

In rare cases, MBPS is not caused by a parent or family member, but by a medical professional (such as a nurse or doctor), who induces illness in a child who is hospitalized for other reasons.

What Happens to the Child?

In the most severe instances, parents or caregivers with MBPS may go to great lengths to make their children sick. When cameras were placed in some children's hospital rooms, some perpetrators were filmed switching medications, injecting kids with urine to cause an infection, or placing drops of blood in urine specimens.

In most cases, hospitalization is required. And because they may be deemed a "medical mystery," hospital stays tend to be longer than usual. Whatever the cause, the child's symptoms—whether created or fabricated—ease or completely disappear when the perpetrator isn't present.

According to experts, common conditions and symptoms that are created or fabricated by parents or caregivers with MBPS can include: failure to thrive, allergies, asthma, vomiting, diarrhea, seizures, and infections.

The long-term prognosis for these children depends on the degree of damage created by the illness or impairment and the amount of time it takes to recognize and diagnose MBPS. Some extreme cases have been reported in which children developed destructive skeletal changes, limps, mental retardation, brain damage, and blindness from symptoms caused by the parent or caregiver. Often, these children require multiple surgeries, each with the risk for future medical problems.

If the child lives to be old enough to comprehend what's happening, the psychological damage can be significant. The child may come to feel that he or she will only be loved when ill and may, therefore,

149

help the parent try to deceive doctors, using self-abuse to avoid being abandoned. And so, some victims of MBPS are at risk of repeating the cycle of abuse.

Getting Help for the Child

If MBPS is suspected, health care providers are required by law to report their concerns. However, after a parent or caregiver is charged, the child's symptoms may increase as the person who is accused attempts to prove the presence of the illness. If the parent or caregiver repeatedly denies the charges, the child would likely be removed from the home and legal action would be taken on the child's behalf.

In some cases, the parent or caregiver may deny the charges and move to another location, only to continue the behavior. Even if the child is returned to the perpetrator's custody while protective services are involved, the child may continue to be a victim of abuse while the perpetrator avoids treatment and interventions.

Getting Help for the Parent or Caregiver

To get help, the parent or caregiver must admit to the abuse and seek psychological treatment.

But if the perpetrator doesn't admit to the wrongdoing, psychological treatment has little chance of helping the situation. Recognizing MBPS as an illness that has the potential for treatment is one way to give hope to the family in these rare situations.

Chapter 12

Sexual Abuse of Children

Chapter Contents

Section 12.1

Statistics and Indicators of Sexual Abuse in Children

Sexual abuse is any sexual contact with a child or the use of a child for the sexual pleasure of someone else. This may include exposing private parts to the child or asking the child to expose him or herself, fondling of the genitals or requests for the child to do so, oral sex or attempts to enter the vagina or anus with fingers, objects or penis, although actual penetration is rarely achieved.

Statistics

- One in four girls and one in six boys is sexually abused in some way by the age of 18 (Kinsey, 1953; Finkelhor, 1979)

- 10% of those children are preschoolers (Children's Hospital, D.C.)

- 85–90% involve a perpetrator known to the child (Groth, 1982; DeFrancis, 1969; Russell, 1983)

- 35% involve a family member (King County Rape Relief, Washington)

- Only 10% of the offenses involve physical violence (Jaffee, 1975)

- 50% of all assaults take place in the home of the child or the offender (Sanford, 1980)

- The average offender is involved with over 70 children in his or her "career" of offending (Sanford, 1980, Abel and Becker, 1980)

Physical Indicators

- Difficulty walking or sitting

- Torn clothing

- Stained or bloody underwear
- Pain or itching in genital area
- Venereal disease, especially in preteens
- Pregnancy

Behavioral Indicators in Child

Children often do not tell us with words that they have been sexually abused, or that they have successfully resisted an assault. They hesitate to talk about what has happened for many reasons, including their relationship to the offender, fear of the consequences, retaliation, or uncertainty about whether or not they will be believed.

Any one of the following signs or changes in behavior could indicate that there has been a sexual assault or it could be indicative of another problem. Whatever has caused a child's change in behavior should be explored.

- Sudden reluctance to go someplace or be with someone
- Inappropriate displays of affection
- Sexual acting out
- Sudden use of sexual terms or new names for body parts
- Discomfort or rejection of typical family affection
- Sleep problems, including: insomnia, nightmares, refusal to sleep alone, or suddenly insisting on a night light
- Regressive behaviors, including: thumb-sucking, bed-wetting, infantile behaviors, or other signs of dependency
- Extreme clinginess or other signs of fearfulness
- A sudden change in personality
- Problems in school
- Unwilling to participate in or change clothing for gym class at school
- Runs away from home
- Bizarre or unusual sophistication pertaining to sexual behavior or knowledge, including sexual acting out
- Reports sexual assault by parent or guardian

153

Indicators of Sexually Abusive Parent/Guardian

- Overly protective or jealous of child and friends
- Abuses alcohol or other drugs
- Encourages exhibitionism in child
- Voyeuristic, seductive to child
- Exposes child to pornographic and sexually stimulating pictures
- Encourages the child in promiscuous and/or prostitute acts
- Freely talks or boasts about sexual themes with child

Who Are Abusers?

Abusers can be family, friends, neighbors, teachers, clergy or coaches. As described by the National Committee for the Prevention of Child Abuse: Child abuse happens in all socioeconomic, racial, ethnic, and religious groups although it is now known that it does not occur equally over all groups (Fryer, 1990).

What Abuse Does to Children

Children who have been physically, sexually, and/or emotionally abused not only suffer a wide range of effects from their victimization, but are at greater risk to be abused again. Abuse commonly produces feelings of guilt, violation, loss of control, and lowered self-esteem.

Even those who seem to be handling their abuse are concerned that it might happen again, they did something wrong, and future relationships might be abusive.

Long-Term Effects of Abuse

Common problems for abused children include emotional problems, behavioral problems, poor performance in school, and further abuse. While these effects are not always obvious, they are important.

Long-term studies of low achievers, runaways, drug abusers, prostitutes and incarcerated individuals paint a disturbing picture. Abuse is a consistent and pervasive element in their backgrounds. Low self-esteem and poor self-concept are ever-present.

Knowing this, there can be little doubt that children who are abused, as well as adults who were abused as children, need assistance to resolve the questions that the abuse experience has raised, even if that assistance does not come until years after the abuse.

Section 12.2

The Nature and Consequences of Child Sexual Abuse

Definition of Child Sexual Abuse

Child sexual abuse is defined as inappropriately exposing or subjecting a child to sexual contact, activity, or behavior. Sexual abuse includes oral, anal, genital, buttocks, and breast contact. It also includes the use of objects for vaginal or anal penetration, fondling, or sexual stimulation. Exploitation of a child for pornographic purposes, making a child available to another as a child prostitute, and stimulating a child with inappropriate solicitation, exhibitionism, and erotic material are also forms of sexual abuse. Non-contact behaviors, such as voyeurism, indecent exposure, and sexual remarks to children, also constitute sexual abuse.

Scope of Child Sexual Abuse

In 2008, approximately 69,184 children (9.1 percent of all substantiated cases of child maltreatment) in the United States were officially counted as victims of child sexual abuse. These figures may actually under-represent the number of child sexual abuse victims. One study indicates that at least 12–35 percent of American women and 4–9 percent of American men experienced some form of sexual abuse as children.

Nature of Child Sexual Abuse

Child sexual abuse occurs in all populations. It happens to children in all socioeconomic and educational levels, across all racial and cultural groups, and in both rural and urban areas. The vast majority of child sexual abusers include someone the child knows such as a parent or other relative, teacher, clergy, neighbor, or friend. Approximately 60 percent of boys and 80 percent of girls who were sexually victimized were abused by someone the child knew.

Only a fraction of those who commit sexual assault are apprehended and convicted for their crimes. According to Center for Sex Offender Management, only 33.9 percent of sexual assaults against persons 12 years or older were reported to law enforcement. Current research does not track the rate of reporting for child sexual abuse for children younger than 12 years of age. Most experts, however, assume such rates are similar to those for children older than 12 years of age.

Child sexual abuse is perpetrated by juveniles as well as adults. Forty percent of reported sexual assaults against children ages six and under are attributable to juvenile abusers, as are thirty-nine percent of reported sexual assaults against children ages six through 11. Adolescent boys make up approximately 23 percent of sexual offenders. Research findings indicate that from 40 to 80 percent of juvenile sex offenders have themselves been victims of sexual abuse.

Common warning signs of those who sexually abuse children include excessive talk about the sexual activities of children or teens; excessive masturbation; talk about sexual fantasies including children; encouraging a child to keep secrets; viewing of child pornography; requests to adult partners to dress or act like a child during sexual activity; excessive time spent with children or teens, not with adults; and the identification of children with sexual slang terms. However, sexual offenders often do not display such overt indicators of their sexual abuse of children. Therefore, in addition to being attuned to warning signs, parents and caregivers should routinely employ risk reduction strategies, which minimize, to the extent possible, the child's risk exposure for sexual abuse. Such basic measures as refraining from public display of the child's printed name on the outside of clothing or backpacks, providing parental supervision calibrated to the level of opportunity a given circumstance may present for the occurrence of child sexual abuse, and observing and monitoring relationships the child has with adolescents and adults are routine practices that parents and caregivers can adopt to reduce the child's risk exposure for sexual abuse.

Consequences of Child Sexual Abuse

The physical signs of child sexual abuse are often hard to detect, as most perpetrators avoid physically harming their victims so they can repeat the activities over time. Because of this dynamic and the fact that children generally disclose long after the last contact, few children will have diagnostic findings. Child sexual abuse can be very different from rape, where force and restraint are used and signs of injury are generally present.

When children are injured as a result of sexual contact, they may present with vaginal or rectal bleeding; genital pain, itching, swelling, or discharge; difficulty with bowel movements; painful urination; and recurring complaints of stomachaches and/or headaches. Few children present with extragenital trauma to the breasts, buttocks, lower abdomen or extremities. Children can also contract sexually transmitted diseases or become pregnant as a result of sexual abuse.

Behavioral and emotional consequences/warning signs include: extreme changes in behavior such as loss of appetite, eating disorder, withdrawal, or aggressiveness; disturbed sleep patterns or a sudden fear of the dark; regression to infantile behavior; multiple personality disorders; and delinquent behavior or a drop of grades in school. Additional indicators may include intrusive thoughts, nightmares, heightened startle response, poor concentration, and hyper-vigilance, and in some cases the child may appear depressed, withdrawn, or lethargic. Children will commonly respond to their victimization with sexualized behaviors and/or age inappropriate knowledge of sexual activities.

Long-term consequences of sexual abuse may include a chronic self-perception of helplessness, hopelessness, depression, impaired trust, self-blame, self-destructive behavior, and low self-esteem.

Other long-term consequences for victims of child sexual abuse include:

- **Increased likelihood of teen pregnancy:** In one study, men who were sexually abused at aged 10 or younger were 80 percent more likely than non-abused men to later engage in sexual activity resulting in teen pregnancy.

- **Increased likelihood of homelessness:** A study of homeless women found that childhood maltreatment, including physical, verbal, and sexual abuse, was a "pervasive and devastating predictor of dysfunctional outcomes," including chronic homelessness.

- **Increased risk of drug and alcohol abuse:** Research indicates that both women and men who have experienced child sexual abuse have an increased risk of drug and alcohol abuse in their adult life.

It is clear that the consequences of child sexual abuse [extend] far beyond the affected children and families. Enormous societal costs are involved. Prevent Child Abuse America estimated the economic impact of child abuse and neglect at $104 billion in 2007; and this was likely a conservative estimate. Thus, in addition to the compelling human argument to help optimize children's development, health and safety, there is also a financial impetus to help prevent the neglect of children. The aphorism that "our children are our nation's most valuable resource" should be more than a slogan. Finally, at the heart of child neglect is a concern with their basic rights, their human rights.

The costs associated with the pervasive and long-lasting effects of child abuse and neglect are as undeniable as our obligation to prevent—not just respond to—this problem. In 2007, $33 billion in direct costs for foster care services, hospitalization, mental health treatment, and law enforcement were supplemented by over $70 billion in indirect costs like loss of individual productivity, chronic health problems, special education, and delinquent and criminal justice services.

For more information contact Prevent Child Abuse America at 312-663-3520 or at mailbox@preventchildabuse.org.

Chapter 13

Incest

Chapter Contents

Section 13.1

How Does Incest Differ from Other Child Sexual Abuse?

Incest is sexual contact between persons who are so closely related that their marriage is illegal (for example, parents and children, uncles/ aunts and nieces/nephews, etc.). This usually takes the form of an older family member sexually abusing a child or adolescent.

Laws vary from place to place regarding what constitutes incest, child sexual abuse, sexual assault, and rape.

How common is incest?

There are very few reliable statistics about how often incest occurs. It's difficult to know how many people are affected by incest because many incest situations never get reported. There are many reasons that the victim might not report the abuse.

- The victim has been told that what is happening is normal or happens in every family, and doesn't realize that it is a form of abuse.

- The victim may not know that help is available or who they can talk to.

- The victim may be afraid of what will happen if they tell someone: The abuser may have threatened the victim; the victim may care about the abuser and be afraid of what will happen to the abuser if they tell; the victim may be afraid of what will happen to them if they tell.

- The victim may also be concerned about how many people will react when they hear about the abuse: They may be afraid that no one will believe them or that the person they confide in will tell the abuser; the victim may be afraid that people will accuse them of having done something wrong.

What makes incest different than child sexual abuse?

All forms of child sexual abuse can have negative long-term effects for the victim. You can read about some of those effects at http://www .rainn.org/get-information/types-of-sexual-assault/child-sexual-abuse.

Incest is especially damaging because it disrupts the child's primary support system, the family.

- When a child is abused by someone outside the family, the child's family is often able to offer support and a sense of safety. When the abuser is someone in the family, the family may not be able to provide support or a sense of safety. Since the children (especially younger children) often have limited resources outside the family, it can be very hard for them to recover from incest.

- Incest can damage a child's ability to trust, since the people who were supposed to protect and care for them have abused them. Survivors of incest sometimes have difficulty developing trusting relationships.

- It can also be very damaging for a child if a non-abusing parent is aware of the abuse and chooses—for whatever reason—not to take action to stop it. There are many reasons that a non-abusing parent might not stop the abuse:

  - The non-abusing parent may feel that they are dependent on the abuser for shelter or income.

  - If the non-abusing parent was the victim of incest as a child, they may think that this is normal for families.

  - The non-abusing parent may feel that allowing the incest to continue is the only way to keep their partner.

  - The non-abusing parent may feel that their child was "asking for it" by behaving in ways that the parent perceives as provocative or seductive. Unfortunately, many non-abusing parents are aware of the incest and choose not to get their child out of the situation, or worse, to blame their child for what has happened. This makes the long-term effects of incest worse.

Section 13.2

What Should I Do If I Am a Victim of Incest?

"What Should I Do if I Am a Victim of Incest?" © 2012 RAINN (Rape, Abuse & Incest National Network), www.rainn.org. All rights reserved. Reprinted with permission. Immediate crisis help and information is available 24 hours per day/7 days per week from the National Sexual Assault Hotline, 800-656-HOPE (4673), or the National Sexual Assault Online Hotline at http://online.rainn.org.

First, know that this is not your fault. No one deserves to be abused. Get some help. You do not have to handle this on your own.

- Tell a trusted adult.
  - If you can't talk to a parent, can you talk to... A teacher? A school counselor? A friend's parent? Your doctor? Your minister (or pastor, priest, rabbi, imam, etc.)?

- If you do not have any trusted adults in your life, you can also call Child Protective Services (CPS) for your area. (Even if you are over 18, CPS may still be able to offer assistance.)
  - You can find the number for CPS in Rape, Abuse and Incest National Network (RAINN)'s mandatory reporting database (http://www.rainn.org/public-policy/laws-in-your-state). Information is listed by state.
  - You can also find the number for Child Protective Services in the Blue Pages of your phone book.
  - Your local police department can also help you contact CPS.

- Be prepared. Not every adult, even trusted adults, are able to help. You may need to tell more than one person before you find someone who can help.

- If you need some help thinking through these options, call the National Sexual Assault Hotline any time at 800-656-HOPE or contact the Online Hotline at http://www.rainn.org/get-help/national-sexual-assault-online-hotline.

Remember that no one deserves to be abused. Help is available.

Section 13.3

What Should I Do If Someone I Know Is a Victim of Incest?

Listen

One of the most important things that you can do for a victim is to listen to their story and believe them.

Help Keep the Victim Safe

This may mean different things depending on who you are and what your relationship is to the victim.

- There may be legal considerations. Depending on where you live and your role in the victim's life, you may be required to report their situation to the authorities.

    - Teachers, ministers, counselors and other professionals are often "mandated reporters," or people who are required by law to report child abuse, including incest.

    - Check RAINN's mandatory reporting database (http://www .rainn.org/public-policy/laws-in-your-state) if you are not sure whether you are required to make a report.

Even if you are not a mandated reporter, calling Child Protective Services (CPS) may be the best way you can help protect the victim.

- You can find the number for CPS in RAINN's mandatory reporting database. Information is listed by state.

- CPS workers will be able to investigate the situation in greater detail and take steps to protect the victim.

• You can make reports to CPS anonymously if you are concerned about the victim's family knowing who made the report.

You may also contact the local police department, particularly if you have concerns about the victim's safety at the time you find out about the incest.

Follow Up

• Let the victim know that you still care.

• Listen. Even after the victim is out of the incest situation, they will still need support.

Remember to take care of yourself. Being involved with an incest situation can be scary or upsetting.

Section 13.4

Incest and the Non-Abusive Parent

If you have recently learned that your child is a victim of incest, you may be experiencing a range of emotions. You might feel...

• **Shock**

    • If you had no idea that incest was occurring, you may be very surprised to hear what has happened.

    • You may have difficulty figuring out how to respond to your child or to the abuser.

• **Anger**

    • You may feel angry at the abuser for hurting your child.

- If you weren't aware of the abuse, you may feel angry at your child for not telling you.
- You might feel angry at your child for disclosing the abuse.

- **Sadness**
  - You may feel sad for your child, for what this means to your family, or for yourself because you need to deal with this situation.

- **Anxiety**
  - You might feel anxiety about responding the "right" way to your child.
  - You might feel anxiety about how this will impact your relationship with your child or the abuser.
  - You may worry that this has legal consequences for you.

- **Fear**
  - Depending on your family circumstances, you may be afraid that the abuser will find a way to harm you or your child.
  - If the abuser was responsible for supporting the family, you may be afraid of being on your own.

There is no "wrong" way to feel. What is important is that you are able to support your child and help them through this situation without blaming them. Remember that abuse is never the victim's fault.

Once you and your child are safe and the abuser no longer has access to your child, you can both begin the process of healing.

To support your child in their healing process, you need to take care of yourself. Good self-care is not selfish. It is essential to take care of yourself so that you can support your child.

- Manage your emotions.
  - You may consider talking to a counselor: After many incest situations, the family may be in counseling. You might also consider individual counseling. The advantage of individual counseling is that the focus can be entirely on you and it will give you the opportunity to work through your feelings and concerns about the situation without needing to worry about how your child will hear those concerns. Local rape crisis centers often provide counseling or can connect you with a provider. Call (800) 656-HOPE or go to http://centers.rainn .org/ to find a center near you.

- Develop your support system: Reach out to friends and family who are supportive and who you feel comfortable talking to about your family situation. Consider joining a support group for non-abusing parents of incest victims.

- Keep a journal: It may be helpful to write down some of the feelings that you are experiencing.

- Practice meditation or relaxation exercises: Relaxation techniques or meditation may help maintain your emotional balance.

- Set limits.

  - Make sure that you spend time doing activities that have nothing to do with the incest situation.

  - Set aside time as needed to cope with the incest situation, whether that means dealing with the legal situation, counseling appointments, visitation or other tasks. When that time is up, move on to other activities.

- Make sure that you are involved in some activities that don't revolve around the incest situation.

You may find that supporting your child is a challenge. Victims have a wide range of reactions to abuse. Your child...

- Might want to talk about the abuse all the time.

- Might not want to talk at all.

- Might not want to talk to you, but may be confiding in someone else.

- Might be angry at you for not protecting them.

- Might be angry at you for ending the abuse.

- They might be experiencing a range of other reactions. It is difficult to predict how a victim will respond, and it may change over time.

Remember that there is no "right" way for a victim to respond to abuse. The process of healing from incest can take a long time, and can be very frustrating. Sometimes it can feel like there is no progress at all. This can be especially frustrating for people who are trying to support the victim.

If you or your child is still in an incest situation, do not hesitate to ask for help.

- You can call Child Protective Services (CPS) for your area.
  - You can find the number for CPS in RAINN's mandatory reporting database (http://www.rainn.org/public-policy/laws-in-your-state). Information is listed by state.
  - You can also find the number for Child Protective Services in the Blue Pages of your phone book.
  - Your local police department can help you contact CPS.
  - If you believe that the child is in immediate danger, call 911.

Chapter 14

Teen Dating Abuse

Dating violence is a type of intimate partner violence. It occurs between two people in a close relationship. The nature of dating violence can be physical, emotional, or sexual.

- **Physical:** This occurs when a partner is pinched, hit, shoved, or kicked.

- **Emotional:** This means threatening a partner or harming his or her sense of self-worth. Examples include name calling, shaming, bullying, embarrassing on purpose, or keeping him/her away from friends and family.

- **Sexual:** This is forcing a partner to engage in a sex act when he or she does not or cannot consent.

- **Stalking:** This refers to a pattern of harassing or threatening tactics used by a perpetrator that is both unwanted and causes fear in the victim.

Dating violence can take place in person or electronically, such as repeated texting or posting sexual pictures of a partner online. Unhealthy relationships can start early and last a lifetime. Dating violence often starts with teasing and name calling. These behaviors are often thought to be a "normal" part of a relationship. But these behaviors can lead to more serious violence like physical assault and rape.

"Understanding Teen Dating Violence," Centers for Disease Control and Prevention (www.cdc.gov), 2012.

Why is dating violence a public health problem?

Dating violence is a serious problem in the United States. Many teens do not report it because they are afraid to tell friends and family.

- Among adult victims of rape, physical violence, and/or stalking by an intimate partner, 22.4% of women and 15.0% of men first experienced some form of partner violence between 11 and 17 years of age.[1]

- Approximately 9% of high school students report being hit, slapped, or physically hurt on purpose by a boyfriend or girl-friend in the 12 months before surveyed.[2]

How does dating violence affect health?

Dating violence can have a negative effect on health throughout life. Teens who are victims are more likely to be depressed and do poorly in school.[3] They may engage in unhealthy behaviors, like using drugs and alcohol[3], and are more likely to have eating disorders.[4] Some teens even think about or attempt suicide.[5] Teens who are victims in high school are at higher risk for victimization during college.[6]

Who is at risk for dating violence?

Studies show that people who harm their dating partners are more depressed and are more aggressive than peers. Other factors that increase risk for harming a dating partner include:[7]

- Trauma symptoms
- Alcohol use
- Having a friend involved in dating violence
- Having problem behaviors in other areas
- Belief that dating violence is acceptable
- Exposure to harsh parenting
- Exposure to inconsistent discipline
- Lack of parental supervision, monitoring, and warmth

Note: These are just some risk factors. To learn more, go to www.cdc.gov/violenceprevention.

How can we prevent dating violence?

The ultimate goal is to stop dating violence before it starts. Strategies that promote healthy relationships are vital. During the preteen and teen years, young people are learning skills they need to form positive relationships with others. This is an ideal time to promote healthy relationships and prevent patterns of dating violence that can last into adulthood.

Prevention programs change the attitudes and behaviors linked with dating violence. One example is Safe Dates, a school-based program that is designed to change social norms and improve problem solving skills.[7]

How does CDC approach prevention?

The Centers for Disease Control and Prevention (CDC) uses a four-step approach to address public health problems like dating violence (for a list of CDC activities, see www.cdc.gov/violenceprevention/pub/ipv_sv_guide.html).

Step 1. Define the problem: Before we can prevent dating violence, we need to know how big the problem is, where it is, and who it affects. CDC learns about a problem by gathering and studying data. These data are critical because they help us know where prevention is most needed.

Step 2. Identify risk and protective factors: It is not enough to know that dating violence is affecting a certain group of people in a certain area. We also need to know why. CDC conducts and supports research to answer this question. We can then develop programs to reduce or get rid of risk factors and increase protective factors.

Step 3. Develop and test prevention strategies: Using information gathered in research, CDC develops and evaluates strategies to prevent violence.

Step 4. Ensure widespread adoption: In this final step, CDC shares the best prevention strategies. CDC may also provide funding or technical help so communities can adopt these strategies.

Where can I learn more?

- CDC's Dating Matters: Strategies to Promote Healthy Teen Relationships: www.cdc.gov/violenceprevention/datingmatters

- National Dating Abuse Helpline: 866-331-9474

- National Domestic Violence Hotline: 800-799-SAFE (7233)
- National Sexual Assault Hotline: 800-656-HOPE (4673)
- National Sexual Violence Resource Center: www.nsvrc.org
- Dating Matters: Understanding Teen Dating Violence Prevention: www.vetoviolence.org/datingmatters

References

1. Black MC, Basile KC, Breiding MJ, Smith SG, Walters ML, Merrick MT, Chen J, Stevens MR. *The National Intimate Partner and Sexual Violence Survey (NISVS): 2010 Summary Report.* Atlanta, GA: National Center for Injury Prevention and Control, Centers for Disease Control and Prevention, 2011. Available from www.cdc.gov/ViolencePrevention/pdf/NISVS_Report2010-a.pdf.

2. Centers for Disease Control and Prevention. Youth risk behavior surveillance—United States, 2011. *MMWR, Surveillance Summaries* 2012; 61(no. SS-4). Available from www.cdc.gov/mmwr/pdf/ss/ss6104.pdf

3. Banyard VL, Cross C. Consequences of teen dating violence: Understanding intervening variables in ecological context. *Violence Against Women* 2008; 14(9):998-1013.

4. Ackard DM, Neumark-Sztainer D. Date violence and date rape among adolescents: Associations with disordered eating behaviors and psychological health. *Child Abuse and Neglect* 2002; 26:455-473.

5. Centers for Disease Control and Prevention. Physical Dating Violence Among High School Students—United States, 2003. *MMWR* 2006; 55:532-535.

6. Smith PH, White JW, Holland LJ. A longitudinal perspective on dating violence among adolescent and college-age women. *American Journal of Public Health* 2003; 93(7):1104–1109.

7. Foshee VA, Matthew RA. Adolescent dating abuse perpetration: A review of findings, methodological limitations, and suggestions for future research. In: Flannery DJ, Vazjoni AT, Waldman ID, editors. *The Cambridge Handbook of Violent Behavior and Aggression.* New York: Cambridge; 2007: 431-449.

Chapter 15

Statutory Rape

Chapter Contents

Section 15.1

State Laws on Statutory Rape

Excerpted from "Statutory Rape: A Guide to State Laws and Reporting Requirements," Office of the Assistant Secretary for Planning and Evaluation, U.S. Department of Health and Human Services, last updated October 10, 2008; accessed September 25, 2012. The complete text of this document, including references can be found online at http://aspe.hhs.gov/hsp/08/sr/ statelaws/summary.shtml. Information in this section discusses laws in specific states; legal information varies by state, but the issues raised are pertinent in most U.S. jurisdictions.

Statutory Rape—Criminal Offenses

Few states use the term statutory rape in their codes. Instead, criminal codes specify the legality of specific sexual acts. The applicable laws are often embedded in the section of the code dealing with other sexual offenses (for example, sexual assault, forcible rape). This section summarizes some key provisions of state statutory rape laws.

Sexual Intercourse with Minors

States' statutory rape offenses detail the age at which an individual can legally consent to sexual activity. This section focuses on laws addressing sexual intercourse. Table 15.1 summarizes, where applicable, each state's laws about the following items:

- **Age of consent:** This is the age at which an individual can legally consent to sexual intercourse under any circumstances.

- **Minimum age of victim:** This is the age below which an individual cannot consent to sexual intercourse under any circumstances.

- **Age differential:** If the victim is above the minimum age and below the age of consent, the age differential is the maximum difference in age between the victim and the defendant where an individual can legally consent to sexual intercourse.

- **Minimum age of defendant in order to prosecute:** This is the age below which an individual cannot be prosecuted for

174

engaging in sexual activities with minors. The table notes those states in which this law only applies when the victim is above a certain age.

As the first column in Table 15.1 shows, the age of consent varies by state. In the majority of states (34), it is 16 years of age. In the remaining states, the age of consent is either 17 or 18 years old (6 and 11 states, respectively).

A common misperception about statutory rape is that state codes define a single age at which an individual can legally consent to sex. Only 12 states have a single age of consent, below which an individual cannot consent to sexual intercourse under any circumstances, and above which it is legal to engage in sexual intercourse with another person above the age of consent. For example, in Massachusetts, the age of consent is 16.

In the remaining 39 states, other factors come into play: age differentials, minimum age of the victim, and minimum age of the defendant. Each is described below.

Minimum age requirement: In 27 states that do not have a single age of consent, statutes specify the age below which an individual cannot legally engage in sexual intercourse regardless of the age of the defendant (see the second column in Table 15.1). The minimum age requirements in these states range from 10 to 16 years of age. The legality of sexual intercourse with an individual who is above the minimum age requirement and below the age of consent is dependent on the difference in ages between the two parties and/or the age of the defendant.

In New Jersey, the age of consent is 16, but individuals who are at least 13 years of age can legally engage in sexual activities if the defendant is less than four years older than the victim.

Age differential: In 27 states, the legality of engaging in sexual intercourse with minors is, at least in some circumstances, based on the difference in age between the two parties (see the third column in Table 15.1). In 12 of these states, the legality is based solely on the difference between the ages of the two parties. For example, in the District of Columbia it is illegal to engage in sexual intercourse with someone who is under the age of consent (16) if the defendant is four or more years older than the victim.

Although it is less common, the age differentials in some states vary depending on the age of the victim. In Washington, sexual intercourse with someone who is at least 14 years of age and less than 16 years

Table 15.1. State Age Requirements

State	Age of con- sent	Mini- mum age of victim	Age differential between the vic- tim and defendant (if victim is above minimum age)	Minimum age of defendant in order to prosecute
Alabama	16	12	2	16
Alaska	16	N/A	3	N/A
Arizona	18	15	2 (defendant must be in high school and < 19)	N/A
Arkansas	16	N/A	3 (if victim is < 14)	20 (if victim is > 14)
California	18	18	N/A	N/A
Colorado	17	N/A	4 (if victim is < 15), 10 (if victim is < 17)	N/A
Connecticut	16	N/A	2	N/A
Delaware	18	16	N/A	N/A
District of Co- lumbia	16	N/A	4	N/A
Florida	18	16	N/A	24 (if victim is > 16)
Georgia	16	16	N/A	N/A
Hawaii	16	14	5	N/A
Idaho	18[13]	18	N/A	N/A
Illinois	17	17	N/A	N/A
Indiana	16	14	N/A	18 (if victim is > 14)
Iowa	16	14	4	N/A
Kansas	16	16	N/A	N/A
Kentucky	16	16	N/A	N/A
Louisiana	17	13	3 (if victim is < 15), 2 (if victim is < 17)	N/A
Maine	16	14	5	N/A
Maryland	16	N/A	4	N/A
Massachusetts	16	16	N/A	N/A
Michigan	16	16	N/A	N/A
Minnesota	16	N/A	3 (if victim is < 13), 2 (if victim is < 16)	N/A
Mississippi	16	N/A	2 (if victim is < 14), 3 (if victim is < 16)	N/A

Table 15.1. State Age Requirements, continued

State	Age of con- sent	Mini- mum age of victim	Age differential between the vic- tim and defendant (if victim is above minimum age)	Minimum age of defendant in order to prosecute
Missouri	17	14	N/A	21 (if victim is > 14)
Montana	16	16	N/A	N/A
Nebraska	16	16	N/A	19
Nevada	16	16	N/A	18
New Hampshire	16	16	N/A	N/A
New Jersey	16	13	4	N/A
New Mexico	16	13	4	18 (if victim is >13)
New York	17	17	N/A	N/A
North Carolina	16	N/A	4	12
North Dakota	18	15	N/A	18 (if victim is >15)
Ohio	16	13	N/A	18 (if victim is > 13)
Oklahoma	16	14	N/A	18 (if victim is > 14)
Oregon	18	15	3	N/A
Pennsylvania	16	13	4	N/A
Rhode Island	16	14	N/A	18 (if victim is >14)
South Carolina	16	14	Illegal if victim is 14 to 16 and defendant is older than victim	N/A
South Dakota	16	10[19]	3	N/A
Tennessee	18	13	4	N/A
Texas	17	14	3	N/A
Utah	18	16	10	N/A
Vermont	16	16	N/A	16
Virginia	18	15	N/A	18 (if victim is >15)
Washington	16	N/A	2 (if victim is < 12), 3 (if victim is < 14), 4 (if victim is < 16)	N/A
West Virginia	16	N/A	4 (if victim is >11)	16, 14 (if victim is < 11)
Wisconsin	18	18	N/A	N/A
Wyoming	16	N/A	4	N/A

Note: Some states have marital exemptions. This Table assumes the two parties are not married to one another.

of age is illegal if the defendant is four or more years older than the victim. The age differential decreases in cases where the victim is less than 14 years of age (three years), further decreasing if the victim is less than 12 years of age (two years).

Minimum age of defendant in order to prosecute: Sixteen states set age thresholds for defendants, below which individuals cannot be prosecuted for engaging in sexual intercourse with minors (see the last column in Table 15.1).

In Nevada, the age of consent is 16; however, sexual intercourse with someone who is under 16 years of age is illegal only if the defendant is at least 18 years of age (the age at which the defendant can be prosecuted).

States that set a minimum age of the defendant also tend to have minimum age requirements for the victim. Often, the age of the defendant is only relevant if the victim is above the minimum age requirement.

In Ohio, sexual intercourse with someone under 13 years of age is illegal regardless of the age of the defendant. However, if the victim is above this minimum age requirement (13) and below the age of consent (16), it is only illegal to engage in sexual intercourse with that individual if the defendant is at least 18 years of age.

Some states define minimum age thresholds for defendants and age differentials. In North Carolina, for example, the age of consent is 16. Sexual intercourse with someone who is under the age of consent is only illegal if the defendant is: (1) at least four years older than the victim and (2) at least 12 years of age (the age at which the defendant can be prosecuted).

Definition of Offenses

States' laws addressing sexual activity involving minors are usually included in the section of the criminal code devoted to sexual offenses.

As noted above, most states do not have laws that specifically use the term "statutory rape;" only five include the offense of statutory rape. More often, state statutes include a variety of offenses addressing voluntary sexual activity involving minors. In New Jersey, for example, sexual activities involving minors is addressed in three offenses: criminal sexual contact, sexual assault, and aggravated sexual assault. The ages of the victim and the defendant as well as the nature of the sexual activity dictate under which offense the conduct falls.

In some cases, provisions addressing statutory rape are embedded in rape or sexual assault laws that typically apply to violent offenses.

178

For example, New Hampshire defines "felonious sexual assault" as voluntary sexual penetration with someone who is at least 13 years of age and under 16 years of age, as well as acts involving the use of physical force irrespective of the age of either party. Other states have separate offenses specifically concerned with sexual crimes involving a minor. For example, Alaska's statute includes four offenses that deal specifically with the sexual abuse of a minor.

State statutes also use a variety of terms when referring to sexual acts (for example, sexual intercourse, sexual penetration, sexual contact, indecent contact), and the definitions of these terms are not always consistent across states.

Understanding the different terms used in a state statute is especially important in those states where an individual may be able to legally consent to one type of sexual activity but not another. For example, Alabama's laws regarding the legality of sexual activities with individuals who are under 16 years of age and more than 12 years of age differ depending on the nature of the activities. In cases involving sexual intercourse, defendants over 16 years of age who are at least two years older than the victim are guilty of rape in the second degree. However, sexual contact is only illegal in cases where the defendant is at least 19 years of age.

More often though, all of the acts will be illegal (with the same age requirements), but the severity of the punishment will differ based on the type of sexual activity. In Kentucky for example, sexual activities with children under 12 years of age are illegal regardless of the age of the defendant. If the activities amount to sexual contact, the defendant is guilty of first degree sexual abuse (a Class D felony); if they amount to sexual intercourse, the defendant is guilty of first degree rape (a Class A felony).

Depending on the state, defendants may be exempt from prosecution if they are married to the victim. In some states, marriage is a defense to all of the crimes listed (for example, Alaska, District of Columbia, West Virginia); other states exclude some of the more aggravated offenses from this exemption (for example, Arkansas, Louisiana, Mississippi). In a few states, the criminal statutes identify age limits for the marriage exemptions.

Child Abuse Reporting Requirements

Statutory rape reporting requirements are generally found in the sections of states' codes that deal with juveniles, children and families, domestic relationships, or social services, whereas the criminal or penal codes address the legality of specific offenses. This section of the report summarizes states' child abuse reporting requirements and the extent to which they address the issue of statutory rape.

State statutes vary in the extent to which statutory rape is included in the reporting requirements. In approximately one-third of the states, mandated reporting is limited to those situations where the abuse was perpetrated or allowed by a person responsible for the care of the child. Consider the example of Virginia. Child abuse, a reportable offense, is defined to include any sexual act that is in violation of the state's criminal law, but it is limited to those acts perpetrated by the victim's parent or other person responsible for the child's care.

In two-thirds of the states, the statutes specify circumstances under which child abuse is a reportable offense irrespective of the defendant's relationship to the victim. In some states, the definition of child abuse includes all of the statutory rape offenses detailed in the criminal code (for example, North Dakota, Ohio, and Wyoming). In such cases, mandated reporters are required to notify the proper authorities if they suspect that a child has been a victim of any of these offenses. More often, states vary in terms of the applicability of the reporting requirements. The following examples illustrate the variation among these states.

In some states, there are only a few specific circumstances under which offenses not involving a person responsible for a child are considered reportable offenses. In Minnesota, for example, such a case is only a reportable offense if the reporter suspects that a defendant has sexually abused two or more children not related to the defendant in the past ten years. Rhode Island law only requires reports of non-familial cases in two situations: (1) if the defendant is less than 18 years of age; or (2) if the mandated reporter is a physician or nurse practitioner who treats a child who is less than 12 years of age and has been infected with a sexually transmitted disease. In Iowa, the reporting requirements only pertain to cases involving someone responsible for the care of the child in question. However, a separate provision requires mandated reporters to notify the proper authorities of all cases of sexual abuse involving a victim under 12 years of age regardless of the defendant's relationship to the victim.

In other states there are fewer limits on the applicability of reporting requirements to statutory rape. Often, such limitations are based on the age of the victim and/or the defendant. For example, in California all sexual activity involving minors is illegal. However, the reporting requirements only apply to the violations of certain criminal offenses—namely, those addressing situations involving victims under

16 years of age where there is an especially large difference in the age of the two parties.

In those states where the definition of child abuse does not explicitly refer to statutory rape, discrepancies between the legality of certain sexual activities and whether they are reportable offenses are more common. Take the following examples:

Georgia: The reporting requirements in Georgia are less strict than the state's statutory rape laws. Even though all sexual activities involving someone who is less 16 years of age are illegal (per the criminal code), such acts only constitute a reportable offense if the defendant is more than five years older than the victim.

Utah: In contrast, Utah's reporting requirements define as reportable offenses some activities that are legal according to the state's criminal code. For example, sexual conduct with someone who is at least 16 years of age and less than 18 years of age is only illegal if the defendant is ten or more years older than the victim. However, sexual abuse, a reportable offense, is defined to include all acts of sexual intercourse, molestation, or sodomy directed towards someone under 18 years of age regardless of the age of the defendant.

Connecticut: Due to some confusion on the part of providers in the state, the Attorney General's office issued an opinion addressing this issue. Specifically, the Commissioner of the Department of Children and Families sought clarification with respect to the reporting laws as they relate to cases involving defendants under 21 years of age who engage in sexual activities with teenagers under the age of consent. The Attorney General concluded that, although such relationships are illegal if the defendant is more than two years older than the victim, mandated reporters are not required to make a report if no other evidence of abuse exists. In justifying the opinion, the Attorney General cited the statute related to the treatment of minors for sexually transmitted diseases, which only requires providers to report cases where the minor seeking treatment is less than 13 years of age.

Mandatory Reporters

Each state's reporting requirements identify certain individuals who are required to notify the authorities of suspected abuse. Although it varies by state, mandated reporters are typically individuals who encounter children through their professional capacity. In Pennsylvania, the statute requires all individuals who encounter a case of abuse through their professional capacity to make a report. More often, a state's statute will refer to a number of specific professions. Common professions include: physical and mental health providers, teachers, child care workers, legal professionals (for example, judges, magistrates, attorneys, law enforcement officers), clergy members, and employees of state agencies that deal with children and families. In addition, some states designate any individual who provides care or treatment to children as a mandatory reporter (for example, Alabama, Missouri, Montana). In 18 states, any individual who suspects that a child has been the victim of abuse is required to notify the proper authorities.

In terms of physical and/or mental health providers (for example, physicians, nurses, psychologists, psychiatrists, dentists, surgeons, osteopaths), statutes often make specific reference to providers who treat adolescents who are pregnant or infected with sexually transmitted diseases. For example, in Texas any individual who suspects child abuse is required to notify the proper authorities. However, the law also includes more specific reporting requirements for individuals who work with children in a professional capacity, including employees of a clinic or health care facility that provides reproductive services.

In some states, a child who is pregnant or infected with a sexually transmitted disease is sufficient to cause reasonable suspicion of abuse, thereby necessitating a report. In Rhode Island, as noted above, the law requires reports of non-familial cases in two situations, one of which is if the mandated reporter is a physician or nurse practitioner who treats a child less than 12 years of age who is infected with a sexually transmitted disease. Michigan also requires medical providers to report all cases where a child under 12 years of age is pregnant or has a sexually transmitted disease. In contrast, California law states that "the pregnancy of a minor does not, in and of itself, constitute a basis for a reasonable suspicion of sexual abuse." The California Court of Appeals has similarly found that mandated reporters are not required to report cases in which a minor is found to have a sexually transmitted disease.

Few states allow mandated reporters to exercise discretion in deciding which cases to report. Consider the following three exceptions:

Florida: The criminal code includes a law stating that anyone 21 years of age or older who impregnates a child under 16 years of age is guilty of contributing to the delinquency or dependency of a minor. However, the reporting requirements state that health care professionals and other individuals who provide medical or counseling services to pregnant children are not required to report abuse when the only violation is impregnation of a child under the circumstances described above if such reporting would interfere with the provision of medical services.

Tennessee: A 1996 law addressing statutory rape added a number of provisions to the state statutes with respect to reporting requirements. One such provision addresses cases in which a physician or other person treating pregnant minors learns that the alleged father of the patient's child is at least four years older than the patient and not her spouse. The provision encourages the provider to notify the appropriate legal authorities. However, such a report can only be made with the consent of the patient or the patient's parent, legal guardian, or custodian.

Wisconsin: Health care practitioners who provide family planning services, pregnancy testing, obstetrical health care or screening, or diagnosis and treatment for sexually transmitted diseases to minors are exempted from the reporting requirements with the following exception: If providers judge that their clients are in a dangerous situation. For example, providers are required to report cases where they believe that: the victim, because of his or her age or immaturity, is incapable of understanding the nature or consequences of sexual activities; the other participant in the sexual acts is exploiting the child; or the child's participation in the sexual acts is not voluntary.

Section 15.2

Adolescent Sexual Behavior and the Law

Excerpted from "Adolescent Sexual Behavior and the Law," by Brittany Longino Smith and Glen A. Kercher (March 2011), Crime Victims' Institute, Sam Houston State University. © 2011 Crime Victims' Institute. All rights reserved. Reprinted with permission. To view the complete text of this publication including references, visit www.crimevictimsinstitute.org. Information in this section discusses laws in specific states; legal information varies by state, but the issues raised are pertinent in most U.S. jurisdictions.

With approximately half of all 17 year olds reporting that they have engaged in sexual intercourse, adults need to acknowledge that teenagers today are participating in the autonomous acts of sexual experimentation. However, in contrast to the high rates of teens admitting to having sexual relationships, and even higher number of the adult population, more than 70%, have stated that adolescents having sex is "always wrong." This public opinion has influenced not only parents but authority figures and the law.

In the state of Texas teenagers under the age of 17 cannot legally give consent to engaging in sexual activities. This is true even if they are a willing participant. However it is not teenagers themselves who can be prosecuted if the law is violated, it is the older person involved, no matter how little the age gap between the two.

Jeff was charged with sexual assault when he was 18 years old. He and his then 15-year-old girlfriend began dating when Jeff was a junior in high school. He and his girlfriend said they were in love and had plans to get married and began a sexual relationship. When Jeff's girlfriend's grades declined, her father blamed him, and after learning they were having sexual relations, he reported Jeff to the police for having sex with a minor.

A case such as the one described above, can be prosecuted in Texas as a sexual assault:

(a) A person commits an offense if the person:

(2) Intentionally and knowingly:

(A) Causes the penetration of the anus or sexual organ of a child by any means;

(B) Causes the penetration of the mouth of a child by the sexual organ of the actor;

(C) Causes the sexual organ of a child to contact or penetrate the mouth, anus, or sexual organ of another person, including the actor;

(D) Causes the anus of a child to contact the mouth, anus, or sexual organ of another person, including the actor; or

(E) Causes the mouth of the child to contact the anus or sexual organ of another person, including the actor.

"Child" in this section means anyone under the age of 17 who is not the spouse of the actor; an offense under this section is considered to be a felony in the second degree. Punishments could include, but are not limited to mandatory jail time, extensive probation, and a life-long registration of the sexual offender registry.

Statutory Rape Laws

The age of consent is set by each state, and used to enforce similar statutory rape laws such as the one described above. While the age of consent varies, currently each state requires a minimum age of consent of at least 16 years old and no older than 18. The ages of consent have changed over the years, as have the statutory rape laws to which they apply.

Although "statutory rape" is rarely used in the language of the laws, the term is typically recognized as encompassing the intent of several other named laws such as sexual assault, sexual assault of a minor, rape of a child, corruption of a minor, carnal knowledge of a minor, unlawful carnal knowledge, sexual misconduct, or child molestation, to name a few. The predominant rationale of statutory rape laws is to protect minors who are said to be incapable of consenting to sexual intercourse or other sexual activities, due to their lack of experiences to make mature, informed decisions. It is believed that youth below the age of consent are less likely to understand and consider the potential consequences of sexual activities, such as sexually transmitted diseases and pregnancies. These minors are also argued to be unequal to adults, socially, economically, and legally. Because of this, statutory rape laws have been introduced to reduce the power adults may have over minors. These laws do consider that minors will consent to sex.

It is the basis for the laws that even if minors consent, adults cannot engage in sexual activities with them because of the power they have over minors. What the laws do not consider is that minors are consenting to have sex with other minors or slightly older peers who do not have power over them.

The wording of these laws encompass teenage relationships making it equally illegal for, say a 17 year old to be sexually intimate with a 16 year old boyfriend or girlfriend. However, because the laws were not originally written to prosecute such cases, the law was rarely enforced among teen couples. In 1995, however, a study was published that caused many states to toughen their statutory rape laws, widening the net to include more teen romances. D.J. Landry and J.D. Forrest (1995), found that half the teenage pregnancies of girls aged 15–17 were the result of teenagers having sexual relationships with men who were 20 years of age or older. Thus, statutory rape laws took on a dual function: protect minors from being taken advantage of sexually by adults and helping to prevent teen pregnancies. The latter however, may be a misguided attempt in light of additional research that shows these laws have little effect on girls who actually become pregnant.

Due to the number of jurisdictions that began to more aggressively prosecute close-in-age offenders, a backlash was created, based on the belief that it was unfair to punish these sexually active teenage relationships in the same way sexual predators were punished. Some argued that the sentences given to some statutory rape offenders were tantamount to cruel and unusual punishment. Media coverage would often highlight cases that created strong public opinions as to the fairness of these laws and the repercussions they had on offenders.

Genarlow, a 17 year old high school senior, was arrested for engaging in oral sex with a consenting partner who was two years younger than he. Those two years would prove to be crucial in this case, since the victim was below the age of consent which is set at 16 in Georgia where the incident took place. On New Year's Eve, 2003, Genarlow attended a party in a hotel room with a number of friends. During the night, several sexual activities among partygoers were video recorded. There were two females involved in the acts, one, a seventeen year old and the other, 15. Even though the 15 year old participated willingly, since she was below Georgia's age of consent, the males who engaged in oral sex with her had committed a crime as described by Georgia law. The mother of one of the girls contacted authorities to report that her 17 year old daughter had been raped. Evidence from the hotel room was confiscated, including the video tape.

186

While the tape showed that the 17 year old girl was a willing participant in the sexual activities she partook in, determining that she had not been raped, it did convict six of the male partygoers, including Genarlow, of Aggravated Child Molestation for the acts they participated in with the 15 year old female. Eventually, five of the males charged in this case chose to accept a plea bargain which required them to register as sex offenders, but would reduce their prison stay from the mandatory ten years. Genarlow did not accept the plea bargain and was given the minimum sentence. He was sentenced to prison for ten years after which he was to be put on probation for a year and made to register as a sex offender for the rest of his life. This case made national headlines, and there was an outcry that the court sentencing was unjust.

This case and others like it prompted the Georgia legislature to amend their Aggravated Child Molestation Laws which would thereafter classify cases like this as a misdemeanor with a maximum sentence of one year in jail, and would not require the offender to register on the sex offender registration list. However, the bill specifically stated that the new amendment would not apply retroactively. As a result, Genarlow remained in jail. After many failed appeals, he was released from prison in 2007. The Georgia State Supreme Court ruled in his favor, finding that this teenager' sentence was cruel and unusual punishment. He was able to return home to his family, which under his original sentence he would not have been able to do as a registered sex offender since his sister was a minor.

Age Gap Provisions

Ironically, if Genarlow had engaged in sexual intercourse with the 15 year old at the New Year's Eve party, he would have only been convicted of a misdemeanor and not have been made to serve any jail time or register as a sex offender due to Georgia's inclusion of an Age Gap Provision in their Child Molestation law. Because he engaged in an oral sex (sodomy) act, his case was classified as Aggravated Child Molestation, which at the time did not have the Age Gap Provision. Now, the law reads as the following:

§ 16-6-4. Child molestation; aggravated child molestation

(a) A person commits the offense of child molestation when such person:

(1) Does any immoral or indecent act to or in the presence of or **with any child under the age of 16**

(2) years with the intent to arouse or satisfy the sexual desires of either the child or the person; or

(3) By means of an electronic device, transmits images of a person engaging in, inducing, or otherwise participating in any immoral or indecent act to a child under the age of 16 years with the intent to arouse or satisfy the sexual desires of either the child or the person.

(b)

(1) Except as provided in paragraph (2) of this subsection, a person convicted of a first offense of child molestation shall be punished by imprisonment for not less than five nor more than 20 years and shall be subject to the sentencing and punishment provisions of Code Sections 17-10-6.2 and 17-10-7. Upon a defendant being incarcerated on a conviction for a first offense, the Department of Corrections shall provide counseling to such defendant. Except as provided in paragraph (2) of this subsection, upon a second or subsequent conviction of an offense of child molestation, the defendant shall be punished by imprisonment for not less than ten years nor more than 30 years or by imprisonment for life and shall be subject to the sentencing and punishment provisions of Code Sections 17-10-6.2 and 17-10-7; provided, however, that prior to trial, a defendant shall be given notice, in writing, that the state intends to seek a punishment of life imprisonment.

(2) **If the victim is at least 14 but less than 16 years of age and the person convicted of child molestation is 18 years of age or younger and is no more than four years older than the victim, such person shall be guilty of a misdemeanor and shall not be subject to the sentencing and punishment provisions of Code Section 17-10-6.2.**

(c) A person commits the offense of aggravated child molestation when such person commits an offense of child molestation which act physically injures the child or involves an act of sodomy.

(d)

(1) Except as provided in paragraph (2) of this subsection, a person convicted of the offense of aggravated child molestation shall be punished by imprisonment for life or by a split sentence that is a term of imprisonment for not less than 25 years and not exceeding life imprisonment, followed by probation for life, and shall be subject to the sentencing and punishment provisions of Code Sections 17-10-6.1 and 17-10-7.

(2) **A person convicted of the offense of aggravated child molestation when:**

(A) **The victim is at least 13 but less than 16 years of age**;

(B) The person convicted of aggravated **child molestation is 18 years of age or younger and is no more than four years older than the victim; and**

(C) The basis of the charge of aggravated child **molestation involves an act of sodomy shall be guilty of a misdemeanor and shall not be subject to the sentencing and punishment provisions of Code Section 17-10-6.1.**

The Age Gap Provisions can be seen in the (2) subsections of this Georgia Law. In the Child Molestation crime, the law now stipulates that if the victim was at least 14 years of age, the offender 18 years of age or younger and no more than four years older than the victim, the same crime will no longer be considered a felony. The offender can be charged with a misdemeanor and will not be subject to the same punishments as those who commit the crime outside of the age gap provision. In other words, with this provision, close-in-age teenage relationships need not have the same consequences as those of older adults seeking to sexually exploit minors.

Many other states have also included these age gap provisions into their existing laws in order to differentiate cases of young persons in close-in-age relationships. In fact, the majority of states currently have some form of an age gap provision in their statutory rape laws.

The following case is a prime example of how Age Gap Provisions work. In 2007, Damon, a 17 year old from New Hampshire, learned the consequences of having a sexual relationship only after he was charged with a Class A Misdemeanor, Sexual Assault for having intercourse with his 15 year old girlfriend. The New Hampshire law states that no person under the age of 16 can rightfully consent to a sexual experience. Therefore, even though Damon's girlfriend agreed to the act, he had still committed a crime. If he had been a year older, or his girlfriend a year younger, he could have faced felony charges. In the end, Damon only received a three-month suspended sentence and did not have to register as a sex offender thanks to New Hampshire passing an Age Gap Provision earlier that year. Before January 1, 2007, the New Hampshire law read under RSA 632-A:3, Felonious Sexual Assault, that a person is guilty of a Class B Felony if such person engages in sexual penetration with a person other than his legal spouse who is 13 years of age or older and under 16 years of age. The law now has been amended to state:

A person is guilty of a Class B Felony if such person engages in sexual penetration with a person other than his legal spouse who is 13 years of age or older and under 16 years of age where the age difference between the actor and the other person is three years or more.

Romeo and Juliet Clauses

As of 2010, 30 U.S. states are considered to have Age Gap Provisions. However, this does not mean that other states do not have some forms of protection for similar close-in-age relationships. Many states have adopted what are often referred to as Romeo and Juliet Clauses. These clauses are often considered the same as Age Gap Provisions, and it is not uncommon for the two terms to be used interchangeably. However, there are slight differences between the two.

Texas is not recognized as having an Age Gap Provision which either reduces the level of the offense or does not consider a crime to have occurred at all. However, Texas does have a Romeo and Juliet Clause. This clause does not stipulate the law, as do the provisions in the laws referred to above. Rather the law remains the same, except that the defendant is given an affirmative defense if certain qualifications are met. The Texas Penal Code under Sec. 22.011 subsection (e) it states that: It is an affirmative defense to the prosecution under Subsection (a)(2) that:

- The actor cannot be more than three years older than the victim.

- The victim was older than 14 years of age at the time the offense occurred.

- The actor was not at the time registered or required to register for life as a sexual offender.

- The conduct did not constitute incest.

- Neither the actor nor the victim would commit bigamy by marrying the other.

Many states that do not have an Age Gap Provision still make cases in which the participants are close in age a lower level of crime. That said, however, it is still a crime according to their laws. If this is the case, as with Romeo and Juliet Clauses, they are not considered to have an Age Gap Provision. It is important to remember that most states do seek to protect close-in-age teenage offenders, even if the law is not specifically structured for it.

Table 15.2. States and Corresponding Age Spans as allowed in Age Gap Provisions or Romeo and Juliet Clauses.

Alabama	2	New Hampshire	N/A
Alaska	3	New Jersey	4
Arizona	0	New Mexico	4
Arkansas	2	New York	4
California	2	North Carolina	4
Colorado	4	North Dakota	N/A
Connecticut	2	Ohio	4
Delaware	4	Oklahoma	2
Iowa	6	Oregon	N/A
Kansas	N/A	Pennsylvania	3
Kentucky	5	Rhode Island	3
Louisiana	2	South Carolina	N/A
Maine	5	South Dakota	3
Maryland	4	Tennessee	4
Massachusetts	N/A	Texas	3
Michigan	N/A	Utah	3
Minnesota	2	Vermont	N/A
Mississippi	0.5	Virginia	3
Missouri	3	Washington	4
Montana	3	West Virginia	4
Nebraska	3	Wisconsin	N/A
Nevada	5	Wyoming	4

N/A = information could not be confirmed as having an Age Group Provision

Discretion

A common concern with Romeo and Juliet Clauses, as opposed to an Age Gap Provision, is the amount of judicial discretion individual cases face in terms of prosecuting and sentencing. Because of the large number of potential statutory rape cases, it is said that many jurisdictions will "pick and choose" which cases they want to investigate and prosecute. The Georgia Supreme Court reported that over seven million cases of Aggravated Child Molestation are committed yearly in the United states under the terms of the former Georgia law, making it literally impossible to try every case. There are often large inconsistencies in deciding which cases to prosecute and the sentences to impose. For example, Wendy was a 17 year old Georgia high school student when she was convicted of Aggravated Child Molestation for engaging in oral sex with a 15 year old boy. Though unlike Genarlow's case described above, which Wendy's case mirrored, she was only sentenced to five years' probation.

In some states, a gender bias in prosecuting offenders is especially prominent when both partners of a sex act are under the age of consent. Under a number of jurisdictions if both partners are minors then they are both considered to be victims and offenders of the crime at the same time. In these cases, according to the law of their respective states, the prosecution of each teen would have been called for. However, it is more common to see the prosecution of only the male. For example, in California where the age of consent is 18, a 16 year old male was prosecuted for having consensual sex with his 14 year old girlfriend. Moreover, in Arizona a 13 year old boy was convicted of having consensual sex with his older, 15 year old, girlfriend.

Critics have argued that due to the lack of consistency in handling these cases, prosecution often results in a disproportionate number of convictions that involve minority men who have sex with white women or impregnate minority women. Reports from California, which does not have an Age Gap Provision, show that this may be true for all of the 32 men on their Statutory Rape Enforcement's most wanted list. These offenders were either African-American or Hispanic.

It has also been pointed out that when men are prosecuted for impregnating a teenager, some of them will not be able to pay child support if they are sent to prison. This may add to the welfare rolls. Furthermore, those offenders who are made to register as sex offenders have restrictions placed on what jobs they can obtain, thereby decreasing the chance that the men will be able to support their children.

Because of the use of discretion in deciding what to do with close-in-age sexual incidents, many believe that the Model Penal Code (MPC) would be a good alternative. This could reduce arbitrary enforcement and confusion among the public on what is and is not punishable. In the MPC, statutory rape cases are addressed in Sec. 213.3 endorsing the movement to decriminalize sexual relationships (both vaginal and oral) between teenagers who are close-in-age provided that the acts are consensual and the person is no more than four years older than the minor.

Sex Offender Registries

The original intent of sex offender registries was to inform the public of sexual offenders living in their communities, so that they could take safety precautions. However, critics are concerned that the large number of low-risk individuals who are placed on sex offender registries may defeat their original intent. Some argue that by requiring offenders to register when their crimes involved consensual teenager relationships makes the purpose of the registries less relevant to the purpose of warning of potentially dangerous predators that are more likely to reoffend. Research has found that sexual offenders who victimize adult women have the highest rates of recidivism accounting for 40% of all sexual offender re-offences. This number becomes even more significant in light of the percent of total re-arrest rates for sexual offenders, which are estimated to be somewhere between 5–12%. This re-offense rate compares to 35-40% of those who committed nonsexual offences.

Critics suggest that in making outcasts of these low-risk offenders by labeling them through registries may create the opposite effect of what was intended by straining their societal bonds, and, thereby, increasing the likelihood of delinquency. The potential stigmatizing effects of registration may limit their reintegration into society, thereby depriving offenders the ability to lead productive lives. Considerable research in criminology supports these claims, suggesting that the main factors that discourage recidivism are public reintegration, stress management, and a stable lifestyle.

Ten states have enacted a "Tier Classification System" to their registries. The risk level assigned determines the degree of sex offender information that is given to the public about an offender. Many states provide a wide range of public notification, such as access to online registries, notices sent to neighbors, schools, and daycare centers. Minnesota provides the public with information on a need-to-know basis. For a Tier I offender his information is available to the victims, witnesses to the crime, and adult member of the immediate household. The information about offenders whose level of risk is higher can be distributed more broadly. For lower risk offenders this will eliminate the public at large from being able to access the offender's picture, address, or other information, thus furthering the goal of reintegrating the individual back into society. Many see policies such as these as a compromise that benefits the public and the offender. States are reluctant to discontinue registries due to the high approval ratings, even if the public admittedly recognizes there is no proof that the registries make communities safer. This is supported by the fact that 73% of the public stated they would still support the registries even without evidence that they reduced sexual abuse offenses. However, by implementing Tier Classification Systems registries will remain but allow offenders more reintegration possibilities.

The Need for Reform

It should be noted that many of those who support reforming laws to decriminalize close-in-age sexual relationships still agree with the need to have defined ages of consent and to prosecute statutory rape violators. Their only complaint is that laws should specifically target adult offenders who prey on children and pose a threat to society.

M.D. Henry and S. Cunningham (2010) conducted a study to determine if states with a higher age of consent resulted in delaying teenagers' sexual onset. States that had stricter statutory rape laws did in fact show that both male and female sexual debuts were delayed. However, the more significant statistics were associated with setting the age of consent higher, as opposed to the number of years in states' age gap spans. In their study using the age of consent as a starting point, they found that the higher the minimum age of consent laws, the more likely a delay in sexual debut.

However, neither this study nor any other research has shown any significant effect of either statutory rape laws or age of consents on teen pregnancies. The authors theorize that this may be due to the fact that teen girls are having more sexual intercourse with teen boys who fall within their states' age spans. These younger males are less experienced, and have less knowledge about contraceptives, with the result of an increase in teen pregnancies.

While protecting children from coerced sexual activity, preserving morality, and attempting to reduce teen pregnancies have been the most common rationales for statutory rape laws and their enforcement, others also have questioned the psychological and emotional developments of minors when having early sexual experiences. Proponents of stricter statutory rape laws and those who advocate harsher punishments, regardless of close-in-age relationships, argue that the younger the sexually active participant is, the more psychological damage is done. It is suggested that those who lack the maturity to engage in sexual activity but do nevertheless, develop more unhealthy attitudes about the acts, relationships, and themselves. Particularly for females, it is said to invoke insecurity and self-esteem issues, often resulting in girls trading sexual acts for acceptance.

However, others argue that these risks are reduced when teens are at the same level of maturity. A.M. Meier (2007) found no significant relationship between the majority of teenage sexual activity and depression. However, she found that those who engaged in sex earlier than their peers and whose relationships dissolved shortly afterward did report signs of depression. This was especially the case with girls.

Meier makes a point to stress that her study did not suggest that those who did not suffer from mental health problems because of sexual experiences, had any positive effects as a result. She even emphasizes that perhaps policy-makers should focus on creating laws that focus on those who are most vulnerable. However, in contradiction to Meier's study, K.P. Harden, J. Mendle, J.E. Hill, E. Turkheimer, and R.E. Emery (2008) found that minors in healthy teenage relationships that include sex may be protected from becoming involved in delinquent acts later and were reported as having more satisfying relationships as adults.

Rehabilitation

In an effort to further reduce the conviction and punishment of close-in-age teenage relationships many states are adding new policies instead of or in addition to their Age Gap Provisions and Romeo and Juliet Clauses. For example, Wisconsin after evaluating their statutory rape cases and the goals that were served through the forms of punishment applicable to those cases, developed an "alternative disposition program" for young offenders. This new policy applies to those who were convicted of statutory rape for the first time, and consists of offering the offender an opportunity to attend a nine-week education and rehabilitation class. If the offender attended and successfully completed the class, they would not have to serve a prison or jail sentence, and the conviction would not be included on their permanent criminal record.

There have been studies showing that rehabilitating juvenile sex offenders instead of punishing them results in a more positive outcome for the offender and the public. M. Carpentier, J.F. Silovsky, and M. Chaffin (2006) found in a ten year follow up with juvenile sex offenders that those who received short term rehabilitation treatment had a relatively low rate of sexual re-offending. The study reported that only 2–3% of previously classified juvenile sexual offenders went on to offend later in life. Chaffin (2008) argues that this number would have been higher if the minors received treatment but were still made to register as a sex offender.

Offering rehabilitation to low-risk offenders in lieu of the requirement to register as a sex offender, may enhance public safety more than the registry itself does. Critics of the sex offender registry argue that there is little evidence of safety gained by enforcing registration laws, and a majority of convicted sex offenders (75%) admitted that registration laws would not deter them from committing another offense should they chose to offend again. Rather, the motivation to remain offense-free was to "prove something" to friends, family and the public.

Removal of Low-Risk Offenders from Registries

Several states including Florida (Statue 943.04354) and Missouri (Section 589.400.3) have introduced bills that would allow certain sex offenders to be removed from the state registry. Two bills have been introduced in the 82nd session of the Texas Legislature (S.B. No. 198, H.B. No. 227) that would allow qualifying sex offenders to be removed from the Sex Offender Registry or not requiring newly convicted sex offenders to register at all. In parallel to the state's Romeo and Juliet affirmative defense, these bills would enable sex offenders who are required to register, to petition to have their information removed from the Registry. For example, the bill states that the conviction of the sex offender must have been based solely on the ages of the defendant and victim at the time of the offense, meaning no other sexual offense could have taken place, such as using force, or being in a position of authority over the victim. Also, the bill would require that the offender was no more than four years older than the victim or intended victim, and that the victim or intended victim was at least 14 years of age at the time of the offense. This bill further stipulates that for the petition to be approved, the exemption must not threaten public safety and, the act did not occur without the victim's consent, and the exemption is in the best interest of the victim, and justice.

Victim Cooperation

Another suggested reform is that of victim cooperation. Many victims in close-in-age relationships may not feel that they have been victimized at all. In fact, many believe no crime has been committed. In these cases, the victim may often try to protect the offender by refusing to cooperate with police in hopes of saving the offender from punishments.

When a victim refuses to cooperate, they will typically be unable to "save" the offender, and could be prosecuted themselves. For example, 16-year-old Amanda was sent to jail under contempt charges because she refused to testify against her older boyfriend with whom she had engaged in sexual acts. Even though she was released from jail and she and her boyfriend were married, her boyfriend was still prosecuted. Some victims refuse to cooperate because of the potentially devastating effects the punishments of the offender will have on them, the victim. For example, they may be less likely to cooperate with police because of the consequences of losing parenting and financial support. Some suggest that in close-in-age situations, the victim's cooperation should be required. Without this cooperation many critics argue that the charges should be dropped.

Parental Restraining Orders

As stated previously, parents may report cases of statutory rape in an attempt to end their teenager's relationship, even if the participants are close in age. However, even parents who wish to dissolve their minor's relationship for whatever reason, rarely understand the true consequences that are in store for the offender. When Frank, a high school senior, had consensual sex with his girlfriend, a freshman at the school he attended, the girl's mother called the police. The reporting was only meant to scare the young couple, because the girl's mother did not approve of her daughter having sex. However, once reported Frank then faced two to twenty years in prison and registration as a sex offender. Once the mother understood the seriousness of her report, she requested that the charges be dropped. The police told her that once it was reported, it could not be dismissed. Now Frank and his young girlfriend are married and have children. However, the reporting and conviction in this case, still limits this young couple's opportunities to live productive lives.

Parents face a dilemma when believing their child is not mature enough to make adult decisions, and not wanting to ruin someone else's life in the process of making the undesired activity stop. It is made even more confusing in states that require mandatory reporting if parents suspect their child is involved in violating statutory rape laws. Some argue that decriminalizing an act undermines parental authority. In cases like these, D. Olszewski (2006) has proposed the enactment of a parental restraining order. This order would allow parents to seek legal assistance in discouraging their teenager's sexual activity. However, the provision would not lead to a conviction of the person to whom the order was directed. It is argued that this approach would empower parents by giving them an option with less severe consequences for the teenage couple when the parents believe a relationship has gone too far.

Conclusions

Statutory rape laws are intended to punish adults who have sex with minors. The assumption behind these laws when they were originally enacted was that only teenagers who exceeded the age of consent could make informed decisions about engaging in sexual behavior. However valid that argument may have been, the reality is that an increasing percentage of teenagers are participating consensual sexual activity in close-in-age dating relationships. The issue is whether these cases should be processed through the juvenile or adult justice systems or not prosecuted at all. Few would argue to do away with these laws altogether, but the suggestion is that more be done to exclude unintended offenders from being prosecuted. The response, as has been discussed previously, has been the introduction of Age Gap Provisions and Romeo and Juliet Clauses. However, many of these cases continue to be processed through the courts and can have life-long effects on the perpetrators of these acts. The question remains whether handling these cases in this way protects the public or the supposed victims.

States have not been quick to embrace the Model Penal Code (MPC), Sec. 213.3, according to which sexual relationships (both vaginal and oral) between teenagers who are close- in-age would be decriminalized provided that the acts are consensual and the person is no more than four years older than the minor. Given that many teenagers whose close-in-age sexual behavior violates statutory rape laws but are of little danger to the public (as seen in re-offense rates), considerable time and expense could be saved by adopting the MPC recommendation. Decriminalization could be tied to brief educational programs and providing parents with the option of a restraining order to control their child's behavior. Even failing these efforts, consideration should be given to encouraging judges and prosecutors to use rehabilitation (for example, educational classes), as opposed to punishment, in deciding these cases.

Requiring sex offenders to register and to have their information posted on the publicly available website is designed to protect the public. The offenders who register have been determined by law to be a danger to the public regardless of their risk of re-offending. Such a requirement, particularly with offenders in close-in-age cases, may not be a danger to public safety. Moreover, this requirement imposes wide-ranging restrictions on young people, and can stigmatize their acceptance in society. Not requiring young people whose cases meet carefully crafted criteria should be considered even if their cases are prosecuted. Legislation under consideration in Texas with regard to enabling close-in-age offenders to be removed from the registry reflects public concern that justice is not always well served by this requirement.

Part Three

Child Neglect
and Emotional Abuse

Chapter 16

Child Neglect

Chapter Contents

Section 16.1

Definition and Scope of Neglect

From "Chapter 2: Definition and Scope," *Child Neglect: A Guide for Prevention, Assessment and Intervention*, by Diane DePanfilis, Office on Child Abuse and Neglect, 2006; available from the Child Welfare Information Gateway (www.childwelfare.gov), a service of the Children's Bureau, Administration for Children and Families. U.S. Department of Health and Human Services. Reviewed by David A. Cooke, MD, FACP, January 2013.

Child neglect is the most common type of child maltreatment. Unfortunately, neglect frequently goes unreported and, historically, has not been acknowledged or publicized as greatly as child abuse. Even professionals often have given less attention to child neglect than to abuse. One study found that caseworkers indicated that they were least likely to substantiate referrals for neglect. In some respects, it is understandable why violence against children has commanded more attention than neglect. Abuse often leaves visible bruises and scars, whereas the signs of neglect tend to be less visible. However, the effects of neglect can be just as detrimental. In fact, some studies have shown that neglect may be more detrimental to children's early brain development than physical or sexual abuse.

What Is Neglect?

How neglect is defined shapes the response to it. Since the goal of defining neglect is to protect children and to improve their well-being, not to blame the parents or caregivers—definitions help determine if an incident or a pattern of behavior qualifies as neglect, its seriousness or duration, and, most importantly, whether or not the child is safe.

Definitions of neglect vary among states and across different disciplines, agencies, and professional groups (for example, child protective services, court systems, health care providers), as well as among individuals within these agencies and groups. The definitions also are used for different purposes within the child welfare field. For example, a medical doctor may view a parent as neglectful if the parent repeatedly forgets to give his child a prescribed medication. This may or may not legally be considered neglect, however, depending on the stringency of the neglect criteria of many Child Protective Services (CPS) agencies.

Difficulty Defining Neglect

Defining neglect historically has been difficult to do, leading to inconsistencies in policies, practice, and research. Without a consistent definition of neglect, it is nearly impossible to compare research results. This inconsistency also leads to variability in the way neglect cases are handled.

The debate over a definition of neglect centers on a lack of consensus in answering these questions:

- What are the minimum requirements associated with caring for a child?

- What action or inaction by a parent or other caregiver constitutes neglectful behavior?

- Must the parent's or caregiver's action or inaction be intentional?

- What impact does the action or inaction have on the health, safety, and well-being of the child?

- What constitutes "failure or inability to provide" adequate food, shelter, protection, or clothing?

- Should "failure or inability to protect" be included?

- Is the action or inaction a result of poverty rather than neglect?

Additionally, what is considered neglect varies based on the age and the developmental level of the child, making it difficult to outline a set of behaviors that are always considered neglect. For example, leaving a child unattended for an hour is considered neglect when the child is young, but not when the child is a teenager. Another issue is that many neglect definitions specify that omissions in care may result either in "risk of harm" or in "significant harm" to the child. While the 1996 reauthorization of the Child Abuse Prevention and Treatment Act (CAPTA) (P.L. 104-235) narrowed the definition of child maltreatment to cases where there has been actual harm or an imminent risk of serious harm, these terms often are not defined by law, leaving the local CPS agencies to interpret them. This leads to a lack of consistency in responding to families who may be challenged to meet the basic needs of their children.

Definitions of Neglect

CAPTA, reauthorized again in the Keeping Children and Families Safe Act of 2003 (P.L. 108-36), provides minimum standards for defining child physical abuse, neglect, and sexual abuse that states must incorporate into their statutory definitions in order to receive federal funds. Under this Act, child maltreatment is defined as:

> Any recent act or failure to act on the part of a parent or caregiver, which results in death, serious physical or emotional harm, sexual abuse or exploitation, or an act or failure to act which presents an imminent risk of serious harm.

A "child" under this definition generally means a person who is under the age of 18 or who is not an emancipated minor. In cases of child sexual abuse, a "child" is one who has not attained the age of 18 or the age specified by the child protection law of the state in which the child resides, whichever is younger.

Instances of neglect are classified as mild, moderate, or severe.

- Mild neglect usually does not warrant a report to CPS, but might necessitate a community-based intervention (for example, a parent failing to put the child in a car safety seat).

- Moderate neglect occurs when less intrusive measures, such as community interventions, have failed or some moderate harm to the child has occurred (for example, a child consistently is inappropriately dressed for the weather, such as being in shorts and sandals in the middle of winter). For moderate neglect, CPS may be involved in partnership with community support.

- Severe neglect occurs when severe or long-term harm has been done to the child (for example, a child with asthma who has not received appropriate medications over a long period of time and is frequently admitted to the hospital). In these cases, CPS should be and is usually involved, as is the legal system.

Viewing the severity of neglect along this continuum helps practitioners assess the strengths and weaknesses of families and allows for the possibility of providing preventive services before neglect actually occurs or becomes severe. There is some controversy over whether "potential harm" should be considered neglect, and, as with the definition of neglect, state laws vary on this issue. Although it is difficult to assess potential harm as neglect, it can have emotional as well as physical consequences, such as difficulty establishing and maintaining current relationships or those later in life.

The seriousness of the neglect is determined not only by how much harm or risk of harm there is to the child, but also by how chronic the neglect is. Chronicity can be defined as "patterns of the same acts or omissions that extend over time or recur over time." An example of chronic neglect would be parents with substance abuse problems who do not provide for the basic needs of their children on an ongoing basis. On the other hand, caregivers might have minor lapses in care, which are seldom thought of as neglect, such as occasionally forgetting to give their children their antibiotics. However, if those children were frequently missing doses, it may be considered neglect. Some situations only need to occur once in order to be considered neglect, such as leaving an infant unattended in a bathtub. Because some behaviors are considered neglect only if they occur on a frequent basis, it is important to look at the history of behavior rather than focusing on one particular incident.

Types of Neglect

While neglect may be harder to define or to detect than other forms of child maltreatment, child welfare experts have created common categories of neglect, including physical neglect; medical neglect; inadequate supervision; environmental, emotional, and educational neglect; and newborns addicted or exposed to drugs, as well as some newly recognized forms of neglect. The following sections give detailed information on each of these types of neglect.

States' definitions of neglect are usually located in mandatory child maltreatment reporting statutes (civil laws), criminal statutes, or juvenile court jurisdiction statutes. For more information about reporting laws, visit the State Laws on Reporting and Responding to Child Abuse and Neglect section of the Child Welfare Information Gateway website at http://www.childwelfare.gov/systemwide/laws_policies/state/index.cfm?event=stateStatutes.showSearchForm.

Framework for Neglect

Current theory on maltreatment views neglect from a socio-ecological perspective in which multiple factors contribute to child abuse and neglect. From this perspective, one should consider not only the parent's role, but also the societal and environmental variables contributing to the parent's inability to provide for the basic needs of the child. The socio-ecological model is valuable because it "recognizes the shared responsibility among individuals, families, communities, and society, thereby enabling a more constructive approach and targeting interventions on multiple levels." Examples of factors to consider when looking at neglect from a socio-ecological perspective are social isolation and poverty.

It is important to keep in mind that not all incidents in which a person fails to provide for the basic needs for a child are necessarily considered neglect. Factors relating to the parent's health and well-being, such as mental illness, substance abuse, or domestic violence, often contribute to neglect. Any intervention for neglect will need to consider these factors as well.

Federal and state laws often assume that it is possible to determine clearly when parents have control over omissions in care and when they do not. For example, children may be poorly fed because their parents are poor and are unable to provide them with the appropriate type and amount of food. In such cases, it is important to identify factors that may be contributing to this inability to provide, such as mental illness. However, when a family consistently fails to obtain needed support or is unable to use information and assistance that is available, an intervention may be required. Having a comprehensive understanding of what may contribute to neglect can help determine appropriate interventions that address the basic needs of the child and family and also enhances professionals' and communities' abilities to develop and to use interventions, regardless of CPS involvement.

Physical Neglect

Physical neglect is one of the most widely recognized forms. It includes these types of neglect:

- **Abandonment:** The desertion of a child without arranging for his reasonable care or supervision. Usually, a child is considered abandoned when not picked up within two days.

- **Expulsion:** The blatant refusal of custody, such as the permanent or indefinite expulsion of a child from the home, without adequately arranging for his care by others or the refusal to accept custody of a returned runaway.

- **Shuttling:** When a child is repeatedly left in the custody of others for days or weeks at a time, possibly due to the unwillingness of the parent or the caregiver to maintain custody.

- **Nutritional neglect:** When a child is undernourished or is repeatedly hungry for long periods of time, which can sometimes be evidenced by poor growth. Nutritional neglect often is included in the category of "other physical neglect."

- **Clothing neglect:** When a child lacks appropriate clothing, such as not having appropriately warm clothes or shoes in the winter.

- **Other physical neglect:** Includes inadequate hygiene and forms of reckless disregard for the child's safety and welfare (for example, driving while intoxicated with the child, leaving a young child in a car unattended).

Medical Neglect

Medical neglect encompasses a parent or guardian's denial of or delay in seeking needed health care for a child as described below:

- **Denial of health care:** The failure to provide or to allow needed care as recommended by a competent health care professional for a physical injury, illness, medical condition, or impairment. The CAPTA amendments of 1996 and 2003 contained no federal requirement for a parent to provide any medical treatment for a child if that treatment is against the parent's religious beliefs. However, CAPTA also designates that there is no requirement that a state either find or be prohibited from finding abuse or neglect in cases where parents or legal guardians act in accordance with their religious beliefs. While CAPTA stipulates that all states must give authority to CPS to pursue any legal actions necessary 1) to ensure medical care or treatment to prevent or to remedy serious harm to a child or 2) to prevent the withholding of medically indicated treatment from a child with a life-threatening condition (except in the cases of withholding treatment from disabled infants), all determinations will be done on a case by case basis within the sole discretion of each state.

- **Delay in health care:** The failure to seek timely and appropriate medical care for a serious health problem that any reasonable person would have recognized as needing professional medical attention. Examples of a delay in health care include not getting appropriate preventive medical or dental care for a child, not obtaining care for a sick child, or not following medical recommendations. Not seeking adequate mental health care also falls under this category. A lack or delay in health care may occur because the family does not have health insurance. Individuals who are uninsured often have compromised health because they receive less preventive care, are diagnosed at more advanced disease stages, and, once diagnosed, receive less therapeutic care.

Homelessness and Neglect

It is unclear whether homelessness should be considered neglect; some states specifically omit homelessness by itself as neglect. Unstable living conditions can have a negative effect on children, and homeless children are more at risk for other types of neglect in areas such as health, education, and nutrition. Homelessness is "considered neglect when the inability to provide shelter is the result of mismanagement of financial resources or when spending rent resources on drugs or alcohol results in frequent evictions."

Inadequate Supervision

Inadequate supervision encompasses a number of behaviors such as the following:

- **Lack of appropriate supervision:** Some states specify the amount of time children at different ages can be left unsupervised, and the guidelines for these ages and times vary. In addition, all children are different, so the amount of supervision needed may vary by the child's age, development, or situation. It is important to evaluate the maturity of the child, the accessibility of other adults, the duration and frequency of unsupervised time, and the neighborhood or environment when determining if it is acceptable to leave a child unsupervised.

- **Exposure to hazards:** Examples of exposure to in- and out-of-home hazards include:

  - Safety hazards: Poisons, small objects, electrical wires, stairs, drug paraphernalia;

  - Smoking: Second-hand smoke, especially for children with asthma or other lung problems;

  - Guns and other weapons: Guns that are kept in the house that are loaded and not locked up or are in reach of children;

  - Unsanitary household conditions: Rotting food, human or animal feces, insect infestation, or lack of running or clean water;

  - Lack of car safety restraints.

- **Inappropriate caregivers:** Another behavior that can fall under "failure to protect" is leaving a child in the care of someone who either is unable or should not be trusted to provide care for a child. Examples of inappropriate caregivers include a young child, a known child abuser, or someone with a substance abuse problem.

- **Other forms of inadequate supervision:** Additional examples of inadequate supervision include:

  - Leaving a child with an appropriate caregiver, but without proper planning or consent (for example, not returning to pick up the child for several hours or days after the agreed upon pick-up time or not giving the caregiver all the necessary items to take care of the child);

  - Leaving the child with a caregiver who is not adequately supervising the child (for example, the caregiver is with the child, but is not paying close attention to the child due to constantly being distracted by other activities);

  - Permitting or not keeping the child from engaging in risky, illegal, or harmful behaviors (for example, letting a child smoke marijuana).

Another common but complex example is single, working parents who are having difficulty arranging for appropriate back-up child care when their regular child care providers are unavailable. For example, a mother may leave her child home alone when the child care provider fails to show up. If the mother does not go to work, she can lose her job and will not be able to take care of her child. However, if she leaves the child alone, she will be guilty of neglect. It is important that parents in situations similar to this receive adequate support so that they are not forced to make these difficult decisions.

Environmental Neglect

Some of the characteristics mentioned above can be seen as stemming from environmental neglect, which is characterized by a lack of environmental or neighborhood safety, opportunities, or resources. While children's safety and protection from hazards are major concerns for CPS, most attention focuses on the conditions in the home and parental omissions in care. A broad view of neglect incorporates environmental conditions linking neighborhood factors with family and individual functioning, especially since the harmful impact of dangerous neighborhoods on children's development, mental health, and child maltreatment has been demonstrated. CPS workers should be aware of this impact on the family when assessing the situation and developing case plans. For example, they can help parents find alternative play areas in a drug-infested neighborhood, rather than have their children play on the streets.

Emotional Neglect

Typically, emotional neglect is more difficult to assess than other types of neglect, but is thought to have more severe and long-lasting consequences than physical neglect. It often occurs with other forms of neglect or abuse, which may be easier to identify, and includes:

- **Inadequate nurturing or affection:** The persistent, marked inattention to the child's needs for affection, emotional support, or attention.

- **Chronic or extreme spouse abuse:** The exposure to chronic or extreme spouse abuse or other domestic violence.

- **Permitted drug or alcohol abuse:** The encouragement or permission by the caregiver of drug or alcohol use by the child.

- **Other permitted maladaptive behavior:** The encouragement or permission of other maladaptive behavior (for example, chronic delinquency, assault) under circumstances where the parent or caregiver has reason to be aware of the existence and the seriousness of the problem, but does not intervene.

- **Isolation:** Denying a child the ability to interact or to communicate with peers or adults outside or inside the home.

Educational Neglect

Although state statutes and policies vary, both parents and schools are responsible for meeting certain requirements regarding the education of children. Types of educational neglect include the following:

- **Permitted, chronic truancy:** Permitting habitual absenteeism from school averaging at least five days a month if the parent or guardian is informed of the problem and does not attempt to intervene.

- **Failure to enroll or other truancy:** Failing to homeschool, to register, or to enroll a child of mandatory school age, causing the child to miss at least one month of school without valid reasons.

- **Inattention to special education needs:** Refusing to allow
  or failing to obtain recommended remedial education services
  or neglecting to obtain or follow through with treatment for a
  child's diagnosed learning disorder or other special education
  need without reasonable cause.

Newborns Addicted or Exposed to Drugs

As of 2005, 24 states had statutory provisions requiring the reporting of substance-exposed newborns to CPS. Women who use drugs or alcohol during pregnancy can put their unborn children at risk for mental and physical disabilities. The number of children prenatally exposed to drugs or to alcohol each year is between 409,000 and 823,000. One study showed that drug-exposed newborns constitute as many as 72 percent of the babies abandoned in hospitals. Another study found that 23 percent of children prenatally exposed to cocaine were later abused or neglected, compared with three percent who were not prenatally exposed. To address the needs of these children, the Keeping Children and Families Safe Act of 2003 (P.L. 108-36, sec. 114(b)(1)(B)) mandated that states include the following in their CAPTA plans:

> (ii) Policies and procedures (including appropriate referrals to child protection service systems and for other appropriate services) to address the needs of infants born and identified as being affected by illegal substance abuse or withdrawal symptoms resulting from prenatal drug exposure, including a requirement that health care providers involved in the delivery or care of such infants notify the child protective services system of the occurrence of such condition of such infants, except that such notification shall not be construed to (I) establish a definition under federal law of what constitutes child abuse; or (II) require prosecution for any illegal action.

> (iii) The development of a plan of safe care for the infant born and identified as being affected by illegal substance abuse or withdrawal symptoms;

> (iv) Procedures for the immediate screening, risk and safety assessment, and prompt investigation of such reports.

Methamphetamine Use and Child Maltreatment

In addition to the problem of prenatal drug use, the rise in methamphetamine abuse also has had a strong impact on child maltreatment.

U.S. Attorney General Alberto Gonzales recently proclaimed "in terms of damage to children and to our society, meth is now the most dangerous drug in America." Children whose parents use methamphetamine are at a particularly high risk for abuse and neglect. Methamphetamine is a powerfully addictive drug, and individuals who use it can experience serious health and psychiatric conditions, including memory loss, aggression, violence, psychotic behavior, and potential coronary and neurological damage. The drug is relatively easy to make, exposing many children of methamphetamine users to the additional risks of living in or near a methamphetamine lab. In 2003, 3,419 children either were residing in or visiting a methamphetamine lab that was seized, and 1,291 children were exposed to toxic chemicals in these labs. For more information on this epidemic, go to http://www.whitehousedrugpolicy .gov/news/press05/meth_factsheet.

Signs of Possible Neglect

It can be difficult to observe a situation and to know for certain whether neglect has occurred. Behaviors and attitudes indicating that a parent or other adult caregiver may be neglectful include if he or she demonstrates these characteristics:

- Appears to be indifferent to the child

- Seems apathetic or depressed

- Behaves irrationally or in a bizarre manner

- Abuses alcohol or drugs

- Denies the existence of or blames the child for the child's problems in school or at home

- Sees the child as entirely bad, worthless, or burdensome

- Looks to the child primarily for care, attention, or satisfaction of emotional needs

Indicators of neglect are more likely to be visible in the appearance or behavior of the child. Mandatory reporters and concerned individuals should consider reporting possible neglect if they notice that a child displays these characteristics:

- Wears soiled clothing or clothing that is significantly too small or large or is often in need of repair

- Seems inadequately dressed for the weather

- Always seems to be hungry; hoards, steals, or begs for food; or comes to school with little food

- Often appears listless and tired with little energy

- Frequently reports caring for younger siblings

- Demonstrates poor hygiene, smells of urine or feces, or has dirty or decaying teeth

- Seems emaciated or has a distended stomach (indicative of malnutrition)

- Has unattended medical or dental problems, such as infected sores

- States that there is no one at home to provide care

Scope of the Problem

According to the National Child Abuse and Neglect Data System (NCANDS), in 2004, an estimated three million referrals were made to CPS, representing 5.5 million children. From this population, approximately 872,000 children were found to be victims of maltreatment, and 64.5 percent of these children were neglected. In comparison, 18 percent of maltreated children were physically abused, 10 percent were sexually abused, and 7 percent were psychologically maltreated. Additionally, 15 percent of victims were associated with "other" types of maltreatment, such as abandonment or congenital drug addiction. A child could be identified as a victim of more than one type of maltreatment.

From 2000 to 2004, the rates of neglect were nearly stable. In 2004, approximately 7.4 out of every 1,000 children in the general population were reported as being neglected. Medical neglect is listed separately, but it also has experienced nearly stable rates, fluctuating between 0.5 children per 1,000 in 2000 and 0.3 children per 1,000 in 2004. Figure 16.1 shows the victimization rate by maltreatment type from 2000 to 2004.

However, according to the Third National Incidence Study of Child Abuse and Neglect (NIS-3), less than one-third of child abuse and neglect cases are reported to CPS. Data from NIS-3 show that the rates of child neglect may be even higher than noted in the NCANDS data, with 13.1 children per 1,000 being neglected. Within the category of neglect, physical neglect was the most commonly occurring type and included abandonment; medical neglect; inadequate nutrition, clothing, or hygiene; and leaving a young child unattended in a motor vehicle.

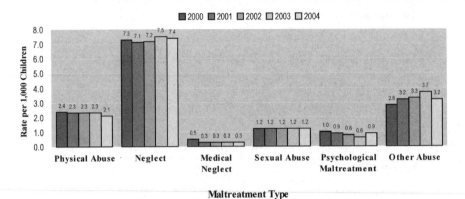

Figure 16.1. *Victimization Rates by Maltreatment Type, 2000–2004.*

Mandatory Reporters

Mandatory reporters are individuals who are required by law to report cases of suspected child abuse or neglect. They can face criminal and civil liability for not doing so. In approximately 18 states, anyone who suspects child abuse or neglect is considered a mandatory reporter. In most states, mandatory reporters are required to make a report immediately upon having suspicion or knowledge of an abusive or neglectful situation. This initial report may be made orally to either CPS or a law enforcement agency. Examples of individuals who typically are listed as mandatory reporters include physicians, social workers, educators, mental health professionals, child care providers, medical examiners, and police. Every state has statutes that specify procedures for mandatory reporters to follow when making a report of child abuse or neglect. For more information about state laws regarding mandatory reporters, see http://www.childwelfare.gov/systemwide/laws_policies/state/.

Spotlight on Chronic Neglect

One issue in defining child neglect involves consideration of "incidents" of neglect versus a pattern of behavior that indicates neglect. Susan J. Zuravin, Ph.D., at the University of Maryland at Baltimore School of Social Work, recommends that if some behaviors occur in a "chronic pattern," they should be considered neglectful. Examples include lack of supervision, inadequate hygiene, and failure to meet a child's educational needs. This suggests that rather than focusing on individual incidents that may or may not be classified as "neglectful," one should look at an accumulation of incidents that may together constitute neglect.

In most CPS systems, however, the criteria for identifying neglect focus on recent, distinct, verifiable incidents. Dr. Zuravin notes that "if CPS focuses only on the immediate allegation before them and not the pattern reflected in multiple referrals, then many neglected children will continue to be inappropriately excluded from the CPS system." For example, a family exhibiting a pattern of behavior that may constitute neglect might have frequent CPS reports of not having enough food in the home or keeping older children home from school to watch younger children. However, since each individual report may not be considered neglect, the family may not receive the appropriate support or be served by the CPS system. Additionally, many definitions of neglect that address chronicity do not identify what it means (for example, what does "frequent reports of not having enough food in the home" mean? Twice per week? Twice per month?). This may prevent CPS caseworkers from consistently applying the child maltreatment laws in these cases.

One study found that many children who had been referred to CPS for neglect did not receive services because their cases did not meet the criteria for neglect. It found, however, that all of these children had, in fact, suffered severe developmental consequences. In recognition of this issue, the Missouri Division of Family Services assigned one of its CPS staff as a chronic neglect specialist and defined chronic neglect as "'a persistent pattern of family functioning in which the caregiver has not sustained and/or met the basic needs of the children, which results in harm to the child." The focus here was on the accumulation of harm. CPS and community agencies are recognizing the importance of early intervention and service provision to support families so that neglect does not become chronic or lead to other negative consequences. For more information on this topic, see "Acts of Omission: An Overview of Child Neglect" at http://www.childwelfare.gov/pubs/focus/acts.

Recurrence

Recurrence of child abuse and neglect remains a very serious problem. It has been shown that subsequent referrals of maltreatment are most often for neglect (and, specifically, lack of supervision), regardless of the type of maltreatment in the initial referral. These findings highlight the need to screen for neglect and to provide preventive services where needed, not just for those cases initially identified as neglect. It is important to know the extent to which children who have been in contact with CPS are victims of repeat maltreatment in order to protect them and to prevent its recurrence.

Through the Child and Family Services Reviews (CFSRs), which are a results-oriented, comprehensive monitoring system designed to assist states in improving outcomes for the children and families they serve, the Children's Bureau set a national standard for recurrence of maltreatment, which is measured using NCANDS data. The percent of states that met the national standard increased from 29.4 percent of all states in 2000 to 42.2 percent of states in 2004. One study on recurrence that followed families for five years defined recurrence as "any confirmed report of physical abuse, sexual abuse, or neglect on any child in the family that occurred at least one day following the index incident report date." Of the 43 percent of families in the study that experienced at least one incident of recurrence of maltreatment within five years of the original incident, 64 percent of them were classified as neglect. This study also found that 52 percent of families who experienced repeated maltreatment had only one recurrence. The highest probability for recurrence was within the first 30 days of the original occurrence of maltreatment.

Child Neglect Fatalities

An estimated 1,490 children died from abuse or neglect in 2004. This is a rate of 2.03 deaths per 100,000 children, which is comparable to the rate of 2.00 per 100,000 children in 2003.

The distinction between child neglect fatalities and child abuse fatalities is that deaths from neglect result from a failure to act, whereas deaths from abuse result from a physical act. Fatalities due to child neglect may offer less obvious clues as to who is responsible and how the death occurred than fatalities due to abuse. Deaths due to child neglect, therefore, often are more difficult to investigate and prosecute. This also causes difficulty in determining the overall number of fatalities due to child neglect. In fact, one study estimated that 85 percent of child maltreatment fatalities are not recorded as such on death certificates. Other studies conducted in Colorado and North Carolina estimated that 50 to 60 percent of deaths due to child maltreatment were not recorded and that child neglect is the most under-recorded form of fatal maltreatment. Differing definitions of child homicide, abuse, and neglect, as well as the lack of thorough investigations into some child fatalities, also may be responsible for this underreporting.

Child neglect fatalities usually result from inadequate supervision, chronic physical neglect, or medical neglect and may result from chronic inaction (for example, malnourishment) or from an acute incident (for example, an unsupervised child drowning in a pool). The child's home is the most common place for a child neglect fatality to occur, and the bathroom is the most common room in which the death occurs. Often these children die from drowning or from fires that occur while they are unsupervised. Other examples of neglect fatalities include dying from falls from unprotected windows, suffocation, poisoning, and not receiving needed medical care.

Figure 16.2 shows the type of maltreatment associated with child fatalities in 2004. As the statistics in Figure 16.1. and 16.2. illustrate, child neglect is the largest form both of child maltreatment and of fatalities due to maltreatment.

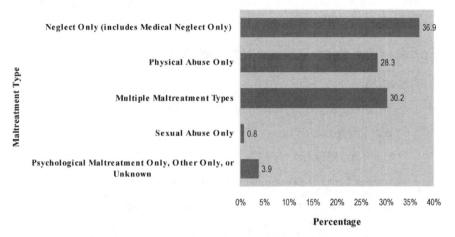

Figure 16.2. Fatalities by Type of Maltreatment, 2004

Section 16.2

Indicators of Neglect in Children

"Indicators of Neglect in Children," July 2008. © Liberty House (http://libertyhousecenter.org). Reprinted with permission. For more information, please contact Liberty House at 503-540-0288. Reviewed by David A. Cooke, MD, FACP, January 2013.

General Neglect: Physical Indicators

The child:

1. is consistently dirty and clothes are unwashed.

2. is hungry, underweight

3. is tired and listless

4. has unattended physical/dental problems.

5. may have accidental injuries due to a lack of supervision

6. is inappropriately/inadequately dressed.

7. has injuries that indicate an unsafe living condition (rat or roach bites, for instance)

General Neglect: Behavioral Indicators

The child:

1. is truant or tardy to school often, or arrives early and stays late.

2. begs or steals food.

3. attempts suicide.

4. is extremely dependent or detached.

5. appears to be exhausted.

6. states that there is frequent or continual absence of parent or guardian.

Behaviors Seen in Infants and Toddlers

1. Withdrawn, apathetic
2. Rocking
3. Fearful
4. Lethargy
5. Failure to thrive
6. Speech and language delays

Behaviors Seen in School-Age Children

1. Withdrawn, apathetic
2. Fearful
3. Learned helplessness
4. Hoarding food
5. Pseudo-independence
6. Regressive behavior
7. Sleeps in class or is unable to concentrate due to fatigue
8. Seems unable to concentrate, preoccupied
9. Parent-child role reversal exists

Behaviors Seen in Adolescents

1. Withdrawn, apathetic
2. Aggressive
3. Unkempt appearance
4. Drug/alcohol abuse
5. Eating disorders
6. Sleeps in class or is unable to concentrate due to fatigue
7. Parent-child role reversal exists
8. Child has been forced out of home

Possible Indicators of Neglectful Parents

1. Delays seeking medical/dental attention for child

2. Is secretive and reluctant to give information about the child's condition

3. Seldom touches, talks to, or makes eye contact with child

4. Becomes impatient about child's crying or need for attention

5. Criticizes or gets angry with the child for being injured or having needs

6. Shows little concern for child's problems, does not respond to inquiries

7. Cannot be found

8. Is using drugs and/or alcohol

9. Has no family or support system to turn to in a crisis or has multiple pressures that diminish capability to accomplish daily tasks

10. Has resources but does not use them to provide adequate care for child

11. Has exposed the child to domestic violence, drug-dealing or use, or knowingly exposed them to unsafe people such as pedophiles

Possible Indicators of Neglect in Housing Conditions

1. Inadequate heat

2. Unsafe use of space heaters

3. Exposed wiring

4. Broken/dangerous furniture or no furniture

5. Missing or broken windows/doors

6. Soiled, urine-soaked bedding

7. Lack of edible food

8. Medicines and cleaning supplies not stored away from reach of children

9. No clean clothing

10. Health dangers such as illegal drugs, feces, urine, rotting/molding food, or clothing

11. Lack of working plumbing

12. Hazards such as broken glass, rotten flooring/railings, vermin

Section 16.3

Recognizing Child Neglect

"Recognizing Child Neglect," reprinted with
permission from the Coalition for Children, www.safechild.org.
© 2012 Sherryll Kraizer, Ph.D. All rights reserved.

Neglect

"Neglected child" means a child less than 18 years of age whose physical, mental, or emotional condition has been impaired or is in danger of becoming impaired as a result of the failure of the child's legal guardian to exercise a minimum degree of care in supplying the child with adequate food, clothing, shelter, or education or medical care. Neglect also occurs when the legal guardian fails to provide the child with proper supervision or guardianship by allowing the child to be harmed, or to be at risk of harm which includes when the guardian misuses drugs or alcohol him/herself.

Please note: Some of these indicators may be attributable to specific life conditions or changes of circumstance such as homelessness, poverty, or other traumatic events. A pattern of conditions or behavior is the strongest indicator of abuse and should not be ignored. Failure to supervise is the leading cause of child death and should never be minimized.

Observable Indicators

- Dirty skin

- Offensive body odor

- Unwashed, uncombed hair

- Tattered, under or oversized, and unclean clothing
- Dressed in clothing that is inappropriate to weather or situation
- Frequently left unsupervised or alone for periods of time

Indicators of Poor Health

- Drowsiness, easily fatigued
- Puffiness under the eyes
- Frequent untreated upper respiratory infections
- Itching, scratching, long existing skin eruptions
- Frequent diarrhea
- Bruises, lacerations, or cuts that are infected
- Untreated illnesses
- Physical complaints not responded to by parent

Indicators of Malnutrition

- Begging for or stealing food
- Frequently hungry
- Rummaging through garbage pails for food
- Gorging self, eating in large gulps
- Hoarding food
- Obesity
- Overeating junk foods

Indicators in Infants and Toddlers

- Listlessness
- Poor responsiveness
- Does not often smile, cry, laugh, play, relate to others
- Lacks interest, curiosity
- Rocks, bangs head, sucks hair, thumb, finger,
- Tears at body

- Is overly self-stimulating, self-comforting
- Does not turn to parent for help or comfort
- Hospitalization for failure to thrive—regresses upon return to home
- Unduly over or under active for no apparent purpose

Indicators in Children

- Cries easily when hurt, even slightly
- Comes to school without breakfast
- Has no lunch or lunch money
- Needs dental care, glasses
- Falls asleep in class
- Often seems in a fog or dream world
- Comes to school early, does not want to go home
- Sees self as failure
- Troublesome at school
- Does no homework, refuses to try
- Destroys completed written work
- Destroys books, assignments, and learning aids or toys
- Is withdrawn, overactive, underactive, and/or lethargic (depressed)
- Is cruel to classmates
- Lies, steals from classmates, school
- Breaks objects or damages school property
- Frequently absent or late for school

Indicators with Parents and Family

- Promises but does not follow up on recommendations
- Fails to keep appointments and/or refuses help from school or other resources
- Abuses alcohol or other drugs

- Lifestyle of relative isolation from relatives, friends
- History of abuse or neglect as a child
- Disorganized, chaotic home life
- History of chronic illness
- Gives impression of resignation and feeling that nothing makes much difference anyway
- Failure to provide supervision of children

Chapter 17

Medical Neglect

Chapter Contents

Section 17.1

Neglect of Children's Health Care

Defining Neglected Health

Neglect of health care occurs when children's basic health care needs are not met. This broad definition focuses on basic needs of children rather than on parental omissions in care. A basic health care need is a need that when it is not met jeopardizes or harms a child's health in a significant way (for example, death of a child with diabetes due to lack of attention to medical recommendations). Many situations do not, however, rise to the level of actual or potential harm (for example, a missed followup appointment for an ear infection in a healthy child).

Implicit in the definition of neglect of health care is the likelihood that treatment will significantly benefit the child. If the benefit of treatment is uncertain (for example, an experimental treatment for cancer), not receiving the treatment should not be construed as neglect.

The definition of neglect used in this text is based on a child's unmet needs, irrespective of what specific factors may contribute to the neglect. From the child's perspective, not receiving necessary care is neglect regardless of the reasons why such care is not provided. Contributing factors, however, are important for planning a response.

The broad definition of neglect of children's health care used here, with its focus on the child, differs from most legal definitions of neglect, which focus on parental failure to obtain medical care for their child. Child protective services (CPS) generally confine its involvement to such legal definitions, with its focus on parental failure.

The broad child-focused definition of neglect has several advantages over the narrow legal approach. The broad definition encourages us to consider the full array of possible contributory factors. Although parents are primarily responsible for their children's care, responsibility extends beyond parents to professionals, community agencies, and social policies, all of which influence children's health. In focusing on a child's needs rather than parental omissions, the broad definition is less blaming and more constructive.

There are several other important dimensions of neglect of children's health care: actual versus potential harm, short-term versus long-term harm, concern with physical and psychological outcomes, and a continuum of care. The following case helps illustrate many of these dimensions:

- Amy is a six-year-old girl with severe asthma. She has been hospitalized four times in the past two years, twice in the intensive care unit. She was discharged from the hospital a week ago and given prescriptions for two medications. She comes to the office for follow-up and appears to be doing well. However, the prescriptions are not filled, and Amy has not received the recommended medications. Amy's mother explains that she is waiting to get her paycheck to fill the prescription. Amy is an only child who lives with her mother. After school, Amy's grandmother cares for her until her mother returns from work. There has been no contact with Amy's father in the past three years, and he makes no financial contribution to Amy or to her mother.

Actual versus Potential Harm

Does there need to be actual harm for there to be neglect, or is the risk of harm sufficient? Most state laws include potential harm in their definitions of child abuse and neglect. CPS agencies, however, overwhelmed by the number of reports, often prioritize the more serious cases, and actual harm is usually viewed as more serious than potential harm. Excluding cases of potential harm is problematic, however, because the sequelae of neglect are often not immediate. In Amy's case, even though Amy appears to be healthy, her history of severe asthma indicates her vulnerability. Without the prescribed medications, her risk for recurrent asthmatic attacks is substantial. Severe asthma can be lethal. In Amy's case, not receiving the recommended medications constitutes neglect. The purpose of defining neglect is to ensure that children's health care needs are met. If we are interested in preventing neglect, a focus on actual harm risks being too narrow, too late.

Short-Term versus Long-Term Harm

As stated above, the impact of neglect may not be immediately apparent, instead manifesting in the long term. Amy may be doing well today, but persistent failures in following recommendations jeopardizes her health and safety.

Physical and Psychological Outcomes

Our concern with children's health and well-being is a broad one. Accordingly, medical, dental, and mental health are all important aspects of health. Thus, a child is experiencing neglect if she has a history of hospitalizations due to severe dental or psychological problems and is not receiving prescribed medication or treatment. There could well be psychological problems related to Amy's asthma being inadequately treated.

A Continuum of Care

We artificially categorize cases as "neglect" or "not neglect" when the reality is that adequacy of care for basic needs falls on a continuum from optimal to grossly inadequate. The child welfare system is most often involved when we encounter situations that cross a threshold into "grossly inadequate." For example, few pediatricians would report Amy to CPS for neglect if the lapse in treatment occurred once or twice. More typically, neglect comes into focus when there is a pattern of repeated episodes that persist despite efforts to help and when harm results or is very likely to result.

How Do We Determine That a Child's Health Is Being Neglected?

Determining whether basic needs are met is at the core of assessing whether neglect exists. This section discusses factors that are relevant to this determination.

Severity

Severity is generally rated in terms of the actual or estimated potential harm as well as the degree of harm involved. For example, Amy's untreated asthma that results in admission to the intensive care unit would be rated as most severe, a regular hospital admission less so, a visit to the emergency department still less so, followed by mild symptoms not requiring professional attention, and, finally, no symptoms. Regarding potential harm, some risks entail only minor consequences, but others might be life threatening. Consideration of severity includes assessing the number of times the condition has occurred and its duration.

Likelihood of Harm

The likelihood of the harm occurring is important to consider. Missing a follow-up appointment for a child with eczema is very different from not seeking care for an infant who has been vomiting and had diarrhea for days. Both the potential medical and psychological ramifications should be considered. Although longitudinal research may help estimate the likelihood and nature of long-term outcomes associated with specific lapses in care (for example, prenatal drug exposure), many neglectful situations are complicated by ongoing environmental challenges such as poverty.

Frequency/Chronicity

Neglect is usually inferred when there is a pattern of unmet needs. A dilemma arises regarding single or rare incidents that may constitute neglect. In some instances, omissions in care are unlikely to be harmful unless they are recurrent. For example, there may be serious risks for a child with a seizure disorder who repeatedly does not get medication but not if there is only an occasional lapse. However, an infant left unattended in a bath once, briefly, could drown. Thus, this single lapse could be construed as neglect. The intervention is likely to be different if there is a pattern of neglect.

Measuring the frequency or chronicity of a problem is difficult. In some instances, medical or pharmacy records show appointments not kept or prescriptions not filled. At times, parents or children may disclose how long they have had food shortages or problems accessing health care. In sum, neglect can be defined as occurring when a child's basic need is not met. Actual and potential harm are both of concern.

Incidence/Prevalence

It is difficult to estimate the extent of neglected health care. Health care providers do not identify many cases of health care neglect, and they may not report identified cases to CPS. In 2008, 71% of the 772,000 substantiated CPS reports were for neglect, less than 1% for medical neglect, 16% for physical abuse (PA), 9% for sexual abuse, and 7.3% for psychological maltreatment (PM). It should be noted that most states do not separately record medical neglect.

In 2008, it is estimated that 39.7% of fatalities were caused by multiple forms of maltreatment. Neglect was responsible for nearly 32% of fatalities. Most fatalities attributable to neglect were caused by lapses in supervision. One study documented 172 known deaths of children in the United States in which medical care was withheld on religious grounds; in most cases medical care would likely have saved their lives.

There is also research that focuses on societal neglect—that is, circumstances where children's basic needs are not adequately met due largely to gaps in services and inadequate policies and programs. For example, children's mental health needs are often not met. One study of youth between ages 9 and 17 years found that only 38% to 44% of children meeting stringent criteria for a psychiatric diagnosis in the prior six months had had a mental health contact in the previous year. Neglected dental care is widespread. For example, a study of preschoolers found that 49% of four-year-olds had cavities, and fewer than 10% were fully treated. Another study found that 8.6% of kindergarteners needed urgent dental care. Neglected health care is not rare. If access to health care and health insurance is viewed as a basic need, then 8.7 million children experienced this form of neglect in 2006.

Etiology

There is no single cause of child neglect. J. Belsky (Child maltreatment: An ecological integration, *American Psychologist*, 35, 320–35; 1980) proposed an ecological theory of multiple and interacting factors at the individual (parent and child), familial, community, and societal levels. A toddler with a chronic, toxic blood lead level illustrates this theory. This child's health is being neglected by a lack of protection from lead and a lack of satisfactory treatment. Contributory factors may include the parents' unwillingness to allow treatment, the parents' inability to move to a lead-free home, a landlord's refusal to have the home deleaded, a city's inability to ensure an adequate lead abatement program, and society's limited investment in low-income housing. Understanding a neglectful situation requires an appreciation of all contributory factors so we can intervene optimally. Regardless of which contributory factors are responsible, a child with a high lead level experiences neglect.

Context—Society and Community

Context refers to the environment in which children live, including poverty, culture, and religion, as well as the community. The context shapes the attitude, knowledge, and behavior of parents and the quality of health care children receive. Poverty has been strongly associated with neglect: Neglect was identified 44 times more often in families with annual incomes under $15,000 compared with those earning above $30,000. It should be noted, however, that most children raised in poor families do not experience neglect. They do, however, experience the adverse effects of poverty, arguably a form of societal neglect.

Another aspect of context concerns culture and religion. Different cultures differ in their beliefs regarding health care. For example, children from Southeast Asia may receive the folkloric remedy of Cao Gio for a fever. A hard object is vigorously rubbed over the chest and may cause bruising. It is unclear whether this practice results in any benefit or significant harm, but there is the risk of not receiving appropriate care for a serious illness (for example, meningitis). Some cultural differences are less dramatic, such as segments of the population that have little interest in psychotherapy. Variations in beliefs pose sensitive dilemmas as health care professionals strive to avoid an ethnocentric approach ("My way is right") and to respect cultural relativism (cultures differ and all should be accepted). When a practice clearly harms children, and when good alternatives exist, society should ensure that children's needs for health care are adequately met.

Some parents hold religious views that are antithetical to Western medicine, believing in alternative approaches to health. For example, sick children may receive prayer from a Christian Scientist faith healer. Many illnesses (for example, colds) are self-limiting, and satisfactory outcomes result regardless of treatment; other illnesses, however, can lead to serious harm without effective health care.

The community and its resources influence parent-child relationships and are strongly associated with maltreatment. A community with a rich array of services such as parenting groups, child care, and good public transportation enhances the ability of families to nurture and protect children. Informal support networks, safety, and recreational facilities are important in supporting healthy family functioning. Families in a high-risk environment are less able to give and share and might be mistrustful of neighborly exchanges. Neglect is strongly associated with social isolation. In one large study, mothers of neglected children perceived themselves as isolated and as living in unfriendly neighborhoods. In summary, communities can either offer valuable support to families or add to the stresses families experience.

Family

Disorganization of the home is characteristic of families of neglected children. A. Kadushin (Neglect in families. In *Mental Illness, Delinquency, Addictions, and Neglect*, E. W. Nunnally et al. eds., Newbury Park, CA: Sage, 1988) described chaotic families of neglected children, with impulsive mothers who repeatedly showed poor planning. Deficient problem-solving skills, poor parenting skills, and inadequate knowledge of children's needs are associated with neglect. The absence of fathers or their limited involvement in their children's lives may be factors in neglect. Several studies have found more negative interactions between mothers and their young children in families of neglected children. Some cases of failure to thrive (FTT) are rooted in "a poor fit" between mother and child. A child's passive or lively temperament may displease a parent. In addition, family problems such as spousal violence or lack of social support may contribute to a difficult parent-child relationship. In contrast, a supportive family can buffer the stresses that impair parenting, illustrating the importance of considering both risk and protective factors in assessing families for possible neglect.

Stress also has been associated with child maltreatment. One study found the highest level of stress—concerning unemployment, illness, eviction, and arrest—among families of neglected children, compared with abusive and control families. J. Lapp (A profile of officially reported child neglect. In *The Dilemma of Child Neglect: Identification and Treatment*, C.M. Trainer, ed., Denver, CO: American Humane Association, 1983) found stress to be frequent among parents reported to CPS for neglect, particularly regarding family relationships and financial and health problems.

Parents

Many of the characteristics of mothers of neglected children may contribute to children's health care needs not being met. Mothers' emotional problems, intellectual deficits, and substance abuse are associated with neglect. Emotional disturbances, especially depression, are found among mothers of neglected children. Intellectual impairment including mental retardation and a lack of education is associated with neglect. High rates of substance abuse are found among families of neglected children. Maternal drug use during pregnancy has become a pervasive problem. Most illicit drugs pose definite risks to the fetus and child. The compromised caregiving abilities of drug-abusing parents are a major concern.

Most decisions regarding children's health care are made by parents, including when to seek professional care. P.M. Crittenden's model (Characteristics of neglectful parents: An information processing approach. *Criminal Justice and Behavior*, 20, 27–48; 1993) helps refine our understanding of parental difficulties by considering four steps: (1) perception of the child's problem, (2) interpretation of the problem, (3) response, and (4) implementation. Difficulties at any of these steps may lead to unmet health care needs. The parent first needs to perceive the problem. Subtle signs such as decreased urination may go undetected. Inadequate knowledge about children and health and inappropriate expectations contribute to neglect. At times, parents may be in denial about a child's condition. Parents of neglected children are less knowledgeable about developmental milestones and have limited knowledge about parenting, poor skills, and low motivation to be a good parent.

Parents may perceive the problem but interpret it incorrectly. For example, based on the parent's prior experience, a child's poor growth may seem normal. A parent may believe moodiness is common in children, unaware that children can be depressed. Popular interpretations of a symptom such as an infant crying because "he's spoiled" may lead to a problem being missed. Again, parents with limited cognitive abilities or emotional problems may have difficulty interpreting their child's cues, determining the care needed, and understanding and implementing the treatment plan.

After recognizing and interpreting the problem, parents choose their response. Initially, they may hope the problem will resolve spontaneously or with a home remedy. For example, parents may hope a small burn will heal without professional care—a reasonable assumption. If the condition deteriorates, only then may it be clear that medical care is needed. Such delays have been viewed suspiciously, but it is important not to misjudge reasonable delays. In considering delay, the context should be considered. If care was obtained at a point when a reasonable layperson could be expected to have recognized the need for professional help then it is not a neglectful situation. An inappropriate response, including delay, may result from inadequate knowledge, parental distress, and cultural or religious beliefs. For example, a depressed youngster may not receive psychotherapy if the parents hold such treatment in disdain.

Finally, the problem may be with implementing recommendations the family has received from health care providers. A parent's inaction may occur because the parent is distracted by other priorities (for example, an eviction notice, obtaining drugs), depression, or difficulty accessing health care.

Other influences on parents' behavior may be useful for professionals to consider. Confidence in the remedy or in one's ability to implement the treatment is important. Thus, a parent's belief that a medicine works enhances compliance. Motivation to address a health problem is important and may be influenced by the chronicity of the problem. With chronic problems, some parents become complacent. For all families, there is a need to balance many needs and to prioritize. For example, paying an electricity bill before filling a prescription may be appropriate in some circumstances. In other circumstances, however, such as Amy's asthma, the decision to delay implementing recommended treatment may place the child at risk, thereby constituting neglect.

Child

Children may contribute to their own neglect, directly and indirectly. A direct example is an adolescent's denial of diabetes, refusing to adhere to the treatment plan despite excellent efforts by caring parents. Some children give no or few cues that they need help. Children's age may influence perceptions of their vulnerability, with more concern directed to younger children. The unmet needs of adolescents may not evoke the same level of concern. J. Belsky and J. Vondra (Lessons from child abuse: The determinants of parenting. In *Child Maltreatment: Theory and Research on the Causes and Consequences of Child Abuse and Neglect*, D. Cicchetti and V. Carlson, eds., New York: Cambridge University Press, 1989) described how children's health status could affect their parents' ability to provide care. For example, premature infants may require extended care in neonatal intensive care units, which may impair bonding and the baby's attachment to the parents. Caring for a child born with low birth weight can be challenging, and studies have found low birth weight to be a risk factor for neglect.

Children with chronic health problems or disabilities have special needs that place them at added risk. Many parents of such children are dedicated caregivers; others may be so stressed that they are unable to provide adequate care. L.J. Diamond and P.K. Jaudes (Child abuse and the cerebral palsied patient. *Developmental Medicine and Child Neurology*, 25, 169–74, 1983) found cerebral palsy to be a risk factor for neglect, but another study found no increase in maltreatment among 500 moderately to profoundly mentally retarded children. P.M. Sullivan and J.E. Knutson (Maltreatment and disabilities: A population-based epidemiological study. *Child Abuse and Neglect*, 24, 1257–73, 2000) found in a population-based study that disabled children were 3.4 times more likely to be identified as maltreated than nondisabled peers (9% vs.

31%). Families of children with special health care needs are often involved with multiple professionals, and increased surveillance may bias reports of neglect. A study found that children with mental health problems were at higher risk for maltreatment but not those children with developmental disabilities. Overall, it appears that the special health care needs of children with disabilities may overwhelm some caring and competent parents, thus contributing to neglect.

The Disorder and the Treatment

The nature of the disorder may influence children's and parents' responses to recommendations or treatment. For example, a disorder that is highly visible (for example, an ugly rash) often evokes more of a response than a disorder that is not visible (for example, lead poisoning). Children and parents who do not perceive that the disorder is serious or do not have confidence in the treatment are less likely to adhere to recommendations. Professionals can prevent neglect by ensuring that children and families are well informed about the disorder and the effectiveness of treatment.

The severity of symptoms makes a difference. Chronic health problems may be accepted without much alarm. For example, Amy's mother may accept that her daughter is a severe asthmatic who will periodically need to be hospitalized. This may be a valuable coping strategy, but undue complacency may result. Alternatively, a chronic and severe disease may evoke great distress that contributes to denial, such as is sometimes seen in adolescents with diabetes.

Neglect is also more likely to occur if the goals of treatment are not consistent with the goals of the child or family. For example, improving pulmonary function tests (a health professional's goal) may mean little to Amy, compared with being able to play sports (a child's goal). Thus, communication about the goals of the child and family and the impact of the disorder and treatment on those goals should help professionals frame the reasons for the treatment in a way that resonates with the goals of the child and family.

Concerns about side effects of treatment or doubts of its effectiveness may dissuade a parent from seeking care. Obesity is an example in which a parent may recognize the problem but be reluctant to engage in treatment that they see as burdensome. In addition to questions about the treatment, families may doubt their ability to implement recommended treatments. For example, the likelihood of neglect may be increased if a parent is anxious about injecting a child who has insulin-dependent diabetes. Professionals should help ensure that parents have both the competence and confidence to follow through with treatment.

The cost of treatment may contribute to the likelihood of neglect. For example, Amy's mother did not fill the prescriptions because she was waiting to receive her paycheck. Sensitive questioning is necessary to determine if a family is able to purchase recommended medications or to implement recommendations. When financial resources are a problem, professionals may consider less expensive options or look for strategies to minimize costs.

Poor communication may be a problem, with the treatment not being clearly conveyed or understood. Finally, simply remembering to take a medication several times in a busy day may be a challenge contributing to neglect. Working with families to help them incorporate recommended treatment into their daily routine helps families adhere to recommendations and avoid neglect.

The nature of health care includes the relationship between a professional and family. Ideally, there is a relationship of mutual trust and respect. Families are more likely to follow recommendations if they have confidence that the recommendations are sound, will be beneficial, and are possible to implement. Without a trusting relationship, families may be discouraged from seeking help or from following recommendations. Ideally, pediatric primary care professionals focus on prevention to avoid serious health problems, including neglect. However, primary care professionals often have many issues to cover and not enough time, compromising their ability to offer comprehensive care. If the clinic or office is not perceived as friendly and supportive, families may feel discouraged from seeking care.

Manifestations of Neglected Health Care

This section discusses the more common forms of neglected health care.

Nonadherence (Noncompliance) with Health Care Recommendations

The most common form of neglected health care involves a lack of adherence with health care appointments, treatment, or recommendations, resulting in actual or potential harm (for example, Amy not getting prescribed treatment). Nonadherence with medical recommendations is common. For example, one study found that half of adolescents were nonadherent with medical regimens. Another study found only 25% of parents of children with attention deficit disorder adhered to the treatment plan; fewer than 10% consulted the physician before stopping medication. The pervasiveness of noncompliance does not minimize its importance.

Noncompliance is not restricted to patients. Researchers have studied how well physicians manage medical conditions that have clear guidelines for treatment. Studies reveal that between 48% and 72% of doctors occasionally fail to adhere to treatment guidelines.

Failure or Delay in Seeking Health Care

Delay in seeking medical care for a child sometimes constitutes neglect. Consider this situation:

- Joe is a 10-month-old infant brought to the emergency department following four days of vomiting, diarrhea, decreased appetite, lethargy, and fever. On the second day, his father spoke with their pediatrician, who recommended an electrolyte solution, fever management, and followup if Joe's condition should worsen. The pediatrician mentioned that he would be leaving town for the holiday weekend, but a partner would be on call. Joe had had this problem once before, and it resolved after a few days. The emergency department staff found Joe to be at least 10% dehydrated and in need of admission to the intensive care unit. The staff were concerned that medical care had not been obtained earlier, raising a question of neglect.

Parents generally decide on the appropriate care for minor problems (for example, a scrape, a cold, sadness at the death of a pet). As conditions become more serious, the need for professional care increases, and parents are responsible for seeking such care. Neglect occurs when necessary health care is not received or when delay is so significant that a child's health is harmed or jeopardized (for example, Joe). The challenge for professionals is to understand what may be contributing to delay in seeking health care.

Joe's case highlights the importance of clear communication between professionals and caregivers. Although Joe's father contacted the pediatrician on the second day of his son's symptoms, Joe's prior recovery from similar symptoms, together with the holiday weekend, may have led to the decision to recommend home management without an office visit. Daily phone contact may have alerted the pediatrician to Joe's worsening condition prior to his need for hospitalization. Thus, Joe did not receive optimal care, although the family responded reasonably. The "system" was at fault.

Religiously Motivated Medical Neglect

Medical neglect can occur when parents actively refuse medical treatment. In some cases, parents believe an alternative treatment is preferable, perhaps because the treatment recommended by doctors is prohibited by their religion. For example, Jehovah's Witnesses, with their prohibition of blood transfusions, routinely refuse surgery when the need for transfusions is anticipated. Other religions, such as Christian Scientists, rely on faith healers and reject Western medicine.

Situations involving religious beliefs and children's health care can be difficult. How do we balance civil liberties, parental rights, and respect for religious belief against the medical needs of children? The principle of *parens patriae* establishes the state's authority to protect its young citizens. If a child's parents cannot or will not provide adequate care, the state must do so. However, 30 states have religious exemptions from their child abuse statutes. Such exemptions state, for example, "A child is not to be deemed abused or neglected merely because he or she is receiving treatment by spiritual means, through prayer according to the tenets of a recognized religion" (American Academy of Pediatrics, 1988). These exemptions are based on the arguments of religious groups that the U.S. Constitution guarantees the protection of religious practice. This interpretation of the Constitution is challenged by court rulings prohibiting parents from martyring their children based on parental beliefs (Prince *v.* Massachusetts, 1944) and from denying them essential medical care (Jehovah's Witnesses of Washington *v.* King County Hospital, 1968). The American Academy of Pediatrics (AAP) has strongly opposed religious exemptions, arguing that the "opportunity to grow and develop safe from physical harm with the protection of our society is a fundamental right of every child. . . . The basic moral principles of justice and of protection of children as vulnerable citizens require that all parents and caretakers must be treated equally by the laws and regulations that have been enacted by state and federal governments to protect children (American Academy of Pediatrics, 1988).

Inadequate Food

Inadequate food may manifest as repeated hunger and may place a child at risk for impaired growth, including failure to thrive (FTT). Although food insufficiency is related to poverty, more than half of food-insufficient individuals live in employed families. Hunger remains prevalent in the United States and may adversely affect children's growth and development. Inadequate food constitutes a serious form of neglect, and professionals should screen for food insufficiency by asking families if they have adequate food for their children.

FTT can result from inadequate nutrition. The etiology of FTT is multifactorial. The traditional classification of *organic* (that is, medical) and *nonorganic* (that is, psychosocial) FTT has limited usefulness; more often, there is a mixed etiology. Children with medical explanations for poor growth (for example, celiac disease) often experience discomfort while eating and develop feeding problems. A psychosocial contribution should be considered regardless of the presence of a medical condition. In addition, psychosocial conditions should be implicated based on evidence, not simply by excluding medical causes. Inadequate food in a context of psychosocial problems jeopardizes children's health and development.

Obesity

Pediatric obesity has dramatically increased. Over 17% of American children have a body mass index (BMI) above the 95th percentile. There is a long list of complications of obesity during childhood and adulthood.

There are multiple contributors to obesity including genetic factors. Because environmental and family factors often contribute, some cases of morbid obesity may be a form of neglect in that the child's need for healthful food and physical activity is not being met. Not addressing the concern of obesity can constitute neglect, especially when a suitable program is available. In a 10-year study, children who were neglected (received little parent support) were sevenfold more likely to become obese as young adults than were children who were not neglected.

Exposure to Environmental Hazards

The health risks associated with environmental hazards are firmly established. Hence, exposure to these hazards inside or outside the home is a form of neglect. Examples inside the home include poisonous substances and dangerous objects within easy reach of young children, smoking around children with pulmonary conditions, exposure to domestic violence, and access to a loaded gun. Hazards outside the home include riding a bike without a helmet, failure to use a car seat or seat belt, and neighborhood violence. Exposure to lead may be a problem both in and out of the home.

Drug-Exposed Newborns and Older Children

The prevalence of maternal drug use during pregnancy as well as high rates of substance abuse among families of neglected children were mentioned earlier. In addition, use of illicit drugs and being raised in a drug-using environment jeopardize children's health and development.

The response to prenatal drug exposure varies. I.J. Chasnoff and L.A. Lowder (Prenatal alcohol and drug use and risk for child maltreatment. A timely approach to intervention. In *Neglected Children: Research, Practice, and Policy*, H. Dubowitz, ed., Thousand Oaks, CA: Sage, 1999) describe responses ranging from inducements to engage in drug treatment all the way to criminal prosecution.

The use of legal but dangerous substances (for example, tobacco, alcohol) during pregnancy also raises an important issue: Is such use neglect? Given our knowledge of the risks involved, it is probably not helpful to label use of these substances as neglect. At the same time, their use should be discouraged during pregnancy. Regarding older children, the risk of secondhand smoke, especially for children with pulmonary problems, is clear.

Section 17.2

Medical Neglect Laws and Faith Healing

- **Quotation:** "The free exercise clause of the First Amendment protects religious belief, but not necessarily conduct." Judge Vincent Howard, Marathon County Circuit Court, Wisconsin.[1]

Freedom to Choose Faith Healing

People in North America are guaranteed freedom of religion:

- The First Amendment to the U.S. Constitution prohibits any action by an American government which restricts "the free exercise of religion."

  - Section 2 of the Canadian Charter of Rights and Freedoms guarantees that "Everyone has the following fundamental freedoms: freedom of conscience and religion."

Courts have generally interpreted the concept of freedom of religion very broadly to include both religious belief and most religious practices, for example the personal freedom to choose prayer and/or religious ritual in place of medical treatment for a disease or disorder. When faced with a medical problem, an adult can seek medical attention, use faith healing, try herbal or other alternative medical treatment, or pursue no treatment at all, and let nature takes its course. Some parents or guardians may wish to exercise the same options for their children. The result is sometimes a conflict with civil authorities: should parents have the right to follow their religion and withhold medical attention from their children, even if the child will probably die needlessly? The problem is aggravated by the teachings of some faith groups which create a culture in which seeking medical health is viewed as rejecting God.

Problems sometimes occur in cases involving a minor or other person who is incapable of giving informed consent for their own treatment. Parents and guardians are generally given almost complete freedom in providing or denying health care to their children. But, in the case of life-threatening medical conditions, the courts and Child Protective Services have occasionally intruded, and ordered treatment of a child against the wishes of its parent(s).

J. Gordon Melton, director of the Institute for the Study of American Religions in Santa Barbara, California has stated that at the start of the 20th century, there were many faith groups that advocated prayer in the place of medicine. Their teaching was largely motivated by a backlash directed against the inroads of modern medicine. The number of groups that still advocate prayer has been dropping ever since.[2]

Dr. Seth Asser, co-author of an article on medically preventable child fatalities commented: "You can't beat, sexually abuse, or starve your kids, but the law allows a parent to refuse medical care in favor of magic. This is not just a social phenomenon, but a public-health issue."[3]

Why Do Parents Choose Prayer in Place of Medical Attention?

Thousands of children die every year in America as a result of neglect or abuse. Often abuse is the result of spanking or other forms of corporal punishment that simply got out of hand. However, this essay deals with a different phenomenon: a sick child who is denied medical attention—often for an easily treated problem—because of the parents' reliance on prayer. On the order of one child a month in the U.S. is known to die as a result of a disease or disorder that is almost certainly curable with medical attention. The full number is unknown.

The root cause of the problem is the parents' concept of truth. In the case of Christians, truth is typically based on four considerations:

1. What the Bible says and means, according to their faith group's interpretation.
2. Their faith group's traditional beliefs.
3. Personal experience.
4. Scientific findings.

Among many fundamentalists, Pentecostals, evangelicals, Roman Catholics, Jehovah's Witnesses and other religious conservatives, as well as Christian Scientists, the first two criteria vastly outweigh the fourth in importance. Some parents are willing to ignore medical and other scientific knowledge and make decisions largely or solely on their religious beliefs.

A major factor is not necessarily what the Bible says, or even what it meant at the time. It is what the Bible means today. Two examples are:

- Jehovah's Witnesses are taught that the dietary rules in the Hebrew Scriptures (Old Testament) requiring that blood be fully drained from meat before it is eaten are literally true. Hebrews are forbidden to eat meat containing blood. The Witnesses interpret these passages as being still binding on modern-day Christians. They also teach that these passages prohibit a member from accepting a blood transfusion, even if it is necessary to save their life. Few other Christian denominations teach either of these beliefs.

- "Pastor Bob" is reported as having once written in the *Unleavened Bread Ministries* web site: "Jesus never sent anyone to a doctor or a hospital. Jesus offered healing by one means only! Healing was by faith."[1] The New Testament does not recommend that people seek medical attention for themselves or their family. It does talk about medical cures through prayer, sometimes involving the elders in the church and anointing with oil. That might have been a useful teaching in the first century CE Galilee, because there were no hospitals available and medical knowledge was so primitive that going to the doctor, on average, endangered your health more than just letting nature take its course. It was only in the early 20th century that medical techniques improved to the point where physician care was beneficial, on average. To some deeply devout parents, the 1st century approach is still the path to take.

Here again, the question is not what the Bible passages say, or even what they meant at the time. It is whether they still have the same meaning today. Some small faith groups teach that because hospitals and modern medicine are not mentioned in the Bible, that modern-day Christians must not take advantage of them today. Prayer, anointing, and the laying on of hands are the only acceptable treatment. With the exception of the U.S., hospital and physician care is now universally accessible throughout the developed world. Most Christian denominations urge their members to take advantage of medical help. A few small faith groups teach that the Bible requires their members to avoid doctors and hospitals.

Religious Exemptions in Child Abuse Laws

In 1974, the U.S. Department of Health, Education and Welfare first required states to have clauses in their child abuse and neglect legislation that permits exemptions from prosecution of parents on religious grounds. If a state refused, they would not receive federal child abuse protection grants.

In 1983, the federal government allowed states to repeal these clauses. However, most state still allow parents to use a religious defense if their child dies because prayer was used instead of medical treatment.

Some recent activity at the state level:

- **1994 Oregon:** Legislature committees heard testimony on two House bills that would require all parents to obtain medical help for their seriously sick or injured children. The bills had strong backing from both major parties, law enforcement, physicians, social workers and child advocates. "...there was limited testimony from Christian Scientists who warned that eliminating the so-called spiritual defense from Oregon's homicide statutes and other areas of the law would unfairly impose upon their religious rights."[4] The House later endorsed a compromise faith healing bill that allows defendants to claim faith healing as a defense.

- **1994 Minnesota:** The state passed a law which requires parents or guardians to alert child protection services if they have withheld medical treatment and that their children were endangered by their decision. Few if any parents or guardians report under this law.

- **1998 Texas:** Critical-care pediatrician Seth Asser said "Kids die from accidental deployment of air bags, and you get hearings in Congress. But this goes on, and dozens die and people think there's no problem because the deaths happen one at a time. But the kids who die suffer horribly. This is Jonestown in slow motion." The American Medical Association, the National District Attorneys Association, the Academy of American Pediatrics and a growing number of local and state legislators agree with him.

- **2001:** The Academy of American Pediatrics went on record in opposition to these exemption laws.[5] Colorado as well as Oregon had experienced an increase in juvenile death rates that paralleled the growth of anti-medical faith groups.[5] Amanda Bates, 13, suffered a horrendous, lingering and painful death from diabetes and gangrene in early 2001. She and her family attended the General Assembly and Church of the First Born. She was the third child to die in that church in three years. This motivated legislators to eliminate an exemption from the child abuse law that had protected parents from abuse charges if they withheld medical attention from children.

- **2002:** 38 states had laws that shield parents from persecution if they reject medical treatment for their children in favor of faith healing. However, most of these state laws specify that if a child's condition is life-threatening, then a physician must be consulted.[6]

- **2009:** Rita Swan is the executive director of the Iowa-based Children's Health Care Is a Legal Duty. They advocate charging parents who do not seek medical help when their children need it. She reports that about 300 children have died in the United States during the previous 25 years after medical care was withheld on religious grounds. Child abuse laws in 30 states still provide some form of protection for practitioners of faith healing in cases of child neglect and other matters.[1]

Some state laws exempt parents only if their children are faced with a non-life threatening condition or disease. The Oregon law covering criminally negligent homicide requires that the prosecution prove that the defendant failed to be aware of a substantial and unjustifiable risk that is "a gross deviation" from what a reasonable person would observe in a similar situation.[7] Both are difficult to prove in court. Parents can claim that they did not realize that their child's condition was very serious; they can claim lack of medical knowledge. A British law requires parents to seek medical help for their children, if the child's condition does not improve after 72 hours of non-medical treatment. That type of legislation may be more effective.

References Used

The following information sources were used to prepare and update the above essay. The hyperlinks are not necessarily still active today.

1. Dirk Johnson, "Trials for Parents Who Chose Faith Over Medicine," *New York Times*, 2009-JAN-20, at: http://www.nytimes.com.

2. "State, church clash over faith healing beliefs," *Beloit Daily News*, Beloit WI, 1997-APR-21 at: http://www.beloitdailynews.com.

3. S.M. Asser & R. Swan, "Child fatalities from religion-motivated medical neglect," *Pediatrics*, 1998; 101(4), pages 625–29.

4. Home in Zion Ministries has a home page at: http://users .southeast.net.

5. Jessica Reaves, "Freedom of Religion or State-Sanctioned Child Abuse? Rising death toll fuels debate over parents who choose prayer over medical treatment on behalf of their children," Time.com, 2001-FEB-21, at: http://www.time.com.

6. "No Cure for Cancer: Tenn. Mom, Preacher Accused of Letting Girl Die by Turning to God," ABCNews.com, 2002-OCT-3, at: http://abcnews.go.com.

7. Steven Mayes, "Fate of Oregon City faith healers now with jury," *Oregon Live*, 2009-JAN-29, at: http://www.oregonlive.com.

Chapter 18

Educational Neglect and Truancy

Chapter Contents

Section 18.1

Children's Educational Needs and the Problem of Educational Neglect

Excerpted from Kelly, Phillip. "Where Are the Children? Educational Neglect across the Fifty States." *The Researcher*, 23 (1), 41–58, Fall 2010. Copyright © 2010 Northern Rocky Mountain Educational Research Association (www.nrmera.org). Reprinted with permission. The complete text of this article is available at http://www.nrmera.org/PDF/Researcher/Researcherv23n1Kelly.pdf.

In an era of increasing educational accountability and economic demands, failure of a child to receive an adequate education generates tremendous costs both for the child and the larger society. Such failure constitutes educational neglect. Since the mid-19th century, it has been the responsibility of states to ensure that students meet compulsory education requirements. Currently, even with our country focused on the federal policy *No Child Left Behind*, most states cannot even identify all of their students of compulsory school age. This study sheds light on this phenomenon at the national level as well as state level.

One unaddressed loophole within *No Child Left Behind* is that it addresses schoolchildren—only. If the goal of leaving no child behind and closing the achievement gap between various groups is to be realized, we must ensure the education of all children. This study examines the incongruence between children identified as living in the federal census and those identified as educated by state departments of education. Some states have abandoned educational oversight of many of the children "missing" from school districts' enrollment lists. These conditions provide a fertile breeding ground for educational neglect.

Educational neglect is phenomenon with tremendous costs. Unfortunately, in a world full of social ills and societal needs, educational neglect often fails to reach the policy threshold at which attention and resources are allocated to address the problem. This study helps to illuminate this phenomenon at the national level as well as for a northwest state specifically.

When addressing educational neglect, policymakers, social workers and educators must overcome several impediments. First is the problem of definition. Within the fields of social work and education, and certainly within statute, there appears to be no commonly agreed upon definition of educational neglect. Second, educational neglect exists as a problem between the jurisdictions of Departments of Health and Welfare and Departments of Education. Unfortunately for the neglected children, as in any endeavor involving multiple parties, where each "is responsible," no one is. Hence, educational neglect is not addressed adequately by either department. Third, social service institutions have more pressing issues such as physical and/or sexual abuse and neglect. Their limited resources are directed to those children who are most in need. Fourth, educational neglect's co-occurrence with other forms of neglect/abuse greatly complicates identification and treatment of educational neglect. Lastly, educational neglect is a phenomenon of non-occurrence, a lack of appropriate education. Documenting that an activity is not occurring is very difficult, especially when those guilty of educational neglect often actively avoid any governmental interaction.

Compulsory Education Laws

Compulsory education laws have a very long and uneven history in the United States. In competition to states' educational authority are parental claims to the same, or superior, authority to guide a student's development.

As compulsory education has progressed, struggles between the state and parents over the right to educational authority have established a system with some balance. While the voice of the individual student is limited, parents and the state hold established roles that complement each other, albeit contentiously. The state requires, enforces, and to some extent regulates education. However, parents hold the ability to choose from a limited range of alternative educational arrangements, providing the opportunity to educate their children in a manner compatible with their lifestyle or belief system. Thus, compulsory education laws have and continue to evolve toward a more democratic state of education in which all interested parties control a sphere of educational authority.

Methodology

This study was designed to investigate educational neglect along three different paths. Our research team simultaneously worked on a national policy review, an examination of the current state of educational neglect in a northwest state and nationwide, and an extensive literature review.

Results

Compulsory Education—A National Perspective

Compulsory education statutes mandate a range of ages during which a child must be educated. The age ranges vary from state to state. Beginning ages range from five to eight years old, while ending ages vary between 16 and 18 years old

Forty-eight of the 50 states require the local school district to report violations of compulsory education statutes. Mississippi relieves the local districts of this duty by locating primary reporting responsibility at the state level, while Hawaii only has one statewide district. When shifting focus from reporting to enforcing, a different grouping of 48 states locate primary responsibility within Departments of Education, while Kansas and North Carolina rely upon their Departments of Health and Human Services. However, all states allow exemptions to compulsory education requirements for a multiple of reasons, with medical exemptions constituting 62% of the states.

Educational Neglect—A National Perspective

Within the Third National Incidence Study of Child Abuse and Neglect (NIS-3) A. Sedlak and D. Broadhurst (*Third National Incidence Study of Child Abuse and Neglect.* Washington, DC: U.S. Department of Health and Human Services, 1996) offer a three part definition of educational neglect that includes failure to enroll, permitted chronic (habitual) truancy, and inattention to special education needs.

If identified, states vary in their treatment of educational neglect. Unfortunately, almost half of the states (48.0%) do not hold any agency responsible for reporting neglect. In other states, agencies responsible for reporting such neglect vary primarily between the local district (36.0%) and the local school (12.0%). A quarter of states rely on the court system to enforce educational neglect provisions, while 18.0% rely on the local district.

If a person is found guilty of educational neglect in one of the 26 states that pursue enforcement, penalties range from being undefined in Colorado and Kansas to a general misdemeanor charge with no clearly described penalty in 16 other states to jail time being imposed in Montana.

Habitual Truancy—A National Perspective

Truancy is any unexcused absence from school. Habitual truancy results when a child accumulates more unexcused absences than is allowed by the local authorities, either school, district, local prosecutor or state officials. Unfortunately, no common definition of habitual truancy exists. Eighty percent of the states define habitual truancy, while ten states fail to define it at the state level. Among those with definitions, the largest portion (36%) define according to some academic time marker, either absences per semester or academic year. Other states (16%) refer to absences per calendar period such as 90 days or one month. Some states (28%) simply refer to the state compulsory education statutes, which is problematic because of the generality of such statutes.

According to NIS-3 (Sedlak and Broadhurst, 1996), the effects of truancy are profound and carry a high cost for both the truant student and the larger society. Chief among these are:

- **Academic achievement:** Students with 95% attendance were more than twice as likely to pass state achievement tests than those with 85% attendance.

- **Drug use:** Truancy is a more accurate predictor of drug use than GPA or sexual activity.

- **Financial effect of dropouts:** Each dropout will lose between $535,800 and $855,000 in lifetime earnings.

- **Criminal effect of dropouts:** Dropouts comprise 80% of the prison population, which produces a significant fiscal burden upon state and federal funds.

Home-Based Education—A National Perspective

Home-based education or home schooling is a growing phenomenon within the United States. Home education is a way for parents to exert more influence in the education and development of their children. It constitutes one way in which the educational authority may be shared between the state and the parents. However, fifteen state departments of education do not report home-educated children in any manner. This greatly inflates the number of children unaccounted for within officially recognized, or accredited educational institutions.

A review of legal code and home schooling statutes paints a different picture than that gleaned from departments of education. According our review of the relevant statutes, only 12.0% or six states do not provide oversight of home educated students. Over half of the states report multiple levels of oversight. Another 18.0% of states require registration with either the local district (16.0%) or the state (2.0%).

Section 18.2

Truancy Prevention

"Truancy Prevention," National Center for Mental Health Promotion and Youth Violence Prevention, www.promoteprevent.org. © 2008 Education Development Center, Inc. All rights reserved. Reprinted with permission. The complete text of this document including references is available at http://www.promoteprevent.org/publications/prevention-briefs/truancy-prevention.

Compulsory school attendance is a reflection of the importance our nation places on education as well as a recognition that regular attendance is necessary if education is to effectively prepare a child for adulthood. Truancy and chronic absenteeism which are often stepping-stones to dropping-out of school before graduation have consequences for children, the adults these children will become, and the society in which they live. Truancy reduction programs that promote consistent attendance by addressing the underlying causes of truancy can also improve academic achievement while reducing problem behaviors, including substance abuse and delinquency.

Definitions and Extent of Truancy

Although the age at which children can legally leave school differs by state, every state requires that children attend school—or substitute an authorized equivalent, such as home schooling. These state mandates are accompanied by regulations describing how state education and juvenile justice agencies should respond to truancy. It should be noted that the number of days absent to be considered truant varies by jurisdiction. While the school often has first responsibility for responding to truancy (often in the form of a call to parents), truancy ultimately involves the possibility of action by juvenile or family courts, sometimes in the form of detention for the children and fines or jail for the parents (although the latter seems to be extremely unusual). The juvenile justice system usually only becomes involved in cases of "habitual truancy," which is usually defined in terms of a specific number of consecutive unexcused absences from school or a total number of unexcused absences over a semester or school year. The majority of students who meet this definition are probably not called before a judge or other court officer.

Reliable national or state data on truancy are difficult to find. State and district attendance records often do not differentiate truancy from excused absences. Schools sometimes do not, or cannot, take the time to ascertain whether an absence is excused or unexcused, creating a third category (sometimes called unverified absences). The No Child Left Behind (NCLB) Act requires states to report truancy rates by school beginning with the 2005–2006 school year. Attendance rates will also play a role in measuring whether a school has fulfilled NCLB Adequate Yearly Progress requirements. At the time of this writing (early 2007), NCLB attendance data are not yet available.

The attendance data that is available is incomplete.

- A study using data from a large national survey of drug use found that about 11 percent of eighth grade students and about 16 percent of tenth grade students reported having been truant at least once in the previous four weeks.

- Another national survey found that the percentage of students who did not go to school at least once during the 30 days prior to the survey because they felt unsafe rose from 4.4 percent in 1993 to 6 percent in 2005. These data do not indicate how many of these students were considered truant by their schools.

- A survey conducted in 1996–1997 found that principals considered tardiness, absenteeism, and class cutting, and physical conflicts to be the three most serious discipline issues in their schools.

While consistent definitions of truancy limit the ability to collect consistent, meaningful national data, some information is available on individual school districts. An unpublished study found that almost 20 percent of the students in Denver's public schools met the state definition of truant (that is, each had at least 10 unexcused absences during a single school year).

Consequences and Causes of Truancy

A review of the research literature review commissioned by the Office of Juvenile Justice and Delinquency Prevention (OJJDP) found correlates between truancy and four categories of risk factors:

1. Family factors (lack of supervision, poverty, alcohol or drug abuse, lack of awareness of attendance laws, attitude toward education)

2. School factors (school size, attitudes of students, staff, teachers, inflexibility toward meeting different learning styles, inconsistent procedures for dealing with chronic absenteeism)

3. Economic factors (employed students, single parent home, high mobility, parents with multiple jobs, lack of transportation)

4. Student factors (drug and alcohol abuse, lack of understanding of attendance laws, lack of social competence, mental and physical health problems)

The broad range of risk factors related to truancy has important implications for programs and activities (discussed below).

Truancy has a number of unfortunate consequences—not just for students, but for schools and communities. It is not surprising that truancy affects academic achievement. A National Center for School Engagement literature review found that truants have lower grades, need to repeat grades, drop out of school, are expelled from school, or just do not graduate from high school, at higher rates than students with fewer unexcused absences. The review reported that there is evidence that at least some schools and districts expel or otherwise "push out" students who are both truant and low-achieving. This removal can raise the school's overall level of academic achievement (as measured by grades, grade promotion, and graduation rates). The review also pointed out that some researchers claim that not enforcing truancy laws can be a form of classroom management, as students who are consistently truant sometimes have behavioral issues that disrupt classrooms, making it difficult for teachers to teach and other student to learn and causing administrators to spend time on disciplinary issues.

The research literature also concludes that truancy is a risk factor for other problems, including substance abuse, delinquency, gang activity, serious criminal behavior (such as car theft and burglary), and dropping out of school. Other research found that truancy itself can lead to (or reinforce existing) risk behaviors, given that children who are not in school are unsupervised and removed from the influence of positive peers and adults. There are a number of studies showing that effective truancy reduction programs can produce a marked decline in delinquency and crimes committed by school age youth.

The OJJDP literature review also concluded that truancy does not just effect young people but also the adults they will become. Adults who were chronically truant from school when young are at elevated risk for a host of problems, including poor physical and mental health, poverty and welfare, incarceration, and raising children who themselves exhibit problem behaviors.

Truancy has long-term economic consequences for both schools and communities. State aid is often distributed to schools or districts based on their average daily attendance. Truancy can thus affect a school's bottom line. Several municipalities have had remarkable success at increasing state aid to their school through truancy reduction programs. The use of attendance as an indicator of a school's effectiveness under NCLB has implications for the distribution of federal resources to schools and districts. And given that truancy is a risk factor for dropping out of school, it has a long-term effect on public finance. One study estimated that each individual who does not complete high school costs a lifetime average of $200,000 in public monies over and above similar costs for high school graduates. These excess public costs include lost tax revenues and the costs of social services and incarceration.

Traditional Approaches to Truancy Reduction

The most basic traditional response by schools to truancy was to call or meet with parents after students did not provide the proper documentation (the almost proverbial "note from home") after being absent. Some schools called parents if a child did not show up at school to make sure the student was not "playing hooky." Police departments would sometimes question students of school age who were found not in school during school hours, bringing them either home or to the school (a practice made more difficult in recent years by open campuses and the amount of serious crime requiring police attention).

In the past, schools often suspended or even expelled habitually truant students. Little thought was given to preventing truancy by means other than the threat of suspension—the logic of which went relatively unquestioned until the last decade. Suspending or expelling truants essentially rewards their desire to avoid school, causes them to fall behind in their school work, and does little to encourage more consistent attendance.

Schools can take habitual truants to juvenile or family court. Six hundred twenty-nine of every 1,000 truants petitioned to the courts are adjudicated as status offenders. (A status offense is an act that becomes an offense by virtue of the person's age. For example, it is illegal for minors to not be in school, buy alcohol, or run away from home. None of this is the case for adults.) Of the adjudicated youth, 491 are placed on probation, 65 are placed in group or foster homes, 55 receive other sanctions, and 17 are released. In many states, parents can be fined or jailed if their children are habitually truant, which has not proven effective. Parents are rarely called into court unless a young child is involved. Schools can be reluctant to file truancy petitions against children or parents because of the time school staff will need to spend in court. Police are similarly disinclined to initiate prosecution of children or their parents. Only 10 percent of the truancy cases formally handled by courts from 1985–2000 were referred by police departments.

There are good reasons why courts hesitate to jail parents or place children in foster care or detention for truancy. Removing the parent from the home (or the child from the school) can be counterproductive in terms of attendance. What evidence exists shows that the threat of such sanctions—and the sanctions themselves—do not reduce truancy. There is also no evidence that placing youth in detention deters truancy.

In the last two decades, school districts, juvenile and family courts, and police departments have begun to take more sophisticated approaches to truancy, approaches that seek to prevent rather than punish truancy, that question the logic of out-of-school suspensions, and that respond to all four categories of truancy-related risk factors (family, school, economic, and student factors). These new approaches are discussed below.

Effective Approaches to Truancy Reduction

The research indicates that truancy can be reduced by programs and activities designed to improve the overall school environment (and its safety), attach children and their families to the school, and enable schools to respond to the different learning styles and cultures of children. Children are less likely to avoid school if they feel safe, comfortable, cared-for, and engaged in a productive and rewarding activity (that is, effective education). The National Dropout Prevention Center/Network recommends the following strategies that fall into these categories as effective in reducing truancy:

- Systemic renewal
- School-community collaboration
- Safe learning environments
- Family engagement
- Early childhood education
- Early literacy development
- Mentoring/tutoring
- Service learning

- Alternative schooling
- After-school opportunities
- Professional development
- Active learning
- Educational technology
- Individualized instruction
- Career and technical education

The Northwest Regional Educational Laboratories adds a number of other programs and practices to this menu, including the following:

- Personalized learning
- Smaller schools or learning communities within schools (such as learning academies focused on particular topics, house plans, or magnet schools)
- Mentoring
- Student advisory programs
- Interventions targeted at improving educational effectiveness in the classroom

There are also interventions specifically designed to reduce truancy. These include the following types of activities and programs:

Attendance policies are school and district regulations concerning student attendance requirements, excused and unexcused absences, and the consequences for truancy. A review of the research on attendance policies reveals that the most effective attendance policies are those that promote attendance rather than punish absence (especially through out-of-school expulsion). Policies should be clear and consistent across the entire school district. Students, parents, and staff must understand these policies, and especially the difference between excused absences and truancy.

Early intervention programs identify students who have started skipping school and work with these children and their families before they become habitual truants. Early intervention programs might involve calling families after an unexplained absence, explaining the importance of consistent attendance at school, and helping them solve problems that might affect their child's presence in school (for example, transportation issues).

Some programs also seek to promote a pro-attendance culture in the school by, for example, rewarding students for consistent attendance, and holding events and campaigns that reinforce the importance of attendance. Some of these efforts also reach out to parents and the community through public education campaigns and events to create pro-attendance cultures in the family and community that reinforce that of the school.

Alternatives to adjudication for truancy allow students who are truant to avoid formal adjudication. Such alternatives include community truancy boards that negotiate contracts between schools and truant students (and their families) for more consistent attendance or peer or teen (youth) courts composed of other students (in some cases students who have had, and resolved, their own truancy issues). These contracts can include restrictions on student behavior (such as confining the student to the campus during lunch hours) as well as participation by the student and/or the family in specialized services when appropriate.

Court-based truancy reduction programs are based in juvenile or family courts, but attempt to provide services to truants and their families as an alternative to adjudication (while acknowledging the possibility of adjudication as a motivation for becoming involved with these services).

Alternative education programs are specifically for students whose truancy results from a divergence between the school's educational practices and individual student's learning styles. These might include occupational or career education programs or advanced courses in local community colleges, depending on student interest and ability. Some evaluation studies show that targeted truancy reduction programs can work. Given the limited evaluation data, it is difficult to determine exactly what type of truancy prevention program works best (and for whom). However, two recent reports provide an overview of the common elements of programs that effectively reduce truancy and promote school attendance. One found that effective strategies for increasing student attendance fell into four broad categories:

1. Sound and reasonable attendance policies with consequences for missing school

2. Early interventions, especially with elementary students and their families

3. Targeted interventions for students with chronic attendance problems

4. Strategies to increase engagement and personalization with students and families that can affect attendance rates: family involvement, culturally responsive culture, smaller learning community structures, mentoring, advisory programs, maximization and focus on learning time, and service learning

The second report identified critical components necessary for effective truancy prevention programs:

- Collaboration, including a broad-based multidisciplinary collaboration of the agencies and organizations whose involvement can affect truancy (such as schools, juvenile courts, and law enforcement agencies).

- Family involvement: True family involvement values parents "for their advice, experience, and expertise in the community, as clients of our public systems of care, and as experts in the lives of their children."

- Comprehensive approach: Effective programs address, either directly or through partnerships, all the factors that affect truancy, including transportation, mental health issues, academic issues, and school climate.

- Incentives and sanctions: Effective programs combine meaningful sanctions for truancy and meaningful incentives for attendance to change the behavior of students. For example, suspending students from school for truancy is not effective and does not promote pro-school attitudes among students.

- Supportive context: This context includes organizations, community cultures, and policies.

- Rigorous evaluation and assessment, including outcome data.

Both reviews provide evidence that effective truancy reduction programs are comprehensive and respond to the four categories of risk factors shown to be relevant to truancy (that is, family, school, economic, and student factors).

The Cost-Benefits of Reducing Truancy

Although the field of truancy reduction would benefit from more precise evaluation programs—especially evaluations clarifying the effectiveness of the individual components in multimodal programs—it has been the focus of some compelling cost-benefit analysis. Based on a fairly rigorous estimate that, over their lifetime, a person who drops out of high school costs the public more than $200,000 in excess criminal justice, social service, and health care costs, and that habitual truancy is a major risk factor for dropping out of school, one study calculated that two different multimodal truancy reduction programs paid for themselves (that is, saved more public money than it spends) if each prevented one student from dropping out every four years. A larger program in an urban area required successfully preventing four students per year from dropping out to pay for itself (in terms of public monies saved). All three programs had much better success rates than were required to break even (in terms of public expenditures versus public expenditures saved) and thus ultimately represented a savings to the taxpayers.

Chapter 19

Emotional Abuse of Children

Chapter Contents

Section 19.1

Indicators of Emotional Abuse

Emotional abuse is a pattern of behavior that attacks a child's emotional development and sense of self-worth. Emotional abuse includes excessive, aggressive, or unreasonable demands that place expectations on a child beyond his or her capacity. Constant criticizing, belittling, insulting, rejecting, and teasing are some of the forms these verbal attacks can take. Emotional abuse also includes failure to provide the psychological nurturing necessary for a child's psychological growth and development—providing no love, support, or guidance (National Committee for the Prevention of Child Abuse, 1987).

Please note: Any one of these indicators could be attributable to a specific life event or other trauma. A pattern of behavior is the strongest indicator of abuse and should not be ignored.

Observable Indicators

- Child rocks, sucks, bites self
- Inappropriately aggressive
- Destructive to others
- Suffers from sleep, speech disorders
- Restricts play activities or experiences
- Demonstrates compulsions, obsessions, phobias, hysterical outbursts

Behavioral Indicators in Child

- Negative statements about self
- Shy, passive, compliant
- Lags in physical, mental, and emotional development

- Self-destructive behavior
- Highly aggressive
- Cruel to others
- Overly demanding

Family or Parental Indicators

- Blames or puts down child
- Is cold and rejecting
- Indifferent to child's problems or welfare
- Withholds affection
- Shows preferential treatment when there is more than one child in the family

Emotional abuse is an evolving part of the child abuse field. It is rarely recognized by Child Welfare systems and interventions are few. But the impact is profound and this is an area of child abuse that should be called to light and interventions for children experiencing emotional abuse need to be provided.

Section 19.2

The Nature and Consequences of Emotional Abuse

Definition of Child Emotional Abuse

The emotional abuse of children has been difficult to define, and state definitions vary considerably. The following behaviors, however, characterize what many agree constitutes forms of emotional abuse:

- **Rejecting:** The caregiver refuses to acknowledge the child's worth and the legitimacy of the child's needs.

- **Isolating:** The adult cuts the child off from normal social experiences, prevents the child from forming friendships, and makes the child believe that he or she is alone in the world.

- **Terrorizing:** The adult creates a climate of fear, bullies and frightens the child, and makes the child believe that the world is capricious and hostile.

- **Ignoring:** The adult deprives the child of essential stimulation and responsiveness.

- **Corrupting:** The adult encourages the child to engage in destructive and antisocial behavior, reinforces deviance, and impairs a child's ability to behave in socially appropriate ways.

- **Verbally assaulting:** The adult humiliates the child with repeated name-calling, harsh threats, and sarcasm that continually "beat down" the child's self-esteem.

- **Overpressuring:** The adult imposes extreme pressure upon the child to behave and achieve in ways that are far beyond the child's capabilities.

Some states also recognize excessively harsh discipline and exposure of children to family violence as child emotional abuse.

Scope of Child Emotional Abuse

In 2008, approximately 55,196 children (7.3 percent of all substantiated cases of child maltreatment) were officially counted as victims of child emotional abuse. Given the difficulties defining the emotional abuse of children, we lack good ways to measure this problem. Its scope remains uncertain, although many sense that it is quite prevalent.

Nature of Child Emotional Abuse

There is no single cause of emotional abuse. Instead, there are usually multiple and interacting contributors at the levels of the child, parent, family, community, and society. Examples of contributors include a child with a disability, a parent struggling with depression or substance abuse, intimate partner violence, a father who is not involved in their child's life, a lack of community supports (for example, affordable child care), the burdens associated with poverty, and inadequate policies to support families and parents. These characteristics greatly contribute to the intractability of the problem. Combinations of such problems may impair a parent's ability to ensure his or her child's needs are adequately met.

It is apparent that other forms of maltreatment, physical and sexual abuse as well as neglect, may in different ways be emotionally abusive. Indeed, long after bruises have faded and fractures healed, the emotional scars may be long lasting.

Consequences of Child Emotional Abuse

The consequences of child emotional abuse can be devastating and long-lasting, and include: increased risk for a lifelong pattern of depression, estrangement, anxiety, low self-esteem, inappropriate or troubled relationships, or a lack of empathy. During their childhood, victims may experience a delay in their developmental progress. Research also indicates that emotional abuse may be a stronger predictor of psychological, emotional, and behavioral impairments and trauma than accompanying physical abuse.

It is clear that the consequences of child emotional abuse extend far beyond the affected children and families. Enormous societal costs are involved. Prevent Child Abuse America estimated the economic impact of child abuse and neglect at $104 billion in 2007; and this was likely a conservative estimate. Thus, in addition to the compelling human argument to help optimize children's development, health and safety, there is also a financial impetus to help prevent the neglect of children. The aphorism that "our children are our nation's most valuable resource" should be more than a slogan. Finally, at the heart of child neglect is a concern with their basic rights, their human rights.

The costs associated with the pervasive and long-lasting effects of child abuse and neglect are as undeniable as our obligation to prevent—not just respond to—this problem. In 2007, $33 billion in direct costs for foster care services, hospitalization, mental health treatment, and law enforcement were supplemented by over $70 billion in indirect costs like loss of individual productivity, chronic health problems, special education, and delinquent and criminal justice services.

For more information contact Prevent Child Abuse America at 312-663-3520 or at mailbox@preventchildabuse.org.

Chapter 20

Technology and Abuse

Chapter Contents

Section 20.1

Electronic Devices and Aggression

Excerpted from: Hertz MF, David-Ferdon C. "Electronic Media and Youth Violence: A CDC Issue Brief for Educators and Caregivers." Atlanta (GA): Centers for Disease Control; 2008. The complete text of this document, including references, can be found online at http://www.cdc.gov/violenceprevention/pdf/EA-brief-a.pdf. Revised by David A. Cooke, MD, FACP, January 2013.

Overview

Technology and adolescents seem destined for each other; both are young, fast paced, and ever changing. In previous generations teens readily embraced new technologies, such as record players, TVs, cassette players, computers, and VCRs, but the past two decades have witnessed a virtual explosion in new technology, including cell phones, iPods, MP-3s, DVDs, and smartphones. This new technology has been eagerly embraced by adolescents and has led to an expanded vocabulary, including instant messaging ("IMing"), blogging, and text messaging. New technology has many social and educational benefits, but caregivers and educators have expressed concern about the dangers young people can be exposed to through these technologies. To respond to this concern, some states and school districts have, for example, established policies about the use of cell phones on school grounds and developed policies to block access to certain websites on school computers. Many teachers and caregivers have taken action individually by spot-checking websites used by young people, such as Facebook. This section focuses on the phenomena of electronic aggression: any kind of aggression perpetrated through technology—any type of harassment or bullying (teasing, telling lies, making fun of someone, making rude or mean comments, spreading rumors, or making threatening or aggressive comments) that occurs through e-mail, a chat room, instant messaging, a website (including blogs), or text messaging.

Caregivers, educators, and other adults who work with young people know that children and adolescents spend a lot of time using electronic media (blogs, instant messaging, chat rooms, e-mail, text messaging). What is not known is exactly how and how often they use different types of technology. Could use of technology increase the likelihood that a young person is the victim of aggression? If the answer is yes, what should caregivers and educators do to help young people protect themselves? To help answer these questions, the Centers for Disease Control and Prevention, Division of Adolescent and School Health and Division of Violence Prevention, held an expert panel on September 20-21, 2006, in Atlanta, Georgia, entitled "Electronic Media and Youth Violence." There were 13 panelists, who came from academic institutions, federal agencies, a school system, and nonprofit organizations who were already engaged in work focusing on electronic media and youth violence. The panelists presented information about if, how, and how often technology is used by young people to behave aggressively. They also presented information about the qualities that make a young person more or less likely to be victimized or to behave aggressively toward someone else electronically.

Two documents were developed to summarize the presentations and the discussion that followed. One of the documents was developed for researchers to summarize the data, to highlight the research gaps, and to suggest future topics for research to better understand the growing problem of electronic media and youth violence. The other document (this document) was developed for educators and caregivers and summarizes what is known about young people and electronic aggression and discusses the implications of these findings for school staff, educational policy makers, and caregivers.

The expert panel highlighted the fact that a variety of terms are being used to describe and measure this new form of aggression including: internet bullying, internet harassment, and cyberbullying. Accordingly, when specific results from any study or group of studies are discussed, this document uses the wording the researcher used. So, for example, if a researcher surveyed young people and asked about "cyberbullying," when that information is discussed, the term "cyberbullying" is used. In general discussion sections, the phrase "electronic aggression" is used to refer to any kind of aggression perpetrated through technology. Each panelist also expanded upon his or her panel presentation in individual articles. These articles are compiled in the *Journal of Adolescent Health*, Volume 41, Issue 6 and contain more detailed information than what is provided below.

The information presented in this document is based upon what is currently known; we still have a lot to learn about electronic aggression. The research findings described here need to be repeated and validated by other researchers and the possible action steps for educators, educational policy makers, and caregivers need to be evaluated for effectiveness.

How Common Is Electronic Aggression?

Because electronic aggression is fairly new, limited information is available, and those researching the topic have asked different questions about it. Thus, information cannot be readily compared or combined across studies, which limits our ability to make definitive conclusions about the prevalence and impact of electronic aggression.

What we know about electronic aggression is based upon a few studies that measure similar but not exactly the same behaviors. For example, in their studies, some of the panelists use a narrow definition of electronic aggression (e.g., aggression perpetrated through e-mail or instant messaging), while others use a broader definition (e.g., aggression perpetrated through e-mail, instant messaging, on a website, or through text messaging). In addition to different definitions, in their research the panelists also asked young people to report about their experiences over different time periods (e.g., over the past several months, since the beginning of school, in the past year), and surveyed youth of different ages (e.g., 6th–8th-graders, 10–15-year-olds, 10–17-year-olds). As a result, the most accurate way to describe the information we have is to give ranges that include the findings from all of the studies.

We know that most youth (65–91%) report little or no involvement in electronic aggression. However, 9% to 35% of young people say they have been the victim of electronic aggression. As with face-to-face bullying, estimates of electronic aggression perpetration are lower than victimization, ranging from 4% to 21%. In some cases, the higher end of the range (e.g., 21% and 35%) reflects studies that asked about electronic aggression over a longer time period (e.g., a year as opposed to two months). In other cases, the higher percentages reflect studies that defined electronic aggression more broadly (e.g., spreading rumors, telling lies, or making threats as opposed to just telling lies).

When we look at data across all of the panelists' studies, the percentage of young people who report being electronic aggression victims has a fairly wide range (9–35%). However, if we look at victimization over a similar time frame, such as "monthly or more often" or "at least once in the past two months," the range is much narrower, from 8% to 11%.

Similarly, although the percentage of young people who admit they perpetrate electronic aggression varies considerably across studies (4–21%), the range narrows if we look at similar time periods. Approximately 4% of surveyed youth report behaving aggressively electronically "monthly or more often" or "at least once in the past two months."

We currently know little about whether certain types of electronic aggression are more common than other forms. A study that looked at electronic aggression victimization "over the past year," found that making rude or nasty comments was the type of electronic aggression most frequently experienced by victims (32%), followed by rumor spreading (13%), and then by threatening or aggressive comments (14%).

Who Is At Risk?

Whether the rates of electronic aggression perpetration and victimization differ for boys and girls is unknown. Research examining differences by sex is limited, and findings are conflicting. Some studies have not found any differences, while others have found that girls perpetrate electronic aggression more frequently than do boys.

There is also little information about whether electronic aggression decreases or increases as young people age. As with other forms of aggression, there is some evidence that electronic aggression is less common in 5th grade than in 8th- grade, but is higher in 8th grade than 11th grade, suggesting that electronic aggression may peak around the end of middle school/beginning of high school.

Current studies on electronic aggression have focused primarily on white populations. We have no information on how electronic aggression varies by race or ethnicity. It is important to note that there is an overlap between victims and perpetrators of electronic aggression. As with many types of violence, those who are victims are also at increased risk for being perpetrators. Across the studies conducted by our panelists, between 7% and 14% of surveyed youth reported being both a victim and a perpetrator of electronic aggression.

Although the news media has recently devoted a lot of attention to the potential dangers of technology, face-to-face verbal and physical aggression are still far more common than electronic aggression. Verbal bullying is the type of bullying most often experienced by young people, followed by physical bullying, and then by electronic aggression. However, electronic aggression is becoming more common. In 2000, 6% of internet users ages 10–17 said they had been the victim of "on-line harassment," defined as threats or other offensive behavior [not sexual solicitation] sent on-line to someone or posted on-line. By 2005, this percentage had increased by 50%, to 9%. As technology becomes more affordable and sophisticated, rates of electronic aggression are likely to continue to increase, especially if appropriate prevention and intervention policies and practices are not put into place.

271

What Is the Relationship between Victims and Perpetrators of Electronic Aggression?

Electronic technology allows adolescents to hide their identity, either by sending or posting messages anonymously, by using a false name, or by assuming someone else's on-screen identity. So, unlike the aggression or bullying that occurs in the school-yard, victims and perpetrators of electronic aggression may not know the person with whom they are interacting. Between 13% and 46% of young people who were victims of electronic aggression report not knowing their harasser's identity. Similarly, 22% of young people who admit they perpetrate electronic aggression report they do not know the identity of their victim. In the school-yard, the victim can respond to the bully or try to get a teacher or peer to help. In contrast, in the electronic world a victim is often alone when responding to aggressive e-mails or text messages, and his or her only defense may be to turn off the computer or smartphone. If the electronic aggression takes the form of posting of a message or an embarrassing picture of the victim on a public website, the victim may have no defense.

As for the victims and perpetrators who are not anonymous, in one study, almost half of the victims (47%) said the perpetrator was another student at school. In addition, aggression between siblings is no longer limited to the backseat of the car: 12% of victims reported their brother or sister was the perpetrator, and 10% of perpetrators reported being electronically aggressive toward a sibling.

Do Certain Types of Electronic Technology Pose a Greater Risk for Victimization?

The news media often carry stories about young people victimized on social networking websites. Young people do experience electronic aggression in chat rooms: 25% of victims of electronic aggression said the victimization happened in a chat room and 23% said it happened on a website. However, instant messaging appears to be the most common way electronic aggression is perpetrated. Fifty-six percent of perpetrators of electronic aggression and 67% of victims said the aggression they experienced or perpetrated was through instant messaging. Victims also report experiencing electronic aggression through e-mail (25%) and text messages (16%).

The way electronic aggression is perpetrated (for example, through instant messaging, the posting of pictures on a website, sending an e-mail) is also related to the relationship between the victim and the perpetrator. Victims are significantly more likely to report receiving an aggressive instant message when they know the perpetrator from in-person situations (64% of victims), than they are if they only know the perpetrator on-line (34%). Young people who are victimized by people they only know on-line are significantly more likely than those victimized by people they know from in-person situations to be victimized through e-mail (18% vs. 5%), chat rooms (18% vs. 4%), and on-line gaming websites (14% vs. 0%).

In terms of frequency, electronic aggression perpetrated by young people who know each other in-person appears to be more similar to face-to-face bullying than does aggression perpetrated by young people who only know each other on-line. For example, like in-person bullying, electronic aggression between young people who know each other in-person is more likely to consist of a series of incidents. Fifty-nine percent of the incidents perpetrated by young people who knew each other in-person involved a series of incidents by the same harasser, compared to 27% of incidents perpetrated by on-line-only contacts. In addition, 59% of the incidents perpetrated by young people who knew each other in-person involved sending or posting messages for others to see, versus 18% of those perpetrated by young people the victims only knew on-line.

What Problems Are Associated with Being a Victim of Electronic Aggression?

We are just beginning to look at the impact of being a victim of electronic aggression. At this point, we do not have information that shows that being a victim of electronic aggression causes a young person to have problems. However, the information we do have suggests that, as with young people who experience face-to-face aggression, those who are victims of electronic aggression are more likely to have some difficulties than those who are not victimized.

For example, young people who are victims of internet harassment are significantly more likely than those who have not been victimized to use alcohol and other drugs, receive school detention or suspension, skip school, or experience in-person victimization. Victims of internet harassment are also more likely than non-victims to have poor parental monitoring and to have weak emotional bonds with their caregiver. Although these difficulties could be the result of electronic victimization, they could also be factors that increase the risk of electronic victimization (but do not result from it), or they could be related to something else entirely. At this point, the risk factors for victimization through technology and the impact of victimization need further study.

Some research does show that the level of emotional distress experienced by a victim is related to the relationship between the victim and perpetrator and the frequency of the aggression. Young people who were bullied by the same person both on-line and off-line were more likely to report being distressed by the incident (46%) than were those who reported being bullied by different people on-line and off-line (15%), and those who did not know who was harassing them on-line (18%). Victims who were harassed by on-line peers and did not know their perpetrator in off-line settings also experienced distress, but they were more likely to experience distress if the harassment was perpetrated by the same person repeatedly (as opposed to a single incident), if the harasser was aged 18 or older, or if the harasser asked for a picture.

Finally, distress may not be limited to the young person who is victimized. Caregivers who are aware that their adolescent has been a victim of electronic aggression can also experience distress. Caregivers report that sometimes they are even more fearful, frustrated, and angry about the incidents of electronic aggression than are the young victims.

What Are the Problems Associated with Being a Perpetrator of Electronic Aggression?

Consistent with the discussion of victimization, we have limited information about what increases or decreases the chance that an adolescent will become a perpetrator of electronic aggression. One study suggests that young people who say they are connected to their school, perceive their school as trusting, fair and pleasant, and believe their friends are trustworthy, caring, and helpful are less likely to report being perpetrators of electronic, physical, and verbal aggression. We also have some evidence that perpetrators of electronic aggression are more likely to engage in other risky behaviors. For example, like perpetrators of other forms of aggression, perpetrators of electronic aggression are more likely to believe that bullying peers and encouraging others to bully peers are acceptable behaviors. Additionally, young people who report perpetrating electronic aggression are more likely to also report perpetrating face-to-face aggression.

Is Electronic Aggression Just An Extension of School-Yard Bullying?

Are the kids who are victims of electronic aggression the same kids who are victims of face-to-face aggression at school? Is electronic aggression just an extension of school-yard bullying? The information we currently have suggests that the answer to the first question is "maybe," and the answer to the second question is "no." One study found that 65% of young people who reported being a victim of electronic aggression were not victimized at school. Conversely, another study found considerable overlap between electronic aggression and in-person bullying, either as victims or perpetrators. The study found few young people (6%) who were victims or perpetrators of electronic bullying were not bullied in-person.

Evidence that electronic aggression is not just an extension of school-yard bullying comes from information from young people who are home-schooled. If electronic aggression was just an extension of school-yard bullying, the rates of electronic aggression would be lower for those who are home-schooled than for those who attend public or private school. However, the rates of internet harassment for young people who are home-schooled and the rates for those who attend public and private schools are fairly similar.

The vast majority of electronic aggression appears to be experienced and perpetrated away from school grounds. Discussions with middle and high school students suggest that most electronic aggression occurs away from school property and during off-school hours, with the exception of electronic aggression perpetrated by text messaging using cell phones. Schools appear to be a less common setting because of the amount of structured activities during the school day and because of the limited access to technology during the school day for activities other than school work. Additionally, because other teens are less likely to be, for instance, on social-networking websites during school hours, the draw to such websites during the day is limited. Even when electronic aggression does occur at school, victimized students report that they are very reluctant to seek help because, in many cases, they would have to disclose that they violated school policies that often prohibit specific types of technology use (for example, cell phones, social networking websites) during the school day.

Whether electronic aggression occurs at home or at school, it has implications for the school and needs further exploration. As was previously mentioned, young people who were harassed on-line were more likely to get a detention or be suspended, to skip school, and to experience emotional distress than those who were not harassed. In addition, young people who receive rude or nasty comments via text messaging are significantly more likely to report feeling unsafe at school.

What Can We Do?

A common response to the problem of electronic aggression is to use "blocking software" to prevent young people from accessing certain websites. There are several limitations with this type of response, especially when the blocking software is the only option that is pursued. First, young people are also victimized via cell-phone text messaging, and blocking software will not prevent this type of victimization. Second, middle and high school students have indicated that blocking software at school is limited because many students can navigate their way around this software and because most students do not attempt to access social networking websites during the school day. Students can also access sites that may be blocked on home and school computers from another location. Finally, blocking software may limit some of the benefits young people experience from new technology including social networking websites. For instance, the growth of internet and cellular technology allows young people to have access to greater amounts of information, to stay connected with family and established friends, and to connect and learn from people worldwide. Additionally, some young people report that they feel better about themselves on-line than they do in the real world and feel it is easier to be accepted on-line. Thus, while blocking software may be one important tool that caregivers and schools choose to use, the panel emphasized the need for comprehensive solutions. For example, a combination of blocking software, educational classes about appropriate electronic behavior for students and parents, and regular communication between adults and young people about their experiences with technology would be preferable to any one of these strategies in isolation.

What Are the Steps from Here?

Areas for further consideration that were developed by the panel for educators, educational policy makers, and parents/caregivers are detailed below. None of these areas has been tested to determine if it is effective in reducing the occurrence or negative impact of electronic aggression. Regardless, given what is known about other types of youth violence and the information currently available about electronic aggression and other forms of aggression, these are the panel's suggestions for areas educators and caregivers may want to consider as they address the issue of electronic aggression with young people.

Educators/Educational Policy Makers

1. Explore current bullying prevention policies.

Examine current policies related to bullying and/or youth violence to see whether they need to be modified to reflect electronic aggression. If no policies currently exist, examine examples of other state, district, or school policies to see whether they might meet the needs of your population. For information about existing laws on bullying and on harassment, see http://www.nasbe.org/index.php/prjects-separator/shs/healthpolicies-database.

2. Work collaboratively to develop policies.

States, school districts, and boards of education must work in conjunction with attorneys to develop policies that protect the rights of all students and also meet the needs of the state or district and those it serves. In addition, it is also helpful to involve representatives from the student body, students' families, and community members in the development of the policy. The policy should also be based upon evidence from research and on best practices. Developers of policies related to electronic aggression may want to consider following the general outline of steps proposed by the CDC's School Health Guidelines and the expert panelists that are summarized and bulleted below. Although research specifically regarding electronic aggression is limited, the little that exists should be incorporated into policy (see the *Journal of Adolescent Health*, Volume 41, Issue 6 for some of the latest work).

- Include a strong opening statement on the importance of creating a climate that demonstrates respect, support, and caring and that does not tolerate harassment or bullying.

- Be comprehensive and recognize the responsibilities of educators, law enforcement, caregivers, students, and the technology and entertainment industries in preventing electronic aggression from affecting students and the school climate.

- Focus on increasing positive behaviors and skills, such as problem-solving and social competence by students.

- Emphasize that socially appropriate electronic behaviors should be exemplified by faculty and staff members.

- Identify specific people and organizations responsible for implementing, enforcing, and evaluating the impact of the policy. Without accountability, a policy is likely to have a limited impact. For the policy to serve as a deterrent for aggression, it should be clearly communicated to young people, and the consequences of violating it should be clear and concise. These guidelines also serve to provide a framework for the enforcing agency.

- Explicitly describe codes of electronic conduct for all members of the school community, focusing on acceptable behaviors but also including rules prohibiting unsafe or aggressive behavior.

- Explain the consequences for breaking rules and provide for due process for those identified as breaking the rules.

Unfortunately, the work does not end when the policy is approved by policy makers. In order for the policy to be effective, widespread dissemination is critical. Dissemination plans should be developed and include specific strategies to educate students, families, and community members (including law enforcement) about the school policy. In addition, policies should be re-evaluated and modified as more research becomes available. A mechanism for evaluating the impact of the policy should be included in the policy language. Many educational policies have been implemented throughout the years, but only a few have been rigorously evaluated. Districts may be paying a high cost to implement policies that may not be effective. Evaluation is critical because it determines whether the policy is actually protecting students and whether it is cost-effective. Also, data from evaluations can be very useful in justifying ongoing or expanded funding and for modifying policies to make them more effective.

3. Explore current programs to prevent bullying and youth violence.

From a programming perspective, schools and districts should explore many of the evidence-based programs for the prevention of bullying and youth violence that are currently in the field; see "Best Practices in Youth Violence Prevention," the National Youth Violence Prevention Resource Center (www.safeyouth.org), and "The Effectiveness of Universal School-Based Programs for the Prevention of Violent and Aggressive Behavior," (http://www.cdc.gov/mmwr/preview/mmwrhtml/rr5607a1.htm for more information. Many of the programs developed to prevent face-to-face aggression address topics (such as school climate and peer influences) that are likely to be important for preventing electronic aggression.

4. Offer training on electronic aggression for educators and administrators.

The training should include the definition of electronic aggression, characteristics of victims and perpetrators, related school or district policies, information about recent incidents of electronic violence in the district, and resources available to educators and caregivers if they have concerns. The training could also include information about the school's legal responsibility for intervention and investigation. Finally, the training should emphasize to staff that even if they are not technologically savvy, they can have a positive impact on electronic aggression. Students who perceive that teachers are willing to intervene in instances of electronic aggression are less likely to perpetrate—so teacher attitude and response matter.

5. Talk to teens.

While it may be difficult to have individual conversations with all students, providing young people opportunities to discuss their concerns through, for example, creative writing assignments, is an excellent way to begin a classroom dialogue about using electronic media safely and about the impact and consequences of inappropriate use. In addition, technology safety could easily be integrated into the standard health education curricula. In addition, the fascination and skill of young people with electronic media should not be ignored: educators and researchers should explore with adolescents how electronic media can be used as tools to prevent electronic aggression and other adolescent health problems.

6. Work with IT and support staff.

Frequently, classroom teachers are aware of electronic aggression, but this information is not passed on to information technology (IT) services staff. Administrators must create the infrastructure and support necessary for classroom teachers to work with IT staff to keep abreast of issues affecting young people and develop strategies to minimize risk.

7. Create a positive school atmosphere.

Research indicates that students who feel connected to their school, who think their teachers care about them and are fair, and who think the school rules are clear and fair are less likely to perpetrate any type of violence or aggression, including electronic aggression.

8. Have a plan in place for what should happen if an incident is brought to the attention of school officials.

Rather than waiting for a problem to arise, educators and families need to be proactive in developing a thoughtful plan to address problems and concerns that are brought to their attention. Having a system in place may make young people more likely to come forward with concerns and may support the appropriate handling of a situation when it arises. Educators and families should develop techniques for prevention and intervention that do not punish victims for coming forward but instead create an atmosphere that encourages a dialogue between educators and young people and between families and young people about their electronic experiences.

Considerations for Parents/Caregivers

Young people spend a good portion of their day in school, but the most influential people in their lives are their caregivers; peers are a very close second, but caregivers are still first.

1. Talk to your child.

One of the expert panelists insightfully described the challenge facing adults who are trying to communicate with young people about technology: "The problem is that adults view the internet as a mechanism to find information. Young people view the internet as a place. Caregivers are encouraged to ask their children where they are going and who they are going with whenever they leave the house. They should take the same approach when their child goes on the internet—where are they going and who are they with?" Young people are sometimes reluctant to disclose victimization for fear of having their internet and cellular phone privileges revoked. Parents/ caregivers should talk with their teens to come up with a solution to prevent or address victimization that does not punish the teen for his or her victimization.

2. Develop rules.

Together with your child, develop rules about acceptable and safe behavior for all the electronic media they use and what they should do if they become a victim of electronic aggression or they witness or know about another teen being victimized.

3. Explore the internet.

Once you have talked to your child and discovered which websites he/she frequents, visit them yourself. This will help you understand where your child has "been" when he/she visits the website and will help you understand the pros and cons of the various websites. Remember that most websites and on-line activities are beneficial. They help young people learn new information, interact with and learn about people from diverse backgrounds, and express themselves to others who may have similar thoughts and experiences. Technology is not going away, so forbidding young people to access electronic media may not be a good long-term solution. Together, parents and youth can come up with ways to maximize the benefits of technology and decrease its risks.

4. Talk with other parents / caregivers.

Talk to others about how they have discussed technology use with their teens, the rules they have developed, and how they stay informed about their child's technology use. Others can comment on strategies they used effectively and those that did not work very well.

5. Encourage your school or school district to conduct a class for caregivers about electronic aggression.

The class should include a review of school or district policies on the topic, recent incidents in the community, and resources available to caregivers who have concerns.

6. Keep current.

Technology changes rapidly, and so it is important to keep current on what new devices and features your child is using, and in what ways. Many developers of new products offer information and classes to keep people aware of advances. Additionally, existing internet websites change, and new internet websites develop all the time, so continually talk with your teen about "where they are going" and explore these websites yourself. Your adolescent may also be an important resource for information, and having your teen educate you may help strengthen parent-child communication and bonding, which is important for other adolescent health issues as well.

Final Thoughts

Educators, teens, and caregivers are far ahead of researchers in identifying trends in electronic aggression and bringing attention to potential causes and solutions. Adolescents, their families, and the school community have known for several years that electronic aggression is a problem, but researchers have only recently begun to examine this issue. Creating a stronger partnership between schools, caregivers, and researchers would strengthen the activities of all invested persons. However, until research catches up with those "on the front lines," the best advice seems to be: do not rely on just one strategy to prevent your child from becoming a victim or a perpetrator. Although blocking software might be one strategy, especially for younger children, blocking is not likely to be effective without talking—caregivers and young people need to talk to each other on an ongoing basis. We do not discourage young people from going to school because of the potential for in-person bullying. Likewise, we should not discourage young people from using technology because of a fear of electronic aggression. We should work together to draw attention to bullying, in all forms, when it does occur, and figure out how to apply the lessons learned from school-yard bullying to electronic aggression. We send our children out into the world every day to explore and learn, and we hope that they will approach a trusted adult if they encounter a challenge; now, we need to apply this message to the virtual world.

Section 20.2

What Is Cyberbullying?

From "What Is Cyberbullying?" "Prevent Cyberbullying," and
"Report Cyberbullying," U.S. Department of Health and Human
Services (www.stopbullying.gov), April 2012.

What Is Cyberbullying?

Cyberbullying is bullying that takes place using electronic technology. Electronic technology includes devices and equipment such as cell phones, computers, and tablets as well as communication tools, including social media sites, text messages, chat, and websites.

Examples of cyberbullying include mean text messages or e-mails, rumors sent by e-mail or posted on social networking sites, and embarrassing pictures, videos, websites, or fake profiles.

Why Cyberbullying Is Different

Kids who are being cyberbullied are often bullied in person as well. Additionally, kids who are cyberbullied have a harder time getting away from the behavior.

- Cyberbullying can happen 24 hours a day, seven days a week, and reach a kid even when he or she is alone. It can happen any time of the day or night.

- Cyberbullying messages and images can be posted anonymously and distributed quickly to a very wide audience. It can be difficult and sometimes impossible to trace the source.

- Deleting inappropriate or harassing messages, texts, and pictures is extremely difficult after they have been posted or sent.

Effects of Cyberbullying

Cell phones and computers themselves are not to blame for cyberbullying. Social media sites can be used for positive activities, like connecting kids with friends and family, helping students with school, and for entertainment. But these tools can also be used to hurt other people. Whether done in person or through technology, the effects of bullying are similar.

Kids who are cyberbullied are more likely to have these problems:

- Use alcohol and drugs

- Skip school

- Experience in-person bullying

- Be unwilling to attend school

- Receive poor grades

- Have lower self-esteem

- Have more health problems

Frequency of Cyberbullying

The 2008–2009 *School Crime Supplement* (National Center for Education Statistics and Bureau of Justice Statistics) indicates that 6% of students in grades 6–12 experienced cyberbullying.

The 2011 *Youth Risk Behavior Surveillance Survey* finds that 16% of high school students (grades 9–12) were electronically bullied in the past year.

Research on cyberbullying is growing. However, because kids' technology use changes rapidly, it is difficult to design surveys that accurately capture trends.

Prevent Cyberbullying

Parents and kids can prevent cyberbullying. Together, they can explore safe ways to use technology.

Be Aware of What Your Kids are Doing Online

Talk with your kids about cyberbullying and other online issues regularly.

- Know the sites your kids visit and their online activities. Ask where they're going, what they're doing, and who they're doing it with.

- Tell your kids that as a responsible parent you may review their online communications if you think there is reason for concern. Installing parental control filtering software or monitoring programs are one option for monitoring your child's online behavior, but do not rely solely on these tools.

- Have a sense of what they do online and in texts. Learn about the sites they like. Try out the devices they use.

- Ask for their passwords, but tell them you'll only use them in case of emergency.

- Ask to "friend" or "follow" your kids on social media sites or ask another trusted adult to do so.

- Encourage your kids to tell you immediately if they, or someone they know, is being cyberbullied. Explain that you will not take away their computers or cell phones if they confide in you about a problem they are having.

Establish Rules about Technology Use

Establish rules about appropriate use of computers, cell phones, and other technology. For example, be clear about what sites they can visit and what they are permitted to do when they're online. Show them how to be safe online.

Help them be smart about what they post or say. Tell them not to share anything that could hurt or embarrass themselves or others. Once something is posted, it is out of their control whether someone else will forward it.

Encourage kids to think about who they want to see the information and pictures they post online. Should complete strangers see it? Real friends only? Friends of friends? Think about how people who aren't friends could use it.

Tell kids to keep their passwords safe and not share them with friends. Sharing passwords can compromise their control over their online identities and activities.

Understand School Rules

Some schools have developed policies on uses of technology that may affect the child's online behavior in and out of the classroom. Ask the school if they have developed a policy.

Report Cyberbullying

When cyberbullying happens, it is important to document and report the behavior so it can be addressed.

Steps to Take Immediately

- Don't respond to and don't forward cyberbullying messages.

- Keep evidence of cyberbullying. Record the dates, times, and descriptions of instances when cyberbullying has occurred. Save and print screenshots, e-mails, and text messages. Use this evidence to report cyberbullying to web and cell phone service providers.

- Block the person who is cyberbullying.

Report Cyberbullying to Online Service Providers

Cyberbullying often violates the terms of service established by social media sites and internet service providers.

- Review their terms and conditions or rights and responsibilities sections. These describe content that is or is not appropriate.

- Visit social media safety centers to learn how to block users and change settings to control who can contact you.

- Report cyberbullying to the social media site so they can take action against users abusing the terms of service.

Report Cyberbullying to Law Enforcement

When cyberbullying involves these activities it is considered a crime and should be reported to law enforcement:

- Threats of violence

- Child pornography or sending sexually explicit messages or photos

- Taking a photo or video of someone in a place where he or she would expect privacy

- Stalking and hate crimes

Some states consider other forms of cyberbullying criminal. Consult your state's laws and law enforcement for additional guidance.

Report Cyberbullying to Schools

- Cyberbullying can create a disruptive environment at school and is often related to in-person bullying. The school can use the information to help inform prevention and response strategies.

286

- In many states, schools are required to address cyberbullying in their anti-bullying policy. Some state laws also cover off-campus behavior that creates a hostile school environment.

Section 20.3

Protecting Kids from Technology-Related Abuse

From "Protect Your Kids Online: Talk to Your Kids, Kids and Socializing Online, and Kids and Mobile Phones," Federal Trade Commission (www.onguardonline.gov), September 2011.

Talk to Your Kids

When your kids begin socializing online, you may want to talk to them about certain risks:

- **Inappropriate conduct:** The online world can feel anonymous. Kids sometimes forget that they are still accountable for their actions.

- **Inappropriate contact:** Some people online have bad intentions, including bullies, predators, hackers, and scammers.

- **Inappropriate content:** You may be concerned that your kids could find pornography, violence, or hate speech online.

You can reduce these risks by talking to your kids about how they communicate—online and off—and encouraging them to engage in conduct they can be proud of.

Talk Early and Often

The best way to protect your kids online? Talk to them. Research suggests that when children want important information, most rely on their parents.

Start early: After all, even toddlers see their parents use all kinds of devices. As soon as your child is using a computer, a cell phone, or any mobile device, it's time to talk to them about online behavior, safety, and security. As a parent, you have the opportunity to talk to your kid about what's important before anyone else does.

Initiate conversations: Even if your kids are comfortable approaching you, don't wait for them to start the conversation. Use everyday opportunities to talk to your kids about being online. For instance, a TV program featuring a teen online or using a cell phone can tee up a discussion about what to do—or not—in similar circumstances. And news stories about internet scams or cyberbullying can help you start a conversation about your kids' experiences and your expectations.

Create an Honest, Open Environment

Kids look to their parents to help guide them. Be supportive and positive. Listening and taking their feelings into account helps keep conversation afloat. You may not have all the answers, and being honest about that can go a long way.

Communicate Your Values

Be upfront about your values and how they apply in an online context. Communicating your values clearly can help your kids make smarter and more thoughtful decisions when they face tricky situations.

Be Patient

Resist the urge to rush through conversations with your kids. Most kids need to hear information repeated, in small doses, for it to sink in. If you keep talking with your kids, your patience and persistence will pay off in the long run. Work hard to keep the lines of communication open, even if you learn your kid has done something online you find inappropriate.

Kids and Socializing Online

Social networking sites, chat rooms, virtual worlds, and blogs are how teens and tweens socialize online; it's important to help your child learn how to navigate these spaces safely. Among the pitfalls that come with online socializing are sharing too much information or posting comments, photos, or videos that can damage a reputation or hurt someone's feelings. Applying real-world judgment can help minimize those risks.

Remind Kids that Online Actions Have Consequences

The words kids write and the images they post have consequences offline.

Kids should post only what they're comfortable with others seeing: Some of your child's profile may be seen by a broader audience than you—or they—are comfortable with, even if privacy settings are high. Encourage your child to think about the language they use online, and to think before posting pictures and videos, or altering photos posted by someone else. Employers, college admissions officers, coaches, teachers, and the police may view your child's posts.

Remind kids that once they post it, they can't take it back: Even if you delete the information from a site, you have little control over older versions that may exist on other people's computers and may circulate online.

Tell your kids not to impersonate someone else: Let your kids know that it's wrong to create sites, pages, or posts that seem to come from someone else, like a teacher, a classmate, or someone they made up.

Tell Kids to Limit What They Share

Help your kids understand what information should stay private: Tell your kids why it's important to keep some things—about themselves, family members, and friends—to themselves. Information like their Social Security number, street address, phone number, and family financial information—say, bank account or credit card numbers—is private and should stay that way.

Talk to your teens about avoiding sex talk online: Research shows that teens who don't talk about sex with strangers online are less likely to come in contact with predators. In fact, researchers have found that predators usually don't pose as children or teens, and most teens who are contacted by adults they don't know find it creepy. Teens should not hesitate to ignore or block them.

Encourage Online Manners

Politeness counts: You teach your kids to be polite offline; talk to them about being courteous online as well. Texting may seem fast and impersonal, yet courtesies like "pls" and "ty" (for please and thank you) are common text terms.

Tone it down: Using all caps, long rows of exclamation points, or large bolded fonts are the online equivalent of yelling. Most people don't appreciate a rant.

Cc: and Reply all: with care: Suggest that your kids resist the temptation to send a message to everyone on their contact list.

Limit Access to Your Kids' Profiles

Use privacy settings: Many social networking sites and chat rooms have adjustable privacy settings, so you can restrict who has access to your kids' profiles. Talk to your kids about the importance of these settings, and your expectations for who should be allowed to view their profile.

Set high privacy preferences on your kids' chat and video chat accounts, as well. Most chat programs allow parents to control whether people on their kids' contact list can see their status, including whether they're online. Some chat and e-mail accounts allow parents to determine who can send messages to their kids, and block anyone not on the list.

Create a safe screen name: Encourage your kids to think about the impression that screen names can make. A good screen name won't reveal much about how old they are, where they live, or their gender. For privacy purposes, your kids' screen names should not be the same as their e-mail addresses.

Review your child's friends list: You may want to limit your children's online "friends" to people they actually know.

Talk to Kids about What They're Doing Online

Know what your kids are doing: Get to know the social networking sites your kids use so you understand their activities. If you're concerned about risky online behavior, you may want to search the social sites they use to see what information they're posting. Are they pretending to be someone else? Try searching by their name, nickname, school, hobbies, grade, or community.

Ask your kids who they're in touch with online: Just as you want to know who your kids' friends are offline, it's a good idea to know who they're talking to online.

Encourage your kids to trust their guts if they have suspicions: Encourage them to tell you if they feel threatened by someone or uncomfortable because of something online. You can then help them report concerns to the police and to the social networking site. Most of these sites have links for users to report abusive, suspicious, or inappropriate behavior.

Kids and Mobile Phones

What age is appropriate for a kid to have a mobile phone? That's something for you and your family to decide. Consider your child's age, personality, and maturity, and your family's circumstances. Is your child responsible enough to follow rules set by you and the school? When you decide your children are ready for a mobile phone, teach them to think about safety and responsibility.

Phones, Features, and Options

Decide on options and features for your kid's phone: Your mobile phone company and the phone itself should give you some choices for privacy settings and child safety controls. Most carriers allow parents to turn off features, like web access, texting, or downloading. Some cell phones are made especially for children. They're designed to be easy to use, and have features like limited internet access, minute management, number privacy, and emergency buttons.

Be smart about smart phones: Many phones offer web access and mobile apps. If your children are going to use a phone and you're concerned about what they might find online, you can choose a phone with limited internet access, or you can turn on web filtering.

Get familiar with social mapping: Many mobile phones now have GPS technology installed: kids with these phones can pinpoint where their friends are—and be pinpointed by their friends. Advise your kids to use these features only with friends they know in person and trust, and not to broadcast their location to the world, 24/7. In addition, some carriers offer GPS services that let parents map their kid's location.

Develop Cell Phone Rules

Explain what you expect: Talk to your kids about when and where it's appropriate to use their cell phones. You also may want to establish rules for responsible use. Do you allow calls or texting at the dinner table? Do you have rules about cell phone use at night? Should they give you their cell phones while they're doing homework, or when they're supposed to be sleeping?

Don't stand for mobile bullying: Kids can use mobile phones to bully or harass others. Talk to your kids about treating others the same way they want to be treated. The manners and ethics you've taught them apply on phones, too.

Set an example: It's illegal to drive while texting or surfing or talking on the phone without a hands-free device in many states, but it's dangerous everywhere. Set an example for your kids. Talk to them about the dangers and consequences of distracted driving.

Mobile Sharing and Networking

Networking and sharing on-the-go can present unique opportunities and challenges. These tools can foster creativity and fun, but they could cause problems related to personal reputation and safety.

Use care when sharing photos and videos: Most mobile phones now have camera and video capability, making it easy for teens to capture and share every moment. Encourage your teens to think about their privacy and that of others before they share photos and videos via cell phone. Get the okay of the photographer or the person in the shot before posting videos or photos. It could be embarrassing and even unsafe. It's easier to be smart upfront about what media they share at the outset than to do damage control later.

Use good judgment with mobile social networking: Many social networking sites have a feature that allows users to check their profiles and post comments from their phones, allowing access from anywhere. Filters you've installed on your home computer won't limit what kids can do on a phone. If your teens are using a mobile phone, talk to them about using good sense when they're social networking from it.

Chapter 21

What Every Parent Should Know about Athlete Abuse

Abuse of an athlete can take many forms ranging from failing to act to prevent harm when a dangerous situation is recognized in a sport environment to sexual violence such as when a coach rapes an athlete. There are also many subtle and not so subtle forms of mistreatment that athletes and parents need to recognize as misconduct. Abuse is not always easy to define, especially when it appears to be normally acceptable behavior. For instance, it is professional misconduct for a coach to date or have a romantic relationship with an athlete he or she is coaching, even if the athlete is a consenting adult. While it is acceptable for a coach to touch an athlete for the purpose of demonstrating a proper mechanical position, it is not appropriate if the coach doesn't ask the athlete for his or her permission, and it is abusive for a coach to repeatedly touch an athlete when such touching is not for instructional or congratulatory purposes.

It is also important to recognize that abuse can be inflicted by coaches, adult volunteers, staff members, or teammates of the athlete. Sexual abuse is almost always committed by a person known to the athlete who takes advantage of a position of power, is older or bigger, or intentionally manipulates the immaturity of the athlete, often enticing the athlete into what appears to be a consensual situation. It is

"What Every Parent Should Know About Athlete Abuse," © 2012 Safe4Athletes. Reprinted with permission. For additional information, visit www.safe4athletes .org. This information sheet was adapted from "Definitions of Abuse," British Amateur Swimming Association, May 2009, and "Sexual Harassment and Abuse in Sport," a brochure from WomenSport International.

the obligation of parents, coaches, and other adult sport leaders to immediately act to stop improper behaviors whenever they are observed. All adults are responsible for preventing the infliction of harm to our children. No matter how much a parent respects the position of a coach, abusive and improper behavior cannot be condoned.

While it is virtually impossible to define every behavior that might be classified as abusive, it is helpful to review definitions and examples of commonly encountered behaviors.

Physical Abuse

Physical abuse of athletes can take many forms. Some of the more common forms include when a coach: (1) touches an athlete in a non-instructional or non-congratulatory way; (2) touches an improper body part, (3) requires or suggests that an athlete perform a physical act that has no relevance to the sport and which is intended to cause embarrassment, be degrading, or punish; (4) requires or suggests that an athlete continue to perform a physical act, whether it is relevant to the sport or not, that compromises established conditioning and safety guidelines; (5) places an athlete in a situation where he/she is mismatched physically with an opposing athlete causing the possibility of physical harm, (6) requires the athlete to take performance enhancing drugs or any substance not prescribed by a doctor, or (7) fails to stop an activity where an athlete is clearly being subjected to physical harm.

Emotional Abuse

Emotional abuse is the persistent emotional maltreatment of an athlete that causes severe or persistent adverse effects on the athlete's emotional development. Such treatment may involve conveying to athletes that they are worthless, not liked, inadequate, or valued only insofar as they meet the needs of another person or fulfills the coach's performance expectations. Using derogatory or discriminatory language belittling an individual or group based on race, sex/gender, disability, age, sexual orientation, or social or economic background is emotionally abusive to persons from that group and to those overhearing such comments. Emotional abuse can also occur when a coach continuously criticizes an athlete, uses sarcasm, name-calling, generally belittles the athlete, imposes inappropriate expectations that are beyond the developmental capability of a young athlete, or acts to prevent an athlete from participating in normal social interactions with teammates with the intent to isolate and cause harm to that athlete.

Verbal Abuse

Coaches and athletes constantly engage in verbal interactions. It is the coach's responsibility to use such interactions for instructional and motivational purposes. Verbal abuse of athletes can take many forms such as when a coach: (1) excessively, in comparison to treatment of other athletes, singles out an athlete through negative interactions; (2) routinely uses profanity or degrading language; (3) personalizes error correction; (4) yells or screams at a player; (5) constantly blames the team or groups of players for failures or (6) isolates a player by ignoring him or her. Verbal conduct that is unacceptable for a teacher in the classroom is unacceptable for a coach on the playing field or court. Similarly, coaches should immediately call a halt to any bullying, cruel comments, or verbal abuse undertaken by any athlete toward another athlete while in the coach's presence. Coaches should refrain from and disallow their athletes from engaging in verbal discourse that denigrates others.

Sexual Abuse

Sexual abuse involves forcing or enticing an athlete to take part in sexual activities, whether or not the athlete is aware of what is happening. The activities may involve physical contact, including penetrative (for example, rape or oral sex) or non-penetrative acts. Sexual abuse may also include non-contact activities, such as involving athletes in looking at sexual online images, watching sexual activities, or encouraging athletes to behave in sexually inappropriate ways.

Athlete sex abusers can come from any professional, racial, or religious background and can be male or female. They are not always adults. Other athletes can also behave in a sexually abusive way. Usually the abuser is someone known to the athlete, such as a coach, teammate, or staff member. Some individuals become sport club employees specifically to commit acts of sexual abuse because working in sport program allows them access to children.

Abusers may act alone or as part of an organized group like a team. After the abuse, they may put the abused athlete under great pressure not to tell anyone about it. They will often go to great lengths to get close to athletes and win their trust.

Neglect

Neglect is the persistent failure to meet a child's basic physical and/or psychological needs, likely to result in the serious impairment of the athlete's health or development. Neglect may include failure to protect an athlete from physical and emotional harm or danger, such as a coach failing to intervene when an athlete is being bullied or physically abused, or may involve inadequate supervision such as a coach leaving a potentially dangerous sport activity area without any adult monitoring participation. Or neglect may involve a coach ignoring an athlete who is injured or in pain, failing to be responsive to a need for medical attention. In outdoor sports, neglect could be forcing an athlete to engage in stressful physical activity in conditions of high heat and/ or humidity to the extent his/her health is at risk or to participate in the cold without adequate apparel.

Bullying

Bullying often involves physical and emotional abuse and usually occurs when there is an imbalance of power when a person who is older, larger, stronger, in a position of authority, or someone who is more aggressive uses his or her power to control or harm someone in a weaker position. The person bullying has the intent or goal to cause harm (that is, the act is not accidental) and the action is usually repetitious. Examples of bullying include but are not limited to name-calling, teasing, socially spreading rumors, purposely leaving people out of groups by telling them or others they are unwanted, breaking up friendships by threatening others or spreading rumors about a friend, or physically hitting, punching, pinching, or shoving a person. Cyberbullying is using the internet, e-mail, texting, mobile phones, social media, or other digital technologies to do harm to others. The damage inflicted by bullying can frequently be underestimated. Bullying can cause considerable distress to young athletes, to the extent that it affects their health and development. The competitive nature of sport can create unique opportunities for bullying such as when a parent pushes too hard for a better or tougher performance from his or her child, a coach adopts a win-at-all-costs philosophy, or when a coach or parent calls an athlete a "sissy" or other belittling term.

Harassment

Harassment is acting in a way that is unwanted by, or offensive in the opinion of, the recipient. Harassment can be deemed to be a criminal offence in some circumstances and can lead to the use of a restraining order or criminal prosecution. Harassment can range from suggestive sexual remarks and racist insults or jokes to the use of foul language to unwelcome attention. Harassment can lead to the athlete feeling unhappy, demoralized, or undervalued as a person. Sexual harassment is often persistent sexual attention or other behavior with sexual overtones that creates a hostile learning environment. Sexual harassment may include written or verbal abuse or threats, physical contact, sexually graphic literature, sexual advances, demands for sexual favors, sexually oriented comments, jokes, lewd comments or sexual innuendoes, taunts about body, dress, marital status or sexuality, sexual or homophobic graffiti, practical jokes based on sex, intimidating sexual remarks, fondling, kissing, sex-related vandalism, offensive sexually explicit or romantic phone calls or photos, and/or bullying on the basis of sex. Sexual harassment also includes all forms of sexual violence such as sexual assault, sexual battery, rape, and sexual coercion which will be referred to authorities as criminal matters.

Hazing, Initiation Rituals, and Degrading Physical Punishment

Hazing and inappropriate team initiation or bonding activities are defined as any actions, whether physical, mental, emotional, or psychological, which subjects another person, voluntarily or involuntarily, to any outcome that has the intended or unintended effect of abusing, mistreating, degrading, humiliating, harassing, or intimidating the person, or which may in any fashion compromise the inherent dignity of the person, for the purpose of association with, or induction to, a particular group or team. These are forms of harassment or abuse that are often accepted by the recipient because they are convinced that it is a condition of being accepted on the team. Actions and behaviors constituting hazing, initiation rituals or physical punishment commonly used by sports teams are forcing, requiring or pressuring athletes to:

- Consume alcohol or other drugs

- Ingest any substance

- Shave of any part of the body

- Participate in any activity which is illegal, perverse, publicly indecent, or contrary to the individual's genuine moral beliefs

- Tamper with, steal, or damage property

- Restrict their diets in unhealthy ways

- Be deprived of sleep and waking up/disturbing individuals during normal sleep hours

- Purposefully suffer excessive fatigue unrelated to normal training expectations and activities

- Perform calisthenics or any type of physically abusive exercise unrelated to normal training

- Paddle, whip, beat, or commit physical abuse of any kind

- Engage in public stunts and buffoonery

- Be tattooed or branded

- Participate in road trips, kidnapping, drop-offs, or any other such activities

- Work on projects without the full participation of the team

- Perform pranks, such as borrowing or stealing items, painting property or objects, or harassing other individuals or groups

- Subject a teammate to cruel and unusual psychological conditions

- Wear apparel in public which is conspicuous, not normally in good taste, or designed to humiliate the individual(s) wearing it

- Participate in morally degrading or humiliating games or activities

- Participate in line-ups, kangaroo courts, or any interrogation not consistent with the legitimate testing for information about the purposes and history of the team

- Participate in sexual rituals, assaults, and/or required nudity

- March or participate in similar collective behaviors

- Violate state laws or club policies

- "Greet" initiated members

- Answer phones or doors with songs, chants, or riddles

- Yell or scream upon entering or leaving a facility

- Engage in deception or threats contrived to convince the new member that he/she will not be permitted to join

- Endure mentally abusive or demeaning behavior

Inappropriate Professional Conduct

Coaches, staff members, volunteers, or others who have authority over or provide professional services to athletes must exhibit the highest standards of impartiality and professional treatment and are prohibited from engaging in inappropriate conduct with athletes. It is unethical for coaches, other staff and volunteers to have any physical bodily contact with athletes outside of the practice or contest environment. Within the practice or contest environment, coaches may not have any physical bodily contact with athletes except with the athlete's permission to correct physical form or a pat on the head or back when congratulating an athlete for a good performance. Having a sexual, intimate, romantic, or similar close personal relationship with individuals over which a coach has an instructional or service responsibility, even if a consensual relationship between adults, is professionally unethical and unacceptable because it creates the appearance or actuality of favoritism and special treatment. Examples of other professionally inappropriate behaviors expressly prohibited include but are not limited to:

- Coaches performing back rubs or massage on an athlete even if the coach is a licensed allied health professional (must be performed by a licensed allied health professional hired for this specific purpose and approved by the club)

- Kissing

- Commenting on athletes' or employees' bodies or appearance in a sexual manner

- Exchanging romantic gifts or communications

- Showing obscene or suggestive photos

- Videotaping or photographing athletes or employees in revealing or suggestive poses

- Discussing/writing about sexual topics unrelated to work responsibilities of employees

- Making sexual jokes, sexual gestures, and innuendos or engaging in inappropriate sexually oriented banter (for example, discussion of dating behavior)

- Sharing sexual exploits or marital difficulties

- Intentionally invading the athlete's or employee's privacy during non-working hours or outside of regularly schedules practice and competition

- Using e-mail, text-messaging, instant messaging, or other social media to discuss sexual topics with athletes or employees

Such unprofessional behaviors or sexual or romantic personal relationships undermine the trust in the coach or employee and belief that the athlete will be treated impartially.

Indicators of Abuse

The vast majority of athletes do not find it easy to disclose their concerns. Many are afraid of being criticized by teammates. Many will not question a coach's behavior because they believe they will not receive instructional attention or be selected for a team or performance group. Some athletes are afraid of being criticized by parents who they fear will suggest that they have to be stronger. The sport environment contributes to this expectation of athlete "toughness." Often, parents and athletes tolerate abusive coaches thinking that it is acceptable behavior for coaches to "push" athletes to do their best using almost any conceivable means. Our culture often accepts coach use of profanity, physically pulling athletes into position, and other behaviors that would never be tolerated of teachers in a classroom setting. In sport club settings, parents almost blindingly allow the coach carte blanche in the handling of athletes. Such behaviors are simply not acceptable.

Considering these deterrents to reporting abuse in the sport environment, if an athlete does disclose a concern and describes what may be an abusive act or another person, such reports should be taken very seriously. There are other indicators of abuse that parents and sport leaders need to be sensitive to such as:

- Unexplained or recurring injuries such as cuts and bruises situated in areas of the child's body which are not normally prone to injury

- Physical injury where the explanation given is inconsistent

- Unexplained changes in behavior such as a child becoming withdrawn, quiet, aggressive, or verbally violent

- Inappropriate sexual awareness and/or behaving in a sexualized manner

- Disordered eating behaviors, such as the athlete overeating or showing a loss of appetite

- Excessive weight loss or weight gain for no obvious reason

- Physical appearance becomes unkempt

- The athlete becomes withdrawn and isolated from the team and seems unable to make friends

- The athlete begins to display a distrust of adults

- The athlete begins to exhibit behavioral changes such as reduced concentration and/or becoming withdrawn, clingy, depressed, tearful, emotionally up and down, reluctant to go to school, training or sports club

- A drop in performance at school or in the sport

- Physical signs such as stomachaches, headaches, difficulty in sleeping, bed-wetting, scratching and bruising, damaged clothes and bingeing, for example, on food, cigarettes, or alcohol

- A shortage of money or frequent loss of possessions

- A high turnover of club members

This is not an exhaustive list of indicators and the presence of an indicator cannot be seen to be definitive proof that an athlete is being abused. But the response to such indicators should be an investigation of the possibility that abuse is occurring.

What Parents Can Do to Help Prevent Abuse

There are many things that parents can do to help prevent sexual and other forms of misconduct in the amateur sports environment. All of the following should be considered:

- Ask the sports club or program whether all coaches, volunteers, and staff undergo criminal background checks before they are hired.

- Ask whether the club has written policies that clearly define coach misconduct, prohibit romantic or other nonprofessional relationships between coaches and athletes, define and prohibit emotional, verbal, and physical abuse, bullying, hazing, initiation rituals, harassment, and physical punishment by staff or athletes.

- Ask whether the sport club has education sessions for athletes to help them identify inappropriate behaviors and a process to report such behaviors.

- Ask if the sport club has an independent athlete welfare advocate or athlete protection officer who athletes know they can go to in complete confidence to help them address concerns.

- Ask whether the sports club conducts education sessions for coaches, staff, and volunteers regarding professional behavior and behaviors that they must stop if they observe them.

- Talk to your children regarding all inappropriate or abusive behaviors and what they should do if they observe or are subjected to such behaviors.

This information was adapted from two primary resources "Definitions of Abuse" as published in Wavepower, Loughborough, Leicestershire, UK: British Amateur Swimming Association, May, 2009; and, WomenSport International's brochure on "Sexual Harassment and Abuse in Sport" retrieved on October 14, 2011 from http://www.sportsbiz.bz/womensportinternational/taskforces/harassment_brochure.htm.

Part Four

Adult Survivors
of Child Abuse

Chapter 22

Adult Survivors
of Child Abuse

Chapter Contents

Section 22.1

Consequences of Child Abuse in Adulthood

Excerpted from "Effects of Child Abuse and Neglect for Adult Survivors," by Alister Lamont. © 2010 Commonwealth of Australia. Reprinted by permission of the Australian Institute of Family Studies, www.afis.gov.au.

Exposure to child abuse and neglect can lead to a wide range of adverse consequences that can last a lifetime. The purpose of this information is to indicate the potential long-term effects of child abuse and neglect that may extend into adulthood.

Types of Abuse and Neglect

Child abuse and neglect consists of any act of commission or omission that results in harm, potential for harm, or the threat of harm to a child (0–18 years of age) even if harm was unintentional (Gilbert et al., 2009). In the case of all but sexual abuse it is generally perpetrated by a parent or caregiver. The five main types of child maltreatment are: physical abuse; sexual abuse; emotional maltreatment; neglect and witnessing domestic violence.

Evidence suggests that different types of abuse and neglect rarely occur in isolation, and children who experience repeated maltreatment often experience multiple forms of abuse (Higgins, 2004).

For more information on the definitions of child abuse and neglect, see NCPC [National Child Protection Clearinghouse] Resource Sheet, What is Child Abuse and Neglect? (available online at http://www.aifs .gov.au/cfca/pubs/factsheets/a142091/index.html).

Factors Affecting the Consequences of Abuse and Neglect

The consequences of child abuse and neglect that extend into adulthood will vary considerably. For some adults, the effects of child abuse and neglect are chronic and debilitating; others have more positive outcomes as adults, despite their abuse and neglect histories

(Miller-Perrin and Perrin, 2007). Factors that may impact on the way child abuse and neglect affects adults include:

- their age were when maltreatment occurred;
- the severity of maltreatment;
- the frequency and duration of maltreatment;
- the relationship they had with the perpetrator;
- the type/s of abuse/neglect;
- whether the abuse or neglect was detected and action taken to assure the safety of the child (e.g., child protection intervention);
- positive or protective factors that may have mitigated the effects of maltreatment (e.g., a strong relationship with grandparents); and
- whether victims/survivors received therapeutic services to assist them in recovery.

Sometimes, the effects of child abuse and neglect remain largely hidden only to emerge at key times in later life (McQueen, Itzin, Kennedy, Sinason, and Maxted, 2009). Abusive experiences in adulthood can reopen old wounds of past child abuse or neglect that may lead to further adverse outcomes for adult survivors.

Childhood Trauma/Trauma Theory

The impact of childhood trauma is often used to explain the strong associations between past histories of child abuse and neglect and adverse consequences in both children and adults.

Experiences of childhood trauma caused by abuse or neglect can lead to a variety of overwhelming emotions, such as anger, sadness, guilt, and shame. In order to avoid such feelings, children can take refuge in dissociation, denial, amnesia, or emotional numbing (Everett and Gallop, 2001). These coping mechanisms can become over-generalized with time and without protective factors (i.e., positive events or characteristics) to intervene, these negative outcomes may continue throughout life. Adult survivors of childhood trauma may also find it difficult to control emotions and or actions. For adults with a history of childhood trauma, recollections of past trauma can almost be as strongly felt as if it was happening again, which may lead to unexpected reactions, such as lashing out in anger or bursting into uncontrolled weeping in response to what most people would view as relatively minor events (Everett and Gallop, 2001).

Multiple Types of Abuse

Any maltreatment of a child may lead to damaging adverse consequences, however, research indicates that chronicity and experiencing multiple types of abuse and neglect may lead to more severe adverse outcomes in both childhood and adulthood (Arata, Langhinrichsen-Rohling, Bowers, and O'Farrill-Swails, 2005; Ethier, Lemelin, and Lacharite, 2004; Higgins and McCabe, 2001). Chronic abuse and neglect can be defined as "recurrent incidents of maltreatment over a prolonged period of time" (Bromfield, Gillingham, and Higgins, 2007). Chronic experiences of child abuse and neglect occurring over a long period of time increases the probability of more severe adverse outcomes in adult survivors (Gilbert et al., 2009; Sachs-Ericsson, Cromer, Hernandez, and Kendall-Tackett, 2009).

Long-Term Consequences of Child Abuse and Neglect

Experiences of child abuse and neglect may lead to negative physical, cognitive, psychological, behavioral or social consequences in adulthood. Adverse outcomes of abuse and neglect that emerge in children and adolescents may continue in adults with histories of abuse and neglect (Miller-Perrin and Perrin, 2007).

For a more detailed discussion of the impact of child abuse and neglect on children see, "The Effects of Child Abuse and Neglect for Children and Adolescents" (Lamont, 2010).

The following section discusses the long-term effects of child abuse and neglect that may extend into adulthood. The research reviewed included high quality literature reviews/meta-analyses and primary research in English speaking countries. The negative consequences associated with past histories of abuse and neglect are often interrelated, as one adverse outcome may lead to another (e.g., substance abuse problems or engaging in risky sexual behavior may lead to physical health problems). Adverse consequences are broadly linked to all abuse types, however, where appropriate, associations are made between specific types of abuse and neglect and specific negative outcomes.

Physical Health Problems

Adults with a history of child abuse and neglect are more likely to have physical health problems and chronic pain symptoms. Research indicates that adult survivors of childhood abuse and neglect have more health problems than the general population, including diabetes, gastrointestinal problems, arthritis, headaches, gynecological problems, stroke, hepatitis and heart disease (Felitti et al., 1998; Sachs-Ericsson et al., 2009; Springer, Sheridan, Kuo, and Carnes, 2007). In a review of recent literature, Sachs-Ericsson et al. (2009) found that a majority of studies showed that adult survivors of childhood abuse had more medical problems than non-abused counterparts. Using survey data from over 2,000 middle-aged adults in a longitudinal study in the United States, Springer et al. (2007) found that child physical abuse predicted severe ill health and several medical diagnoses, including heart and liver troubles and high blood pressure. Some researchers suggest that poor health outcomes in adult survivors of child abuse and neglect could be due to the impact early life stress has on the immune system or to the greater propensity for adult survivors to engage in high-risk behaviors (e.g., smoking, alcohol abuse and risky sexual behavior) (Sachs-Ericsson et al., 2009; Watts-English, Fortson, Gilber, Hooper, and De Bellis, 2006).

Exposure to abuse and neglect in childhood may also contribute to the development of chronic pain disorders in adulthood (Davis, Luecken, and Zautra, 2005; Sachs-Ericsson et al., 2009). In a meta-analysis by Davis et al. (2005), studies assessing the abuse and neglect history of chronic pain patients indicated that patients were more likely to report having been abused or neglected in childhood than healthy controls.

Mental Health Problems

Persisting mental health problems are a common consequence of child abuse and neglect in adults. Mental health problems associated with past histories of child abuse and neglect include personality disorders, post-traumatic stress disorder, dissociative disorders, depression, anxiety disorders, and psychosis (Afifi, Boman, Fleisher, and Sareen, 2009; Chapman et al., 2004; McQueen et al., 2009; Springer et al., 2007). Depression is one of the most commonly occurring consequences of past abuse or neglect (Kendall-Tackett, 2002). In an American representative study based on the National Co-morbidity Survey, adults who had experienced child abuse were two and a half times more likely to have major depression and six times more likely to have post-traumatic stress disorder compared to adults who had not experienced abuse (Afifi et al., 2009). The likelihood of such consequences increased substantially if adults had experienced child abuse along with parental divorce (Afifi et al., 2009). In a prospective longitudinal study in the United States, Widom, DuMont, and Czaja (2007) found that children who were physically abused or experienced multiple types of abuse were at increased risk of lifetime major depressive disorder in early adulthood.

Suicidal Behavior

Consistent evidence shows associations between child abuse and neglect and risks of attempted suicide in young people and adults. In the Adverse Childhood Experiences (ACE) study in the United States, Felitti et al. (1998) indicated that adults exposed to four or more adverse experiences in childhood were 12 times more likely to have attempted suicide than those who had no adverse experiences in childhood. In a meta-analysis by Gilbert et al. (2009), retrospective studies, which record participants recollections of past traumatic events showed a strong association between child abuse and neglect and attempted suicide in adults. Prospective studies, which trace participant's experiences of traumatic events over several years indicated a more moderate relationship. The higher rates of suicidal behavior in adult survivors of child abuse and neglect has been attributed to the greater likelihood of adult survivors suffering from mental health problems.

Eating Disorders and Obesity

Eating disorders and obesity are common among adult survivors of child abuse and neglect (Johnson, Cohen, Kasen, and Brook, 2002; Kendall-Tackett, 2002; Rodriguez-Srednicki and Twaite, 2006; Rohde et al., 2008; Thomas, Hypponen, and Power, 2008). Prospective research studies have consistently shown links between child abuse and neglect and obesity in adulthood (Gilbert et al., 2009). Using a large population-based survey, Rohde and colleagues (2008) found that both child sexual abuse and physical abuse were associated with a doubling of the odds of obesity in middle-aged women. In a prospective longitudinal study in the United Kingdom, results indicated that severe forms of childhood adversity, such as physical abuse, witnessing domestic violence, and neglect were associated with increased risk of obesity in middle adulthood by 20 to 40% (Thomas et al., 2008). In a community based study, Johnson and colleagues found (2002) that adolescents and young adults with a history of child sexual abuse or neglect were five times more likely to have an eating disorder compared to individuals who did not have a history of abuse. Stress and mental health problems such as depression may increase the likelihood of adults with a history of abuse and neglect becoming obese or having an eating disorder (Rodriguez-Srednicki and Twaite, 2006).

Re-Victimization

Research suggests that adults, particularly women, who were victimized as children are at risk of re-victimization in later life (Mouzos and Makkai, 2004; Whiting, Simmons, Havens, Smith, and Oka, 2009; Widom, Czaja, and Dutton, 2008). Findings from the Australian component of the International Violence Against Women Survey (IVAWS) indicated that 72% of women who experienced either physical or sexual abuse as a child also experienced violence in adulthood, compared to 43% of women who did not experience childhood abuse (Mouzos and Makkai, 2004). In a prospective study by Widom and colleagues (2008), all types of childhood victimization (physical abuse, sexual abuse, and neglect) were associated with increased risk of lifetime re-victimization. Findings indicated that childhood victimization increased the risk for physical and sexual assault/abuse, kidnapping/stalking, and having a family friend murdered or commit suicide (Widom et al., 2008). Women who experience childhood violence or who have witnessed parental violence could be at risk of being victimized as adults as they are more likely to have low self-esteem and they may have learned that violent behavior is a normal response to dealing with conflict (Mouzos and Makkai, 2004).

Alcohol and Substance Abuse

Associations have often been made between childhood abuse and neglect and later substance abuse in adulthood (Simpson and Miller, 2002; Widom, White, Czaja, and Marmorstein, 2007). In a systematic review by Simpson and Miller (2002) of 224 studies, a strong relationship was found between child physical and sexual abuse and substance abuse problems in women. Less of an association was found among men, although men with child sexual abuse histories were found to be at greater risk of substance abuse problems. The authors suggested that it is possible that men are less likely to disclose childhood abuse due to social values and expectations (Simpson and Miller, 2002). In the Adverse Childhood Experiences Study in the United States, adults with four or more adverse experiences in childhood were seven times more likely to consider themselves an alcoholic, five times more likely to have used illicit drugs and ten times more likely to have injected drugs compared to adults with no adverse experiences (Felitti et al., 1998). The higher rates of substance abuse problems among adult survivors of child abuse and neglect may, in part, be due to victims using substances to self-medicate from trauma symptoms such as anxiety, depression and intrusive memories caused by an abusive history (Whiting et al., 2009).

Aggression, Violence, and Criminal Behavior

Violence and criminal behavior is another frequently identified long-term consequence of child abuse and neglect for adult survivors, particularly for those who have experienced physical abuse or witnessed domestic violence (Gilbert et al., 2009; Kwong, Bartholomew, Henderson, and Trinke, 2003; Miller-Perrin and Perrin, 2007). Widom (1989) compared a sample of adults with a history of substantiated cases of child abuse and neglect in the United States with a sample of matched comparisons and found that adults with a history of abuse and neglect had a higher likelihood of arrests, adult criminality, and violent criminal behavior. In a study of 36 men with a history of perpetrating domestic violence, Bevan and Higgins (2002) found that child maltreatment (particularly child neglect) and low family cohesion were associated with the frequency of physical spouse abuse. Witnessing domestic violence (but not physical abuse) as a child had a unique association with psychological spouse abuse and trauma symptomology. Adults with a history of child physical abuse or witnessing domestic violence may be more likely to be violent and involved in criminal activity as they have learned that such behavior is an appropriate method for responding to stress or conflict resolution (Chapple, 2003). Substance abuse problems are also associated with higher rates of criminal behavior (e.g., theft, prostitution) to support addiction (Dawe, Harnett, and Frye 2008).

Intergenerational Transmission of Abuse and Neglect

Evidence suggests that adults who are abused or neglected as children are also more likely to abuse or neglect their own children (Kwong et al., 2003; Mouzos and Makkai, 2004; Pears and Capaldi, 2001). In a study by Pears and Capaldi (2001), parents who had experienced physical abuse in childhood were significantly more likely to engage in abusive behaviors toward their own children or children in their care. Oliver (1993) in a review of the research literature concluded that an estimated one-third of children who are subjected to child abuse and neglect go on to repeat patterns of abusive parenting towards their own children. This is a significant number, however, it is also important to note that Oliver's estimations indicate that a majority of maltreated children do not go on to maltreat their own children. Kwong and colleagues (2003) determined that growing up in an abusive family environment can teach a child that the use of violence and aggression is a viable means for dealing with interpersonal conflict, which can increase the likelihood that the cycle of violence will continue when the child reaches adulthood. Although links have been made between adult survivors of child physical abuse perpetrating the same type of abuse on their own children (Kwong et al., 2003; Pears and Capaldi, 2001), there is little evidence to suggest that maltreating parents who experienced other forms of abuse or neglect, such as child sexual abuse will perpetrate the same type of abuse on their own children.

High-Risk Sexual Behavior

Adults who have experienced childhood abuse and neglect, particularly child sexual abuse are more likely to engage in high-risk sexual behavior. This can lead to a wide range of sexually transmitted diseases or early pregnancy (Cohen et al., 2000; Hillis, Anda, Felitti, Nordenberg, and Marchbanks, 2000; Steel and Herlitz, 2005). Using a random population sample in Sweden, Steel and Herlitz (2005) found that a history of child sexual abuse was associated with a greater frequency of unintended pregnancy, younger age at first diagnosis of a sexually transmitted disease, greater likelihood of participation in group sex, and a greater likelihood of engaging in prostitution. In a large retrospective study in the United States, the prevalence of sexually transmitted diseases was three and a half times higher for men and women who were exposed to three to five adverse childhood experiences compared to adults who had no adverse childhood experiences (Hillis et al., 2000). Steel and Herlitz (2005) determined that factors that may increase the likelihood of engaging in risky sexual behaviors include: the inability to be assertive and prevent unwanted sexual advances, feeling unworthy, and having competing needs for affection and acceptance. These are all feelings that may occur as a consequence of child abuse and neglect.

Homelessness

Strong associations have been made between histories of child abuse and neglect and experiences of homelessness in adulthood. A study by Herman, Susser, Struening, and Link (1997) found that the combination of lack of care and either physical or sexual abuse during childhood was highly associated with an elevated risk of adult homelessness. Adults who experienced a combination of a lack of care and either child physical or sexual abuse were 26 times more likely to have been homeless than those with no experiences of abuse. In a study examining whether adverse childhood events were related to negative adult behaviors among homeless adults in the United States, 72% of the sample had experienced one or more adverse childhood events (Tam, Zlotnick, and Robertson, 2003). Higher rates of homelessness among adult survivors of abuse and neglect could be due to difficulties securing employment or experiences of domestic violence. Although evidence associating past histories of child abuse and neglect and unemployment is limited, a small body of research suggests that children and adolescents affected by abuse and neglect risk poor academic achievement at school, which may lead to difficulties finding employment in adulthood (Gilbert et al., 2009). The relationship between homelessness and adult survivors of abuse and neglect may also be connected to other adverse outcomes linked to child abuse and neglect such as substance abuse problems, mental health problems and aggressive and violent behavior. These consequences may make it difficult to achieve stable housing.

Research Limitations

Research investigating the effects of child abuse and neglect in adulthood is extensive, however in most research studies it is difficult to make casual links between abuse and neglect and adverse consequences due to several limitations. Many research studies are unable to control for other environmental and social factors. This makes it difficult to rule out influences such as socio-economic disadvantage, disability, and social isolation when associating abuse and neglect with negative consequences.

Most research studies on adult survivors are based on retrospective studies and are therefore reliant on participants' recollection of events over long periods. This can limit the data in that participants' recollections may have changed over time. Prospective studies have the advantage of tracing participants with reported experiences of child abuse or neglect over several years. However prospective studies alone are not completely representative of the population, as a high proportion of child abuse and neglect goes undetected and those experiencing abuse and neglect are less likely to participate or remain in a longitudinal study (Kendall-Tackett and Becker-Blease, 2004). Kendall-Tackett and Becker-Blease (2004) argued that there should be a mix of prospective and retrospective studies as both types of research can provide insight into the long-term consequences of child abuse and neglect.

Other limitations in the research included:

- studies focusing solely on one type of abuse (particularly sexual abuse). Focusing research on only one type of abuse or neglect overlooks the effects of children experiencing chronic and multiple types of abuse and neglect. Without assessing chronicity and the effects of other forms of child abuse and neglect, bias and misleading conclusions are often made on the specific impact of that form of maltreatment (Bromfield et al., 2007; Higgins and McCabe, 2001).

- a reliance on recruiting participants already involved in clinical services. Only including participants involved in clinical services excludes adult survivors who have not sought clinical services. This can make negative outcomes appear worse than in reality as participants are only those who have presented with a problem.

- far more studies focusing on the effects of child abuse and neglect in women compared to men. Having more research on the effects of child abuse and neglect in women makes it difficult to compare differences between men and women as less is known on the effects of child abuse and neglect on men (Springer et al., 2007; Widom, DuMont et al., 2007).

In spite of the various limitations, research consistently indicates that adults with a history of child abuse and neglect are more likely to experience adverse outcomes.

Conclusion

The effects of child abuse and neglect can lead to a wide range of adverse outcomes in adulthood. Adverse outcomes associated with past histories of child abuse and neglect are often inter-related. Experiencing chronic and multiple forms of maltreatment can increase the risk of more severe and damaging adverse consequences in adulthood.

References

Afifi, T., Boman, J., Fleisher, W., and Sareen, J. (2009). The relationship between child abuse, parental divorce, and lifetime mental disorders and suicidality in a nationally representative adult sample. *Child Abuse and Neglect*, 33, 139–147.

Arata, C. M., Langhinrichsen-Rohling, J., Bowers, D., and O'Farrill-Swails, L. (2005). Single versus multi-type maltreatment: An examination of the long-term effects of child abuse. *Journal of Aggression, Maltreatment and Trauma*, 11(4), 29–52.

Bevan, E. and Higgins, D. (2002). Is domestic violence learned? The contribution of five forms of child maltreatment to men's violence and adjustment. *Journal of Family Violence*, 17(3), 223–245.

Bromfield, L. M., Gillingham, P., and Higgins, D. J. (2007). Cumulative harm and chronic child maltreatment. *Developing Practice*, 19, 34–42.

Chapman, D., Whitfield, C., Felitti, V., Dube, S., Edwards, V., and Anda, R. (2004). Adverse childhood experiences and the risk of depressive disorders in adulthood. *Journal of Affective Disorders*, 82, 217–225.

Chapple, C. (2003). Examining intergenerational violence: violent role modeling or weak parental controls? *Violence and Victims*, 18(2), 143–162.

Cohen, M., Deamant, C., Barkan, S., Richardson, J., Young, M., Holman, S., et al. (2000). Domestic violence and childhood sexual abuse in HIV-infected women and women at risk of HIV. *American Journal of Public Health*, 90(4), 560–565.

Davis, D., Luecken, L., and Zautra, A. (2005). Are reports of childhood abuse related to the experience of chronic pain in adulthood? A meta-analytic review of the literature. *Clinical Journal of Pain*, 21(5), 398–405.

Dawe, S., Harnett, P., and Frye, S. (2008). *Improving outcomes for children living in families with parental substance misuse: What do we know and what should we do?* (Child Abuse Prevention Issues No. 29). Retrieved from: <www.aifs.gov.au/nch/pubs/issues/issues29/issues29.html>

Ethier, L., Lemelin, J. P., and Lacharite, C. (2004). A longitudinal study of the effects of chronic maltreatment on children's behavioral and emotional problems. *Child Abuse and Neglect*, 28, 1265–1278.

Everett, B., and Gallop, R. (2001). *The link between childhood trauma and mental illness*. Thousand Oaks: Sage Publications, Inc.

Felitti, V., Anda, R., Nordenberg, D., Williamson, F., Spitz, A., Edwards, V., et al. (1998). Relationship of childhood abuse and household dysfunction in many of the leading causes of death in adults. *American Journal of Preventive Medicine*, 14(4).

Gilbert, R., Spatz Widom, C., Browne, K., Fergusson, D., Webb, E., and Janson, J. (2009). Burden and consequences of child maltreatment in high-income countries. *Lancet*, 373, 68–81.

Herman, D., Susser, E., Struening, E., and Link, B. (1997). Adverse childhood experiences: Are they risk factors for adult homelessness? *American Journal of Public Health*, 87(2), 249–255.

Higgins, D. (2004). Differentiating between child maltreatment experiences. *Family Matters*, 69, 50–55.

Higgins, D., and McCabe, M. (2001). Multiple forms of child abuse and neglect: Adult retrospective reports. *Aggression and Violent Behaviour*, 6, 547–578.

Hillis, S., Anda, R., Felitti, V., Nordenberg, D., and Marchbanks, P. (2000). Adverse childhood experiences and sexually transmitted diseases in men and women: A retrospective study. *Pediatrics*, 106(1), 1–6.

Johnson, J., Cohen, P., Kasen, S., and Brook, J. (2002). Childhood adversities associated with risk for eating disorders or weight problems during adolescence or early adulthood. *American Journal of Psychiatry*, 159(3), 394–400.

Kendall-Tackett, K. (2002). The health effects of childhood abuse: four pathways by which abuse can influence health. *Child Abuse and Neglect*, 26(6–7), 715–729.

Kendall-Tackett, K., and Becker-Blease, K. (2004). The importance of retrospective findings in child maltreatment research. *Child Abuse and Neglect*, 28, 723–727.

Kwong, M., Bartholomew, K., Henderson, A., and Trinke, S. (2003). The intergenerational transmission of relationship violence. *Journal of Family Psychology*, 17(3), 288–301.

Lamont, A. (2010). *The Effects of Child Abuse and Neglect for Children and Adolescents* (NCPC Resource Sheet). Melbourne: National Child Protection Clearinghouse, Australian Institute of Family Studies.

McQueen, D., Itzin, C., Kennedy, R., Sinason, V., and Maxted, F. (2009). *Psychoanalytic psychotherapy after child abuse. The treatment of adults and children who have experienced sexual abuse, violence, and neglect in childhood.* London: Karnac Books Ltd.

Miller-Perrin, C., and Perrin, R. (2007). *Child maltreatment: an introduction.* Thousand Oaks: Sage Publications.

Mouzos, J., and Makkai, T. (2004). *Women's experiences of male violence. Findings from the Australian component of the International Violence Against Women Survey (IVAWS).* Canberra: Australian Institute of Criminology. Retrieved 2 September 2009, from <http://www.aic.gov.au/documents/5/8/D/{58D8592E -CEF7-4005-AB11-B7A8B4842399}RPP56.pdf>

Oliver, J. (1993). Intergenerational transmission of child abuse: Rates, research and clinical implications. *American Journal of Psychiatry*, 150(9), 1315–1324.

Pears, K., and Capaldi, D. (2001). Intergenerational transmission of abuse: A two-generational prospective study of an at-risk sample. *Child Abuse and Neglect*, 25, 1439–1461.

Rodriguez-Srednicki, O., and Twaite, J. (2006). *Understanding, assessing, and treating adult victims of childhood abuse*. Lanham: Rowman and Littlefield Publishers Inc.

Rohde, P., Ichikawa, L., Simon, G., Ludman, E., Linde, J., Jeffrey, R., et al. (2008). Associations of child sexual and physical abuse with obesity and depression in middle-aged women. *Child Abuse and Neglect*, 32, 878–887.

Sachs-Ericsson, N., Cromer, K., Hernandez, A., and Kendall-Tackett, K. (2009). A review of childhood abuse, health, and pain-related problems: The role of psychiatric-disorders and current life stress. *Journal of Trauma and Dissociation*, 10(2), 170–188.

Simpson, T., and Miller, W. (2002). Concomitance between childhood sexual and physical abuse and substance use problems. A review. *Clinical Psychology Review*, 22, 27–77.

Springer, K., Sheridan, J., Kuo, D., and Carnes, M. (2007). Long-term physical and mental health consequences of childhood physical abuse: Results from a large population-based sample of men and women. *Child Abuse and Neglect*, 31, 517–530.

Steel, J., and Herlitz, C. (2005). The association between childhood and adolescent sexual abuse and proxies for sexual risk behavior: A random sample of the general population of Sweden. *Child Abuse and Neglect*, 29, 1141–1153.

Tam, T., Zlotnick, C., and Robertson, M. (2003). Longitudinal perspective: Adverse childhood events, substance use, and labor force participation among homeless adults. *American Journal of Drug and Alcohol Abuse*, 29(4), 829–846.

Thomas, C., Hypponen, E., and Power, C. (2008). Obesity and type 2 diabetes risk in midadult life: The role of childhood adversity. *Pediatrics*, 121, 1240–1249.

Watts-English, T., Fortson, B., Gilber, N., Hooper, S., and De Bellis, M. (2006). The psychobiology of maltreatment in childhood. *Journal of Social Issues*, 62(4), 717–736.

Whiting, J., Simmons, L. A., Havens, J., Smith, D., and Oka, M. (2009). Intergenerational transmission of violence: the influence of self-appraisals, mental disorders and substance abuse. *Journal of Family Violence*, 24, 639–648.

Widom, C. (1989). Child abuse, neglect, and violent criminal behaviour. *Criminology*, 27(2), 251–271.

Widom, C., Czaja, S., and Dutton, M. (2008). Childhood victimization and lifetime revictimization. *Child Abuse and Neglect*, 32, 785–796.

Widom, C., DuMont, K., and Czaja, S. (2007). A prospective investigation of major depressive disorder and comorbidity in abused and neglected children grown up. *Archives of General Psychiatry*, 64, 49–56.

Widom, C., White, H., Czaja, S., and Marmorstein, N. (2007). Long-term effects of child abuse and neglect on alcohol use and excessive drinking in middle adulthood. *Journal of Studies on Alcohol and Drugs*, 317–325.

Section 22.2

Effects of Adverse Childhood Experiences Over the Lifespan

"Adverse Childhood Experiences and Health and Well-Being Over the Lifespan," Substance Abuse and Mental Health Services Administration (www.samhsa.gov), April 26, 2010.

This section shows the sequence of events that unaddressed childhood abuse and other early traumatic experiences set in motion. Without intervention, adverse childhood events (ACEs) can result in long-term disease, disability, chronic social problems, and early death. 90% of public mental health clients have been exposed to multiple physical or sexual abuse traumas. Importantly, intergenerational transmission that perpetuates ACEs may continue without implementation of interventions to interrupt the cycle.

Adverse Childhood Experiences (Birth to 18)

Abuse of Child

- Emotional abuse 11%*
- Physical abuse 28%*
- Contact sexual abuse 22%

Trauma in Child's Household Environment

- Alcohol or drug user by household member 27%
- Chronically depressed, emotionally disturbed or suicidal household member 17%
- Mother treated violently 13%
- Imprisoned household member 6%
- Not raised by both biological parents 23% (Loss of parent by separation or divorce, natural death, suicide, abandonment)

320

Neglect of Child*

- Physical neglect 19%
- Emotional neglect 15%

*Above types of ACEs are the "heavy end" of abuse, for example, emotional: recurrent threats, humiliation, chronic criticism; physical: beating vs spanking; neglect: lack of basic needs for attachment, survival/growth

One ACE category = score of 1.

List is limited to ACE study types: Other trauma may include: combat, poverty, street violence, historical, racism, stigma, natural events, persecution, etc.

Impact of Trauma and Adoption of Health Risk Behaviors to Ease Pain of Trauma

Neurobiologic Effects of Trauma

- Disrupted neuro-development
- Difficulty controlling
- Anger, rage
- Hallucinations
- Depression (and numerous other mental health problems—see Notes)
- Panic reactions
- Anxiety
- Multiple (6+) somatic problems
- Sleep problems
- Impaired memory
- Flashbacks
- Dissociation

Health Risk Behaviors

- Smoking
- Severe obesity

- Physical inactivity
- Suicide attempts
- Alcoholism
- Drug abuse
- 50+ sex partners
- Repetition of original trauma
- Self-injury
- Eating disorders
- Perpetrate interpersonal violence (aggression, bullying, etc.).

Long-Term Consequences of Unaddressed Trauma

Disease and Disability

- Ischemic heart disease
- Cancer
- Chronic lung disease
- Chronic emphysema
- Asthma
- Liver disease
- Skeletal fractures
- Poor self rated health
- Sexually transmitted disease
- HIV/AIDS

Social Problems

- Homelessness
- Prostitution
- Delinquency, violence, and criminal behavior
- Inability to sustain employment
- Re-victimization: by rape, domestic violence, bullying, etc.
- Compromised ability to parent

- Negative alterations in self-perception and relationships with others
- Alterations in systems of meaning
- Intergenerational transmission of abuse
- Long-term use of multi human service systems

Cost

- At annual cost of $103,754,017,492.00

Notes

1. Multiple studies reveal the origin of many mental health disorders may be found in childhood trauma, including borderline personality disorder (BPD), anti-social personality disorder, post-traumatic stress disorder (PTSD), schizophrenia, bipolar disorder, dissociative identity disorder (DID), anxiety disorders, eating disorders including severe obesity, attention deficit hyperactivity disorder (ADHD), oppositional defiant disorder (ODD) and others.

2. Sources: *Adverse Childhood Experiences Study* (CDC and Kaiser Permanente, see http://www.ACEstudy.org) *The Damaging Consequences of Violence and Trauma* (see http://www .NASMHPD.org) and *Trauma and Recovery* (J Herman). Cost data: 2007 Economic Impact Study (PCAA). Chart created by Ann Jennings, PhD. http://www.TheAnnaInstitute.org Revision: April 6, 2010

Finding Your ACE Score

While you were growing up, during your first 18 years of life:

1. Did a parent or other adult in the household often or very often swear at you, insult you, put you down, or humiliate you? Or, act in a way that made you afraid that you might be physically hurt? Yes? No?

2. Did a parent or other adult in the household often or very often push, grab, slap, or throw something at you? Or, ever hit you so hard that you had marks or were injured? Yes? No?

3. Did an adult or person at least five years older than you ever touch or fondle you or have you touch their body in a sexual

way? Or, attempt or actually have oral, anal, or vaginal intercourse with you? Yes? No?

4. Did you often or very often feel that no one in your family loved you or thought you were important or special? Or, your family didn't look out for each other, feel close to each other, or support each other? Yes? No?

5. Did you often or very often feel that you didn't have enough to eat, had to wear dirty clothes, and had no one to protect you? Or, your parents were too drunk or high to take care of you or take you to the doctor if you needed it? Yes? No?

6. Were your parents ever separated or divorced? Yes? No?

7. Was your mother or stepmother often or very often pushed, grabbed, slapped, or had something thrown at her? Or, sometimes, often, or very often kicked, bitten, hit with a fist, or hit with something hard? Or, ever repeatedly hit at least a few minutes or threatened with a gun or knife? Yes? No?

8. Did you live with anyone who was a problem drinker or alcoholic or who used street drugs? Yes? No?

9. Was a household member depressed or mentally ill, or did a household member attempt suicide? Yes? No?

10. Did a household member go to prison? Yes? No?

Now count up your "Yes" answers: _____. This is your ACE Score.

Chapter 23

Adult Survivors of Childhood Sexual Abuse

Survivors of childhood sexual abuse experience an array of over-whelming and intense feelings. These may include feelings of fear, guilt, and shame. Abusers have been known to tell children that it is the fault of the child that they are abused, shifting the blame away from the abuser, where it belongs, and placing it on the child. Along with this, abusers may threaten or bribe the child into not speaking up; convincing the child that he or she will never be believed.[1] The re-action of a survivor's friends and family to the disclosure of the abuse also has the potential to trigger immense feelings of guilt, shame and distrust, particularly if those individuals denied that the abuse was taking place, or chose to ignore it.

While each individual's experiences and reactions are unique, there are some responses to child sexual abuse that are common to many survivors:[1]

- Low self-esteem or self-hatred

- Survivors may suffer from depression

- Guilt, shame, and blame

- Survivors may feel guilt or shame because they made no direct attempt to stop the abuse or because they experienced physical pleasure

- Sleep disturbances/disorders

  - Survivors may have trouble sleeping because of the trauma or anxiety, which may directly be related to the experience they had as a child; children may be sexually abused in their own beds.

- Lack of trust for anyone

  - Many survivors were betrayed by the very people they are dependent upon (family, teachers, etc.) who cared for them, who insisted they loved them even while abusing them; learning to trust can be extremely difficult under these circumstances.

  - 93% of victims under the age of 18 know their attacker.[2]

- Revictimization

  - Many survivors as adults find themselves in abusive, dangerous situations or relationships.

  - Woman who were sexually assaulted before the age of 18 [are] twice as likely to report being raped as adults.[3]

- Flashbacks

  - Many survivors re-experience the sexual abuse as if it were occurring at that moment, usually accompanied by visual images of the abuse. These flashes of images are often triggered by an event, action, or even a smell that is reminiscent of the sexual abuse of the abuser.

- Dissociation

  - Many survivors go through a process where the mind distances itself from the experience because it is too much for the psyche to process at the time. This loss of connection with thoughts, memories, feelings, actions, or sense of identity, is a coping mechanism and may affect aspects of a survivor's functioning.

- Sexuality/intimacy

  - Many survivors have to deal with the fact that their first sexual encounter was a result of abuse. Such memories may interfere with the survivor's ability to engage in sexual relationships, which may bring about feelings of fright, frustration, or being ashamed.

Adult survivors of childhood sexual abuse often adopt coping mechanisms (or survival strategies) to guard against feelings of terror and helplessness that they may have felt as a child. These past feelings can still have influence over the life and present behavior of an adult survivor. Here are some common coping mechanisms:[1]

- Grieving/mourning

  - Many things were lost—childhood experiences, trust, innocence, relationships with family members. The survivor may feel a deep sadness, jealousy, anger, or longing for something never had.

- Alcohol or drug abuse

  - The abuse of substances can act as an escape from the intense waves of feelings, the terror, and helplessness.

- Disordered eating/eating disorders

  - Compulsive control of food intake can be a way of taking back control over the body that was denied during the abuse.

- Self-injury

  - There are many ways survivors have coped with the feelings that can cause emotional or physical injury on the self. Burning or cutting are some ways for a survivor to relieve intense anxiety, triggered by memories of the abuse

Treatment[1]

In most instances, the survivor never discussed the abuse with others while it was occurring. In fact, many survivors do not remember the abuse until years after it has occurred, and may never be able to clearly recall it. Usually, after being triggered by a memory, this individual learns how, as an adult, to deal with the effects of the abuse.

It is important to speak with someone, whether it be a friend or counselor, about the abuse and past and current feelings.

Community health centers, mental health clinics and family service centers may have counselors who have worked with survivors before. They may also be able to refer you to a self-help group.

If you are an adult dealing with the effects of childhood sexual abuse, please remember that you are not responsible for the abuse and that you are not alone. You can overcome the effects the abuse may have on your life. Please call the National Sexual Assault Hotline (800-656-HOPE) or visit the Online Hotline (https://ohl.rainn.org/online). It's never too late to get help.

Notes

1. *Adult Survivors of Childhood Sexual Abuse.* Dr.Carol Boulware, MFT, Ph.D. 2006. http://www.psychotherapist.net/adultsurvivors.html

2. U.S. Bureau of Justice Statistics. *2000 Sexual Assault of Young Children as Reported to Law Enforcement.* 2000.

3. *Extent, Nature, and Consequences of Rape Victimization: Findings From the National Violence Against Women Survey.* U.S. Department of Justice: Office of Justice Programs: National Institute of Justice. 2006. http://www.ojp.usdoj.gov/nij

Chapter 24

Reactions to Trauma in Adult Survivors of Child Abuse

Chapter Contents

Section 24.1

Posttraumatic Stress Disorder

"What Is PTSD?" National Center for PTSD (http://www.ptsd.va.gov),
U.S. Department of Veterans Affairs, May 29, 2012.

What is PTSD?

Posttraumatic stress disorder (PTSD) can occur after you have been through a traumatic event. A traumatic event is something terrible and scary that you see, hear about, or that happens to you. These are some examples:

- Combat exposure

- Child sexual or physical abuse

- Terrorist attack

- Sexual or physical assault

- Serious accidents, like a car wreck

- Natural disasters, like a fire, tornado, hurricane, flood, or earthquake

During a traumatic event, you think that your life or others' lives are in danger. You may feel afraid or feel that you have no control over what is happening around you. Most people have some stress-related reactions after a traumatic event; but, not everyone gets PTSD. If your reactions don't go away over time and they disrupt your life, you may have PTSD.

How does PTSD develop?

Most people who go through a trauma have some symptoms at the beginning. Only some will develop PTSD over time. It isn't clear why some people develop PTSD and others don't.

Whether or not you get PTSD depends on many things:

- How intense the trauma was or how long it lasted

- If you were injured or lost someone important to you
- How close you were to the event
- How strong your reaction was
- How much you felt in control of events
- How much help and support you got after the event

What are the symptoms of PTSD?

PTSD symptoms usually start soon after the traumatic event, but they may not appear until months or years later. They also may come and go over many years. If the symptoms last longer than four weeks, cause you great distress, or interfere with your work or home life, you might have PTSD.

There are four types of symptoms of PTSD:

1. **Reliving the event (also called re-experiencing symptoms):** You may have bad memories or nightmares. You even may feel like you're going through the event again. This is called a flashback.

2. **Avoiding situations that remind you of the event:** You may try to avoid situations or people that trigger memories of the traumatic event. You may even avoid talking or thinking about the event.

3. **Feeling numb:** You may find it hard to express your feelings. Or, you may not be interested in activities you used to enjoy. This is another way to avoid memories.

4. **Feeling keyed up (also called hyperarousal):** You may be jittery, or always alert and on the lookout for danger. This is known as hyperarousal.

Can children have PTSD?

Children can have PTSD too. They may have symptoms described above or other symptoms depending on how old they are. As children get older, their symptoms are more like those of adults. Here are some examples of PTSD symptoms in children:

- Children age birth to five may get upset if their parents are not close by, have trouble sleeping, or suddenly have trouble with toilet training or going to the bathroom.

- Children age six to 11 may act out the trauma through play, drawings, or stories. Some have nightmares or become more irritable or aggressive. They may also want to avoid school or have trouble with schoolwork or friends.

- Children age 12 to 18 have symptoms more similar to adults: depression, anxiety, withdrawal, or reckless behavior like substance abuse or running away.

What other problems do people with PTSD experience?

People with PTSD may also have other problems. These include the following:

- Feelings of hopelessness, shame, or despair
- Depression or anxiety
- Drinking or drug problems
- Physical symptoms or chronic pain
- Employment problems
- Relationship problems, including divorce

In many cases, treatments for PTSD will also help these other problems, because they are often related. The coping skills you learn in treatment can work for PTSD and these related problems.

Will I get better?

"Getting better" means different things for different people, and not everyone who gets treatment will be "cured." Even if you continue to have symptoms, however, treatment can help you cope. Your symptoms don't have to interfere with your everyday activities, work, and relationships.

What treatments are available?

When you have PTSD, dealing with the past can be hard. Instead of telling others how you feel, you may keep your feelings bottled up. But treatment can help you get better. There are two main types of treatment, psychotherapy (sometimes called counseling) and medication. Sometimes people combine psychotherapy and medication.

Psychotherapy for PTSD: Psychotherapy, or counseling, involves meeting with a therapist. There are different types of psychotherapy:

- Cognitive behavioral therapy (CBT) is the most effective treatment for PTSD. There are different types of CBT, such as cognitive therapy and exposure therapy.

  - Cognitive processing therapy (CPT) is where you learn skills to understand how trauma changed your thoughts and feelings.

  - Prolonged exposure (PE) therapy is where you talk about your trauma repeatedly until memories are no longer upsetting. You also go to places that are safe, but that you have been staying away from because they are related to the trauma.

- A similar kind of therapy is called eye movement desensitization and reprocessing (EMDR). This therapy involves focusing on sounds or hand movements while you talk about the trauma.

Medications for PTSD: Medications can be effective too. A type of drug known as a selective serotonin reuptake inhibitor (SSRI), which is also used for depression, is effective for PTSD. Another medication called Prazosin has been found to be helpful in decreasing nightmares related to the trauma.

Important: Benzodiazepines and atypical antipsychotics should generally be avoided for PTSD treatment because they do not treat the core PTSD symptoms.

Section 24.2

Questions and Answers about Memories of Childhood Abuse

Can a memory be forgotten and then remembered? Can a 'memory' be suggested and then remembered as true?

These questions lie at the heart of the memory of childhood abuse issue. Experts in the field of memory and trauma can provide some answers, but clearly more study and research are needed. What we do know is that both memory researchers and clinicians who work with trauma victims agree that both phenomena occur. However, experienced clinical psychologists state that the phenomenon of a recovered memory is rare (for example, one experienced practitioner reported having a recovered memory arise only once in 20 years of practice). Also, although laboratory studies have shown that memory is often inaccurate and can be influenced by outside factors, memory research usually takes place either in a laboratory or some everyday setting. For ethical and humanitarian reasons, memory researchers do not subject people to a traumatic event in order to test their memory of it. Because the issue has not been directly studied, we cannot know whether a memory of a traumatic event is encoded and stored differently from a memory of a nontraumatic event.

Some clinicians theorize that children understand and respond to trauma differently from adults. Some furthermore believe that childhood trauma may lead to problems in memory storage and retrieval. These clinicians believe that dissociation is a likely explanation for a memory that was forgotten and later recalled. Dissociation means that a memory is not actually lost, but is for some time unavailable for retrieval. That is, it's in memory storage, but cannot for some period of time actually be recalled. Some clinicians believe that severe forms of child sexual abuse are especially conducive to negative disturbances of memory such as dissociation or delayed memory. Many clinicians who work with trauma victims believe that this dissociation is a person's way of sheltering himself or herself from the pain of the memory. Many researchers argue, however, that there is little or no empirical support for such a theory.

What's the bottom line?

First, it's important to state that there is a consensus among memory researchers and clinicians that most people who were sexually abused as children remember all or part of what happened to them although they may not fully understand or disclose it. Concerning the issue of a recovered versus a pseudomemory, like many questions in science, the final answer is yet to be known. But most leaders in the field agree that although it is a rare occurrence, a memory of early childhood abuse that has been forgotten can be remembered later. However, these leaders also agree that it is possible to construct convincing pseudomemories for events that never occurred.

The mechanism(s) by which both of these phenomena happen are not well understood and, at this point it is impossible, without other corroborative evidence, to distinguish a true memory from a false one.

What further research is needed?

The controversy over the validity of memories of childhood abuse has raised many critical issues for the psychological community. Many questions are at this point unanswered. This controversy has demonstrated that there are areas of research which should be pursued; among them are the following:

- Research to provide a better understanding of the mechanism by which accurate or inaccurate recollections of events may be created;

- Research to ascertain which clinical techniques are most likely to lead to the creation of pseudomemories and which techniques are most effective in creating the conditions under which actual events of childhood abuse can be remembered with accuracy;

- Research to ascertain how trauma and traumatic response impact the memory process;

- Research to ascertain if some people are more susceptible than others to memory suggestion and alteration and if so, why.

Much of this research will profit from collaborative efforts among psychologists who specialize in memory research and those clinicians who specialize in working with trauma and abuse victims.

If there is so much controversy about childhood memories of abuse, should I still seek help from a mental health provider if I believe I have such a memory?

Yes. The issue of repressed or suggested memories has been over-reported and sensationalized by the news media. Media and entertainment portrayals of the memory issue have succeeded in presenting the least likely scenario (that of a total amnesia of a childhood event) as the most likely occurrence. The reality is that most people who are victims of childhood sexual abuse remember all or part of what happened to them. Also true is the fact that thousands of people see a psychologist every day and are helped to deal with such things as issues of personal adjustment, depression, substance abuse, and problems in relationships. The issues of childhood abuse or questionable memory retrieval techniques never enter into the equation in the great majority of therapy relationships.

What should I know about choosing a psychotherapist to help me deal with a childhood memory or any other issue?

The American Psychological Association has released to the public the following advice to consider when seeking psychotherapy services.

First, know that there is no single set of symptoms which automatically indicates that a person was a victim of childhood abuse. There have been media reports of therapists who state that people (particularly women) with a particular set of problems or symptoms must have been victims of childhood sexual abuse. There is no scientific evidence that supports this conclusion.

Second, all questions concerning possible recovered memories of childhood abuse should be considered from an unbiased position. A therapist should not approach recovered memories with the preconceived notion that abuse must have happened or that abuse could not possibly have happened.

Third, when considering current problems, be wary of those therapists who offer an instant childhood abuse explanation, and those who dismiss claims or reports of sexual abuse without any exploration.

Fourth, when seeking psychotherapy, you are advised to see a licensed practitioner with training and experience in the issue for which you seek treatment. Ask the therapist about the kinds of treatment techniques he or she uses and how they could help you.

How can I expect a competent psychotherapist to react to a recovered memory?

A competent psychotherapist will attempt to stick to the facts as you report them. He or she will be careful to let the information evolve as your memory does and not to steer you toward a particular conclusion or interpretation. A competent psychotherapist is likely to acknowledge that current knowledge does not allow the definite conclusion that a memory is real or false without other corroborating evidence.

What credentials should I look for when selecting a mental health provider?

You should choose a mental health professional as carefully as you would choose a physical health provider. For example, licensed psychologists have earned an undergraduate degree and have completed five to seven years of graduate study culminating in a doctoral degree and including a one-year, full-time internship. All psychologists are required to be licensed or certified by the state in which they practice and many states require that they keep their training current by completing continuing education classes every year. Members of the American Psychological Association are also bound by a strict code of ethical standards.

Once the provider's competency has been established, his or her experience dealing with the issues you want help with is important. Also important is your level of comfort with the provider. Psychotherapy is a cooperative effort between therapist and patient, so a high level of personal trust and comfort is necessary. However, you should be concerned if your therapist reports to you that a large number of his or her patients recover memories of childhood abuse while in treatment.

There are a number of good ways to get a referral to a mental health professional. Your state psychological association will be able to provide you with referrals to psychologists in your community. Many state associations are located in their state capital. Also, because so many physical ailments have psychological components, most family physicians have a working relationship with a psychologist. Ask your doctor about a referral. Your church or synagogue and school guidance program or university counseling centers also usually maintain lists of providers in the community.

The American Psychological Association (APA) also has published a brochure of advice about the selection of a mental health provider entitled "How to Choose a Psychologist" (available online at http://www.apa.org/helpcenter/choose-therapist.aspx).

Editor's note [from original document]: This document is being released at the direction of the APA Board of Directors. It is based on numerous reports and documents, including, but not limited to, the work of the APA Working Group on the Investigation of Memories of Childhood Abuse.

Chapter 25

Mental Health Issues in Adult Survivors of Child Abuse

Chapter Contents

Section 25.1

Abuse-Related Mental Disorders

The negative impact of child abuse on adult mental health has been documented for over 150 years, and, over the last thirty years, in particular, numerous research studies have documented the link between child abuse and mental illness in later life. At present, there is no single diagnosis or condition that describes the psychological effects of child abuse. When in contact with mental health services, many adult survivors of child abuse find themselves diagnosed with multiple psychological conditions, many of which have considerable overlap.

The psychological impact of abuse on a child depends on a range of factors, including: the type of abuse, the severity of abuse, the relationship of the child to the abuser/s, the child's family environment and their relationship with their parents or other caregivers, and whether the child has previous experiences of abuse, or a history of support, care and love. These factors can soften, or exacerbate, the impact of abuse on a child's psychological wellbeing, and the likelihood that they will develop mental illness later in life.

Below is a list of a range of psychological conditions that are associated with child abuse. Please read on to find out more about them.

Post-Traumatic Stress Disorder

Post-traumatic stress disorder (PTSD) is a psychological condition that develops after a person has been harmed or exposed to danger, and they have been unable to protect themselves. PTSD is particularly likely to develop when a person experiences fear, helplessness and powerlessness, which are all common features of child abuse.

PTSD has three main symptoms:

- Hyperarousal is similar to the jumpy feeling that drinking too much coffee causes. We might experience it as anxiety, agitation or irritability. It is commonly known as the state of "fight or flight."

- Intrusions occur when traumatic experiences dating from a person's past, break through into their consciousness and are experienced as though they are occurring in the present. They are called "flashbacks."

- Avoidance is an attempt to defend oneself against danger by limiting contact with the world. This can involve withdrawing from others or narrowing the range of thoughts and feelings a person allows him/herself to acknowledge. Avoidance can take the form of repression (locking the memory of a traumatic event away), denial (failing to acknowledge that an event which occurred, actually happened), dissociation (altered perception), or amnesia (memory loss). Survivors subconsciously use any or all of these techniques to survive the trauma of their abuse.

Other indicators of PTSD may include:

- Panic attacks
- Uncontrollable crying
- Uncontrollable rages
- Eating disorders
- Suicidal feelings
- Self mutilation
- Somatic pain
- Terror
- Addictions (alcohol, drugs, sex)
- Overreaction to minor stress
- Sleep disorders
- Sense of defilement or stigma
- Nightmares
- State of fight or flight
- Extreme mood swings
- High risk behaviors
- Shame, guilt and blame

Panic Attacks

Anxiety is a feeling of apprehension associated with symptoms of tension. It is different to fear as fear is a response to perceived present danger. When fear occurs inappropriately anxiety can escalate and a panic attack can occur. People who have experienced childhood abuse are more likely to experience frequent or generalized anxiety or panic attacks than those who haven't.

Panic attacks occur when an individual experiences a sudden period of intense fear or discomfort, in which four or more of the following symptoms rapidly develop:

• Palpitations/ pounding heart or racing heart

• Sweating

• Trembling

• Feeling of choking or trouble breathing

• Chest pain or discomfort

• Nausea or abdominal distress

• Feeling dizzy or faint

• Feelings of unreality or of being detached from oneself

• Fear of losing control or going crazy

• Fear of dying

• Numbness or tingling

• Chills or hot flushes

Depression

Depression is common. People who are depressed can feel discouraged about the future, dissatisfied with life (maybe even wishing they were dead), or isolated from others. They might lack the energy to get things done or to even get out of bed, be unable to concentrate, or to eat or sleep normally. Feeling depressed is often a response to past and current losses. To feel bad as a reaction to a tragedy (such as a significant loss) is to be expected. Major depressive disorder, however, occurs when signs of depression (including lethargy, worthlessness, or loss of interest in family, friends, and activities) last two weeks or more for no apparent reason. Symptoms include:

- Depressed mood
- Feelings of worthlessness or excessive or inappropriate guilt
- Markedly diminished interest in all or almost all activities
- Significant weight loss when not dieting or weight gain, or decrease or increase in appetite
- Insomnia or hypersomnia
- Diminished pleasure from usual activities
- Lethargy
- Feelings of hopelessness
- Lack of motivation
- Diminished ability to think or concentrate, or indecisiveness
- Recurrent thoughts of death, suicidal ideation or attempts
- Psychomotor agitation (observable restlessness) or retardation

Dissociation

Dissociative disorders are characterized by alterations in perception; a sense of detachment from one's own self (depersonalization), from the world (derealization) or from memories. Dissociative amnesia occurs when the individual is unable to remember important personal information. In extreme cases, new identities (alters) are formed (dissociative identity disorder, or DID).

The more severe or protracted the abuse, the more the child will use dissociation to escape the horror or pain of a given situation. Survivors carry this skill into their adult life, continuing to use it as a way of avoiding difficulties in their lives. Many are not aware that they are dissociating as the process has become so automatic. Part of the journey of recovery from the trauma of child abuse involves learning to stay present while facing the reality of one's trauma.

Dissociative Identity Disorder (DID)

People with DID can adopt many new identities, all simultaneously co-existing inside one body and mind. In some cases these identities are well-defined, each with its own behavior, tone of voice, and physical gestures. In other cases, only a few characteristics are distinct, because the identities are only partially independent.

Bipolar Disorder

This condition occurs less commonly than major depression. A person suffering from bipolar disorder will tend to alternate between the hopelessness and lethargy of depression and the hyperactive, wildly optimistic, and impulsive phase of mania. The onset of bipolar disorder is usually in the twenties, although it sometimes starts in adolescence. Treatment for bipolar disease, which may include medication, psychotherapy, and lifestyle changes, tends to be effective. Maintenance treatment between episodes may greatly reduce or even prevent further episodes.

Schizophrenia

Schizophrenia refers to a group of severe disorders in which a person loses touch with reality, experiencing grossly irrational ideas or distorted perceptions. It is a potentially serious mental illness which affects almost one person in 100. The first onset is usually in adolescence or early adulthood but the disorder can develop later. The onset may be rapid, developing over weeks, or slow in which case it develops over months or years. Some people only experience one or more brief episodes and recover fully while others have to deal with schizophrenia throughout their lives. The management of schizophrenia has improved a lot in recent years. Medication, psychotherapy, social, and family support are all helpful and contribute to returning the person to work, education, and personal life. Symptoms of schizophrenia include:

- Disorganized thinking—fragmented or bizarre and distorted by false beliefs called delusions. Thought and speech may be jumbled and difficult to follow, with conversation jumping from one subject to another without any obvious logic.

- Delusions can include ideas of persecution (paranoia) or ideas of grandeur.

- Disturbed perceptions including hallucinations: perceiving things that aren't there—often auditory, that is, hearing voices, although hallucinations can involve any of the five senses.

- Inappropriate emotional responses and actions

- Withdrawal from other people

- Loss of drive, initiative, and motivation

- Lack of insight into own behavior and thinking, and denial of the illness

Eating Disorders

The principle feature of eating disorders is a preoccupation with control over eating, body weight, and food. Anorexia and bulimia nervosa are the most serious of the eating disorders.

Anorexia nervosa includes features such as self-induced weight loss (through starvation, purging, and exercise) and an intense fear of becoming fat.

Bulimia nervosa features repeated bouts of uncontrolled over-eating (bingeing), intense fear of gaining weight, engaging in excessive exercise to prevent weight gain, self-induced vomiting, and the use of laxatives and fluid tablets.

Treatment for eating disorders includes nutritional management, cognitive-behavioral therapy around beliefs and distorted body image, psychotherapies, and medication.

Personality Disorders

Personality disorders are long-lasting, maladaptive patterns of behavior that impair social functioning. They are thought to originate in childhood and then continue into adult years.

Types include (this list is not exhaustive):

- **Paranoid personality disorder:** A pervasive distrust and suspicion of others

- **Antisocial personality disorder:** A pervasive pattern of disregard for and violation of the rights of others

- **Borderline personality disorder:** A pervasive pattern of instability of interpersonal relationships, self-image, affects, and control over impulses. A website—the Borderline Mother (http://www.borderlinemothers.com) explains this disorder in more detail.

- **Narcissistic personality disorder:** A pervasive pattern of grandiosity, need for admiration, and lack of empathy

- **Obsessive-compulsive personality disorder:** A pervasive preoccupation with orderliness, perfectionism, and mental and interpersonal control, at the expense of flexibility, openness and efficiency.

Treating people with personality disorders is often difficult as those with a personality disorder often do have little or no insight into the fact that their difficulties are a result of the way they relate to others.

Section 25.2

Link between Child Abuse and Adult Suicide Risk

What is the link between child abuse and adult suicide risk? A startling new study suggests that physical and emotional child abuse makes dramatic and long-lasting changes to young male victims' brains—increasing the odds that they'll grow up to become men who commit suicide.

In the wake of a suicide, friends, family, and loved ones are left reeling, grappling with the big question: Why? One part of the answer was recently found in research performed by scientists associated with the newly formed Sackler Program for Epigenetics and Psychobiology at McGill University. The researchers discovered a novel biological link to some male suicides. Earlier studies linked physical or emotional childhood abuse to suicide, but the Sackler team found that childhood abuse amongst suicide victims was associated with a distinct epigenetic mark on the DNA. The discovery represents a huge step forward for epigenetics—the study of how environmental factors change gene expression—and holds the promise of better understanding suicide and, perhaps, new treatments.

This discovery grew out of a grim, yet indispensable, resource. The Quebec Suicide Brain Bank is exactly what it sounds like: dozens of brain tissue samples from suicide victims, each preserved in Pyrex containers in a Douglas Mental Health University Institute freezer. Every time the Quebec Coroner's office determines a death to be a suicide, it notifies psychiatry professor Dr. Gustavo Turecki, director of the McGill Group for Suicide Studies at the Douglas. Researchers from the MGSS then contact the next of kin to ask whether they are willing to donate a brain tissue sample. But the researchers are interested in more than just the brain; they want to know the person it came from. Using standardized and validated interviews with friends, family, and spouses, they build a complete psychological and medical history of each victim.

Beginning in 2006, Patrick McGowan, a post-doctoral fellow in medicine professor Michael Meaney's lab, was given access to this wealth of information—and, of course, the brains. McGowan had just returned to Montreal (he did his undergraduate studies at Concordia University) after completing his PhD at Duke University in North Carolina. He was specifically attracted by Meaney's collaborations with Moshe Szyf, the James McGill Professor in the Department of Pharmacology and Therapeutics. In a now-famous 2004 paper published in the journal *Nature Neuroscience*, Meaney and Szyf showed that gene expression in rat pups could be affected by maternal care in infancy. The more licking and grooming from the mother, the less anxious the offspring, behavioral changes that correlated with gene expression. The DNA sequence of the rats was unchanged, of course; what was different was the methylation, a chemical coating on the DNA that determines how our genes work.

Meaney and Szyf worked exclusively with rat models, and McGowan was excited by the prospect of taking epigenetics to the next level. Back at the Douglas, Turecki had been following Meaney and Szyf's research, and saw how the Quebec Suicide Brain Bank could be useful. "It became clear to me that we were in a good position to do translation work," he says. "This was a good opportunity to test the theories from animal work and see if they were applicable to humans."

"I had never expected to have a chance to work with human samples," McGowan says. "But the feeling was that if we can do this in animals, why not in humans? We had the brains, and we had the histories."

McGowan's team used a cohort of 36 brain samples. One third were from suicide subjects who were known to have been abused in childhood, one third from suicides with no known abuse in their childhoods, and one third from a control group. The researchers discovered that those suicides who had suffered abuse as children bore specific epigenetic methylation characteristics absent on specific DNA sites that were in the other two groups. Significantly, those marks were shown to influence the hypothalamic-pituitary-adrenal (HPA) function.

The HPA axis is a critical feature of the stress response. It is managed by a set of genes expressed in the hippocampus, including one that was epigenetically marked by the experience of childhood abuse. Abnormal HPA activity in response to stress is in turn strongly linked to suicidal action. Turecki explains that there was no distinction made in their cohorts between severity or nature of the childhood abuse: "Severity is a subjective thing—the impact is much more important."

The study was published in the February 22, 2009 issue of *Nature Neuroscience*. The McGill research team also includes graduate students Ana C. D'Alessio and Benoît Labonté, research associate Aya Sasaki and research technician Sergiy Dymov.

Suicide's links to stress and childhood abuse were both known before, but this breakthrough demonstrates, at least in part, exactly how it works on a biological level. Turecki is careful to avoid speculation about future treatments, but he allows that this is a significant step "toward understanding how early life experiences have a major impact on mental health."

Epigenetics points to a way forward. McGowan believes that epigenetic patterns could serve as a valuable diagnostic tool, if markers can be detected in blood tests. Better yet, it may be possible to manipulate the methylations themselves, thus reversing their unwanted effects. The drug TSA and l-methionine infusions (directly into the brain) have already proved successful in changing methylation patterns established early in a rat's early life. "The l-methionine infusions are particularly interesting," says McGowan, "because l-methionine is an essential amino acid and a popular nutritional supplement. The studies showed effects in adult animals so it's possible that, at some point in the future, therapies might include drugs that change epigenetic patterns in the brain. The key would be to discover how to target these drugs, which have widespread effects, to the right genes. It would be equally interesting to know whether social interventions have protective effects by changing the methylation of certain key genes."

Moshe Szyf, who was recently appointed to the inaugural GlaxoSmith-Kline-CIHR Professorship in Pharmacology, says that this study is the first that he knew of in which there is a clear link between human social environments and their epigenetic code. "It is dynamic, and it acts through life," he says. "And it's not just chemicals that affect these mechanisms, it's the social, and even political, environment." This recent breakthrough raises many more questions about this mysterious relationship between environment and DNA. If a person's genes can be affected by childhood abuse, then what about the effect on those who've grown up in countries that have endured decades of war and oppression? What effect does diet, or even music, have on our DNA? If the social environment has such an effect on who we are, there is almost no area of human endeavor without a potential impact on our epigenetic code. "To understand human health and disease, we must study humans in their true environmental context."

As for the age-old nature-versus-nurture debate? Well, epigenetics just might offer a third choice: both. Medical research has long known that, despite having identical DNA sequences, the health and personality of identical twins often diverge. Environmental influences are often used to explain such inconsistencies in genes and traits—now this new study shows that the environment can actually directly alter the activity of the genome.

"Nature and nurture has always been a false dichotomy," says Mc-Gowan, before quoting famed McGill neuroscientist Donald Hebb: "It's like asking which is more important to a rectangle's area—length or width?"

This research was funded by the Canadian Institutes for Health Research and the U.S. National Institute of Child Health and Development.

Part Five

Child Abuse Preventions, Interventions, and Treatments

Chapter 26

Child Abuse Prevention Strategies

Chapter Contents

Section 26.1

Identifying Behaviors in Adults That May Put Children at Risk

Behaviors to Watch For

We all have personal likes and things that make us uncomfortable. "Personal space" is the private area of control inside an imaginary line or boundary that defines each person as separate.

Ideally, that boundary helps us stay in charge of our own personal space. It helps keep out the things that make us uncomfortable—unsafe and unwanted feelings, words, images, and physical contact. Solid social rules strengthen the boundary. Behaviors that routinely disrespect or ignore boundaries make children vulnerable to abuse.

Do you know an adult or older child who doesn't seem to understand what's acceptable when it comes to [the following areas]?

Personal Space

- Makes others uncomfortable by ignoring social, emotional, or physical boundaries or limits?

- Refuses to let a child set any of his or her own limits? Uses teasing or belittling language to keep a child from setting a limit?

- Insists on hugging, touching, kissing, tickling, wrestling with, or holding a child even when the child does not want this physical contact or attention?

- Frequently walks in on children/teens in the bathroom?

Relationships with Children

- Turns to a child for emotional or physical comfort by sharing personal or private information or activities, normally shared with adults?

- Has secret interactions with teens or children (e.g., games, sharing drugs, alcohol, or sexual material) or spends excessive time to e-mailing, text messaging, or calling children or youth?

- Insists on or manages to spend uninterrupted time alone with a child?

- Seems "too good to be true," i.e., frequently baby sits different children for free; takes children on special outings alone; buys children gifts or gives them money for no apparent reason?

- Allows children or teens to consistently get away with inappropriate behaviors?

Sexual Conversation or Behavior

- Frequently points out sexual images or tells dirty or suggestive jokes with children present?

- Exposes a child to adult sexual interactions or images without apparent concern?

- Is overly interested in the sexuality of a particular child or teen (e.g., talks repeatedly about the child's developing body or interferes with normal teen dating)?

What You Can Do If You See Warning Signs

- Create a safety plan (see http://www.stopitnow.org/family _safety_plan). Don't wait for "proof" of child sexual abuse.

- Look for patterns of behavior that make children less safe. Keep track of behaviors that concern you. The Sample Journal Page (available online at http://www.stopitnow.org/journal _entry) can be a helpful tool.

- See the Stop It Now! publication, *Let's Talk Guidebook* (available at http://www.stopitnow.org/guidebooks) for tips on speaking up whenever you have a concern.

- If you have questions or would like resources or guidance for responding to a specific situation, visit the Stop It Now! Online Help Center, http://GetHelp.StopItNow.org.

Remember, the most effective prevention takes place before there's a child victim to heal or an offender to punish.

Section 26.2

Child Maltreatment Prevention Initiatives

Excerpted from: Child Welfare Information Gateway. (2011). Child maltreatment prevention: Past, present, and future. Washington, DC: U.S. Department of Health and Human Services, Children's Bureau. The complete text of this document, including references is available online at http://www.childwelfare .gov/pubs/issue_briefs/cm_prevention.pdf.

Introduction

Child abuse prevention efforts have grown exponentially over the past 30 years. Some of this expansion reflects new public policies and expanded formal services such as parent education classes, support groups, home visitation programs, and safety education for children. In other cases, individuals working on their own and in partnerships with others have found ways to strengthen local institutions and create a climate in which parents support each other.

This report underscores the importance of prevention as a critical component of the nation's child protection system. It outlines programs and strategies that are proving beneficial in reducing the likelihood of child maltreatment. Looking ahead, it identifies key issues facing high-quality prevention programs as they seek to extend their reach and impacts.

Scope of the Problem

Recent research documenting the number of child maltreatment cases observed by professionals working with children and families across the country suggests prevention efforts are having an impact. For example, the Fourth Federal National Incidence Study (NIS) on Child Maltreatment (2010) reported a 19% reduction in the rate of child maltreatment as reported in a similar survey conducted in 1993. Substantial and significant drops in the rates of sexual abuse, physical abuse, and emotional abuse observed by survey respondents occurred between 1993 and 2006. Although no significant declines were observed in cases of child neglect, the NIS data mirror a similar drop in the number of physical and sexual abuse cases reported in recent years to local child welfare agencies. Between 1990 and 2009, the number of substantiated cases of physical abuse dropped 55%, and the number of substantiated sexual abuse cases declined 61%.

Despite these promising trends, child maltreatment remains a substantial threat to a child's well-being and healthy development. In 2009, over three million children were reported as potential victims of maltreatment. The risk for harm is particularly high for children living in the most disadvantaged communities, including those living in extreme poverty or those living with caretakers who are unable or unwilling to care for them due to chronic problems of substance abuse, mental health disorders, or domestic violence. In 2009, an estimated 1,770 children—or over 4.8 children a day—were identified as fatal victims of maltreatment. As in the past, the majority of these children—over 80 percent—were under the age of four. While child maltreatment is neither inevitable nor intractable, protecting children remains challenging.

History of Child Abuse Prevention

Modern public and political attention to the issue of child maltreatment is often pegged to Henry Kempe's 1962 article in the *Journal of the American Medical Association* on the "battered child syndrome." In contrast to those early pioneers who had used clinical case studies to explain maltreatment patterns, Kempe and his colleagues examined hospital emergency room X-rays for one year from 70 hospitals around the country and surveyed 77 district attorneys. These efforts painted a vivid and disturbing picture of children suffering physical and emotional trauma as a result of overburdened parents or caretakers using extreme forms of corporal punishment or depressed single mothers failing to provide for their children's basic emotional and physical needs.

Armed with these descriptions, Kempe persuaded federal and state policymakers to support the adoption of a formal child abuse reporting system. Between 1963 and 1967, all states and the District of Columbia passed child abuse reporting laws. Federal reporting guidelines were established in 1974 with the authorization of the first federal Child Abuse and Neglect Prevention and Treatment Act.

The 1980s represented a period of significant expansion in public awareness of child maltreatment, research on its underlying causes and consequences, and the development and dissemination of both clinical interventions and prevention strategies. As more became known of the diversity within the maltreatment population, unique subpopulations were singled out for specific programmatic options and legislative attention. On the prevention front, two distinct program-matic paths emerged:

- Interventions targeting reductions in physical abuse and neglect (including emotional neglect and attachment disorders), including services to new parents, general parenting education classes, parent support groups, family resource centers, and crisis intervention services such as hotlines and crisis nurseries

- Interventions targeting reductions in child sexual abuse, including: universal efforts designed to teach children the distinction between good, bad, and questionable touching, the concept of body ownership, or the rights of children to control who touches their bodies and where they are touched; and educational programs that encouraged children and youth who had been victimized to report these incidences and seek services

The effectiveness of general parent education and support programs during this time was generally limited to parents able to access these options. Prevention efforts were far less successful in attracting and retaining families who did not know they needed assistance or, if they recognized their shortcomings, did not know how to access help.

By the 1990s, emphasis was placed on establishing a strong foundation of support for every parent and child, available when a child is born or a woman is pregnant. And the way to reach new parents centered on home-based interventions. The seminal work of David Olds and his colleagues showing initial and long-term benefits from regular nurse visiting during pregnancy and a child's first two years of life provided the most robust evidence for this intervention. Equally important, however, were the growing number of home visitation models being developed and successfully implemented within the public and community-based service sectors. Although less rigorous in their evaluation methodologies, these models demonstrated respectable gains in parent-child attachment, access to preventive medical care, parental capacity and functioning, and early identification of developmental delays

Prevention Today

After implementing home visitation programs for over a decade, the prevention field is facing an important challenge. Recent federal legislation included in the Patient Protection and Affordable Care Act of 2009 will provide states $1.5 billion over the next five years to expand the provision of evidence-based home visitation programs to at-risk pregnant women and newborns. While research justifies an expansion of several high-quality national home visitation models, it also indicates that not all families are equally well-served by this approach; retention in long-term interventions can be difficult; and identifying, training, and retaining competent service providers is challenging. Even intensive interventions cannot fully address the needs of the most challenged populations—those struggling with serious mental illness, domestic violence, and substance abuse, as well as those rearing children in violence and chaotic neighborhoods.

Faced with the inevitable limitations of any individual program model, increased emphasis is being placed on approaches that seek change at a community or systems level. The current prevention challenge is not simply expanding formal services but rather creating an institutional infrastructure that supports high-quality, evidence-based direct services. In addition, prevention efforts have embraced a more explicit effort to both reduce risks and enhance key protective factors, fostering strong partnerships with other local programs serving young children. Among the most salient investments in promoting protective factors are efforts to strengthen parental capacity and resilience, support a child's social and emotional development, and create more supportive relationships among community residents. Communities where residents believe in collective responsibility for keeping children safe may achieve progress in reducing child abuse and strengthening child well-being.

Identifying and Implementing Quality Programs

All prevention services need to embrace a commitment to a set of practice principles that have been found effective across diverse disciplines and service delivery systems. A suggested list of best practice standards appears below. As a group, these items represent best practice elements that lie at the core of effective interventions. To the extent that direct service providers and prevention policy advocates hope to maximize the return on their investments, supporting service strategies that embrace the following principles will be essential:

- A strong theory of change that identifies specific outcomes and clear pathways for addressing these core outcomes, including specific strategies and curriculum content

- A recommended duration and dosage or clear guidelines for determining when to discontinue or extend services that is systematically applied to all those enrolled in services

- A clear, well-defined target population with identified eligibility criteria and strategy for reaching and engaging this target population

- A strategy for guiding staff in balancing the task of delivering program content while being responsive to a family's cultural beliefs and immediate circumstances

- A method to train staff on delivering the model with a supervisory system to support direct service staff and guide their ongoing practice

- Reasonable caseloads that are maintained and allow direct service staff to accomplish core program objectives

- The systematic collection of information on participant characteristics, staff characteristics, and participant service experiences to ensure services are being implemented with fidelity to the model, program intent, and structure

Promising Prevention Strategies

Several researchers suggest that the more universal or broadly targeted prevention efforts have greater success in strengthening a parent's or child's protective factors than in eliminating risk factors, particularly for parents or children at highest risk. Others argue that prevention strategies are most effective when they focus on a clearly defined target population with identifiable risk factors. In truth, a wide range of prevention strategies has demonstrated an ability to reduce child abuse and neglect reports as well as other child safety outcomes such as reported injuries and accidents. In other cases, prevention efforts have strengthened key protective factors associated with a reduced incidence of child maltreatment such as improved parental resilience; stronger social connections; positive child development; better access to concrete supports such as housing, transportation, and nutrition; and improved parenting skills and knowledge of child development.

Public awareness efforts: In the years immediately following Kempe's 1962 article on battered child syndrome, public awareness campaigns were developed to raise awareness about child abuse and to generate political support for legislation to address the problem. Notably, the nonprofit organization Prevent Child Abuse America (PCA America; formerly, the National Committee to Prevent Child Abuse) joined forces with the Ad Council to develop and distribute nationwide a series of public service announcements (PSAs) for television, radio, print, and billboards.

Between 1975 and 1985, repeated public opinion polls documented a sharp increase in public recognition of child abuse as an important social problem and steady declines in the use of corporal punishment and verbal forms of aggression in disciplining children. More recently, broadly targeted prevention campaigns have been used to alter parental behavior. For example, the U.S. Public Health Service, in partnership with the American Academy of Pediatrics (AAP) and the Association of SIDS and Infant Mortality Programs, launched its "Back to Sleep" campaign in 1994 designed to educate parents and caretakers about the importance of placing infants on their backs to sleep as a strategy to reduce the rate of sudden infant death syndrome (SIDS). Notable gains also have been achieved with universal education programs to prevent shaken baby syndrome.

Child sexual assault prevention classes: In contrast to efforts designed to alter the behavior of adults who might commit maltreatment, a category of prevention programs emerged in the 1980s designed to alter the behavior of potential victims. Often referred to as child assault prevention or safety education programs, these efforts present children with information on the topic of physical abuse and sexual assault, how to avoid risky situations, and, if abused, how to respond. A key feature of these programs is their universal service delivery systems, often being integrated into school curricula or into primary support opportunities for children (for example, Boy Scouts, youth groups, recreation programs). Although certain concerns have been raised regarding the appropriateness of these efforts, the strategy continues to be widely available.

Parent education and support groups: Educational and support services delivered to parents through center-based programs and group settings are used in a variety of ways to address risk factors associated with child abuse and neglect. Although the primary focus of these interventions is typically the parent, quite a few programs include opportunities for structured parent-child interactions, and many programs incorporate parallel interventions for children. For instance, programs may include components such as the following:

- Weekly discussions for 8 to 14 weeks with parents around topics such as discipline, cognitive development, and parent-child communication

- Group-based sessions at which parents and children can discuss issues and share feelings

361

- Opportunities for parents to model the parenting skills they are learning

- Time for participants to share meals and important family celebrations such as birthdays and graduations

Educational and support services range from education and information sharing to general support to therapeutic interventions. Many of the programs are delivered under the direction of social workers or health-care providers.

A meta-analysis conducted by the Centers for Disease Control and Prevention (2009) on training programs for parents of children from birth to age seven identified components of programs that have a positive impact on acquiring parenting skills and decreasing children's externalizing behaviors. These components included the following:

- Teaching parents emotional communication skills

- Helping parents acquire positive parent-child interaction skills

- Providing parents opportunities to demonstrate and practice these skills while observed by a service provider

Home visitation: As noted earlier, home visitation has become a major strategy for supporting new parents. Services are one-on-one and are provided by staff with professional training (nursing, social work, child development, family support) or by paraprofessionals who receive training in the model's approach and curricula. The primary issues addressed during visits include the following:

- The mother's personal health and life choices

- Child health and development

- Environmental concerns such as income, housing, and community violence

- Family functioning, including adult and child relationships

- Access to services

Specific activities to address these issues may include the following:

- Modeling parent-child interactions and child management strategies

- Providing observation and feedback

- Offering general parenting and child development information

- Conducting formal assessments and screenings
- Providing structured counseling

In addition to working with participants around a set of parenting and child development issues, home visitors often serve as gatekeepers to the broader array of services families may need to address various economic and personal needs. Critical reviews of the model's growing research base have reached different conclusions. In some cases, reviewers conclude that the strategy, when well implemented, does produce significant and meaningful reduction in child-abuse risk and improves child and family functioning. Others are more sobering in their conclusions, noting the limitations outlined earlier.

Community prevention efforts: The strategies previously outlined focus on individual parents and children. Recently, increased attention is being paid to prevention efforts designed to improve the community environment in which children are raised. Among other things, these efforts institute new services, streamline service delivery processes, and foster greater collaboration among local service providers. This emerging generation of "community child abuse prevention strategies" focuses on creating supportive residential communities where neighbors share a belief in collective responsibility to protect children from harm and where professionals work to expand services and support for parents.

In 2009, prevention researchers examined five community child abuse prevention programs that seek to reduce child abuse and neglect. Their review concluded that the case for community prevention is promising. At least some of the models reviewed show the ability to reduce reported rates of child abuse, reduce injury to young children, improve parent-child interactions, reduce parental stress, and improve parental efficacy. Focusing on community building, such programs can mobilize volunteers and engage diverse sectors within the community, including first responders, the faith community, local businesses, and civic groups. This mobilization exerts a synergistic impact on other desired community outcomes such as economic development and better health care.

Looking Toward the Future

Achieving stronger impacts with young children and their families will require continued efforts at developing and testing a broad array of prevention programs and systemic reforms. No one program or one approach can guarantee success. Although compelling evidence exists to support early intervention efforts, beginning at a time a woman becomes pregnant or gives birth, the absolute "best way" to provide this support is not self-evident. The most salient protective factors or risk factors will vary across populations as well as communities. Finding the correct leverage point or pathway for change for a specific family, community, or state requires careful assessment in which the final prevention plan is best suited to the needs and challenges presented by each situation.

As the prevention field moves forward, current strategies, institutional alignments and strategic partnerships need to be reevaluated and, in some cases, altered to better address current demographic and fiscal realities. Key challenges and the opportunities they present include the following:

- **Improving the ability to reach all those at risk:** The most common factors used to identify populations at risk for maltreatment include young maternal age, poverty, single parent status and severe personal challenges such as domestic violence, substance abuse, and mental health issues. Although such factors are often associated with elevated stress and reduced capacity to meet the needs of the developing child, no one of these factors is consistently predictive of poor parenting or poor child outcomes. In addition, families that present none of these risk factors may find themselves in need of preventive services as the result of a family health emergency, job loss, or other economic uncertainties. In short, our ability to accurately identify those who will benefit from preventive services is limited and fraught with the dual problems of over identification and under identification. Building on a public health model of integrated services, child abuse prevention strategies may be more efficiently allocated by embedding such services within a universal system of assessment and support.

- **Determining how best to intervene with diverse ethnic and cultural groups:** Much has been written about the importance of designing parenting and early intervention programs that are respectful of the participant's culture. For the most part, program planners have responded to this concern by delivering services in a participant's primary language, matching participants and providers on the basis of race and ethnicity, and incorporating traditional child rearing practices into a program's curriculum. Far less emphasis has been placed on testing the differential effects of evidence-based prevention programs on specific racial or cultural groups or the specific ways in which the concept of prevention is viewed by various groups and supported by their existing systems of informal support. Better understanding of these diverse perspectives is key to building a prevention system that is relevant for the full range of American families.

- **Identifying ways to use technology to expand provider-participant contact and service access:** The majority of prevention programs involve face-to-face contact between a provider and program participant. Indeed, the strength and quality of the participant-provider relationship is often viewed as one of the most, if not the most, important determinant of outcomes. Although not a replacement for personal contact, the judicial use of technology can help direct service providers offer assistance to families on their caseload. For example, home visitors use cell phones to maintain regular communication with parents between intervention visits; parent education and support programs use videotaping to provide feedback to parents on the quality of their interactions with their children; and community-based initiatives use the internet to link families with an array of resources in the community. Expanding the use of these technologies and documenting their relative costs and benefits for both providers and program participants offer both potential costs savings as well as ways to reach families living in rural and frontier communities.

- **Achieving a balance between enhancing formal services and strengthening informal supports:** Families draw on a combination of formal services (for example, health care, education, public welfare, neighborhood associations, and primary supports) and informal support (for example, assistance from family members, friends, and neighbors) in caring for their children. Relying too much on informal relationships and community support may be insufficient for families unable to draw on available informal supports or who live in communities where such supports are insufficient to address their complex needs. In contrast, focusing only on formal services may ignore the limitations to public resources and the importance of creating a culture in which seeking assistance in meeting one's parenting responsibilities is the norm. Those engaged in developing and implementing comprehensive, prevention systems need to consider how they might best draw on both of these resources.

Identifying and testing a range of innovations that address all of these concerns and alternatives is important. Equally challenging, however, is how these efforts are woven together into effective prevention systems at local, state, and national levels. Just as the appropriate service focus will vary across families, the appropriate collaborative partnerships and institutional alignments will differ across communities. In some cases, public health services will provide the most fruitful foundation for crafting effective outreach to new parents. In other communities, the education system or faith community will offer the most promising approach. And once innovations are established, they will require new partnerships, systemic reforms, or continuous refinement if they are to remain viable and relevant to each subsequent cohort of new parents and their children.

Conclusion

Preventing child abuse is not simply a matter of parents doing a better job, but rather it is about creating a context in which "doing better" is easier. Enlightened public policy and the replication of high-quality publicly supported interventions are only part of what is needed to successfully combat child abuse. It remains important to remind the public that child abuse and neglect are serious threats to a child's healthy development and that overt violence toward children and a persistent lack of attention to their care and supervision are unacceptable. Individuals have the ability to accept personal responsibility for reducing acts of child abuse and neglect by providing support to each other and offering protection to all children within their family and their community. As sociologist Robert Wuthnow has noted, every volunteer effort or act of compassion finds its justification not in offering solutions for society's problems but in offering hope "both that the good society we envision is possible and that the very act of helping each other gives us strength and a common destiny" (Wuthnow, R. *Acts of compassion: Caring for others and helping ourselves*. Princeton, NJ: Princeton University Press, 1991, p. 304). When the problem is owned by all individuals and communities, prevention will progress, and fewer children will remain at risk.

Chapter 27

Safe Haven Laws

This brief introduction summarizes how states address the topic of *safe haven* in statute. To access the statutes for a specific state or territory, visit the State Statutes Search (available online at http://www .childwelfare.gov/systemwide/laws_policies/state).

Many state legislatures have enacted legislation to address infant abandonment and infanticide in response to a reported increase in the abandonment of infants. Beginning in Texas in 1999, *Baby Moses laws* or *infant safe haven laws* have been enacted as an incentive for mothers in crisis to safely relinquish their babies to designated locations where the babies are protected and provided with medical care until a permanent home is found. Safe haven laws generally allow the parent, or an agent of the parent, to remain anonymous and to be shielded from prosecution for abandonment or neglect in exchange for surrendering the baby to a safe haven.

To date, approximately 49 states and Puerto Rico have enacted safe haven legislation.[1] The focus of these laws is protecting newborns. In approximately 13 states, infants who are 72 hours old or younger may be relinquished to a designated safe haven.[2] Approximately 16 states

---

"Infant Safe Haven Laws: Summary of State Laws," Child Welfare Information Gateway (www.childwelfare.gov), U.S. Department of Health and Human Services, May 2010. This information is a product of the *State Statutes Series* prepared by Child Welfare Information Gateway. While every attempt has been made to be as complete as possible, additional information on these topics may be in other sections of a state's code as well as agency regulations, case law, and informal practices and procedures.

and Puerto Rico accept infants up to one month old.[3] Other states specify varying age limits in their statutes.[4]

Who May Leave a Baby at a Safe Haven?

In most states with safe haven laws, either parent may surrender his or her baby to a safe haven. In four states, only the mother may relinquish her infant.[5] Idaho specifies that only a custodial parent may surrender an infant. In approximately 11 states, an agent of the parent (someone who has the parent's approval) may take a baby to a safe haven for a parent.[6] In California and Kansas, if the person relinquishing the infant is someone other than a parent, he or she must have legal custody of the child. Seven states do not specify the person who may relinquish an infant.[7]

Safe Haven Providers

The purpose of safe haven laws is to ensure that relinquished infants are left with persons who can provide the immediate care needed for their safety and well-being. To that end, approximately 12 states require parents to relinquish their infants to a hospital or health-care facility.[8] Other states designate additional entities as safe haven providers, including emergency medical services, police stations, and fire stations. In seven states, emergency medical technicians, including personnel responding to 9-1-1 calls, may accept an infant.[9] In addition, four states and Puerto Rico allow churches to act as safe havens, but the relinquishing parent must first determine that church personnel are present at the time the infant is left.[10] Generally, anyone on staff at these institutions can receive an infant; however, many states require that staff receiving an infant be trained in emergency medical care.

Responsibilities of Safe Haven Providers

The safe haven provider is required to accept emergency protective custody of the infant and to provide any immediate medical care that the infant may require. In 12 states, when the safe haven receiving the baby is not a hospital, the baby must be transferred to a hospital as soon as possible.[11] The provider is also required to notify the local child welfare department that an infant has been relinquished.

In 25 states, the provider is required to ask the parent for family and medical history information.[12] In 17 states, the provider is required to attempt to give the parent or parents information about the legal repercussions of leaving the infant and information about referral services.[13] In four states, a copy of the infant's numbered identification bracelet may be offered to the parent as an aid to linking the parent to the child if reunification is sought at a later date.[14]

Immunity from Liability for Providers

Safe haven providers are given protection from liability for anything that might happen to the infant while in their care, unless there is evidence of major negligence on the part of the provider.

Protections for the Parents

In approximately 12 states, anonymity for the parent or agent of the parent is expressly guaranteed in statute.[15] In 24 states and Puerto Rico, the safe haven provider cannot compel the parent or agent of the parent to provide identifying information.[16] In addition, 13 states provide an assurance of confidentiality for any information that is voluntarily provided by the parent.[17]

In addition to the guarantee of anonymity, most states provide protection from criminal liability for parents who safely relinquish their infants. Approximately 33 states and Puerto Rico do not prosecute a parent for child abandonment when a baby is relinquished to a safe haven.[18] In 16 states, safe relinquishment of the infant is an affirmative defense in any prosecution of the parent or his/her agent for any crime against the child, such as abandonment, neglect, or child endangerment.[19]

The privileges of anonymity and immunity will be forfeited in most states if there is evidence of child abuse or neglect.

Consequences of Relinquishment

Once the safe haven provider has notified the local child welfare department that an infant has been relinquished, the department assumes custody of the infant as an abandoned child. The department has responsibility for placing the infant, usually in a preadoptive home, and for petitioning the court for termination of the birth parent's parental rights. Before the baby is placed in a preadoptive home, 13 states require the department to request the local law enforcement agency to determine whether the baby has been reported as a missing child.[20] In addition, five states require the department to check the putative father registry before a termination of parental rights petition can be filed.[21]

Approximately 20 states have procedures in place for a parent to reclaim the infant, usually within a specified time period and before any petition to terminate parental rights has been granted.[22] Five states also have provisions for a nonrelinquishing father to petition for custody of the child.[23] In 16 states and Puerto Rico, the act of surrendering an infant to a safe haven is presumed to be a relinquishment of parental rights to the child, and no further parental consent is required for the child's adoption.[24] To see how your state addresses this issue, visit the State Statutes Search.

To find information on all of the states and territories, view the complete printable file in PDF format, Infant Safe Haven Laws: Summary of State Laws (http://www.childwelfare.gov/systemwide/laws_policies/statutes/safehaven.pdf).

Notes

1. The word *approximately* is used to stress the fact that the states frequently amend their laws. This information is current only through May 2010. Nebraska, the District of Columbia, American Samoa, Guam, the Northern Mariana Islands, and the Virgin Islands currently do not address the issue of abandoned newborns in legislation.

2. Alabama, Arizona, California, Colorado, Hawaii, Kentucky, Michigan, Minnesota, Mississippi, Tennessee, Utah, Washington, and Wisconsin.

3. Arkansas, Connecticut, Idaho, Illinois, Louisiana, Maine, Montana, Nevada, New Jersey, Ohio, Oregon, Pennsylvania, Rhode Island, South Carolina, Vermont, and West Virginia.

4. Other limits include five days (New York), seven days (Florida, Georgia, Illinois, Massachusetts, New Hampshire, North Carolina, and Oklahoma), 10 days (Maryland), 14 days (Delaware, Iowa, Virginia, and Wyoming), 21 days (Alaska), 45 days (Indiana and Kansas), 60 days (South Dakota and Texas), 90 days (New Mexico), and one year (Missouri and North Dakota).

5. Georgia, Maryland, Minnesota, and Tennessee. Maryland and Minnesota do allow the mother to approve another person to deliver the infant on her behalf.

6. Arizona, Arkansas, Connecticut, Indiana, Iowa, Kentucky, New Jersey, North Dakota, Rhode Island, Utah, and Wyoming.

7. Delaware, Hawaii, Illinois, Maine, New Mexico, South Carolina, and Vermont.

8. Alabama, Connecticut, Delaware, Georgia, Iowa, Minnesota, New Mexico, North Dakota, Pennsylvania, Utah, Virginia, and West Virginia.

9. Idaho, Indiana, Louisiana, Michigan, New Hampshire, Vermont, and Virginia.

10. Arizona, New Hampshire, South Carolina, and Vermont.

11. Arizona, Florida, Illinois, Kentucky, Louisiana, Maryland, Missouri, Montana, Nevada, New Jersey, South Carolina, and Wyoming.

12. Alaska, California, Connecticut, Delaware, Hawaii, Iowa, Kentucky, Louisiana, Maine, Massachusetts, Michigan, Minnesota, Montana, North Carolina, North Dakota, Ohio, Oklahoma, Pennsylvania, South Carolina, South Dakota, Tennessee, Texas, Utah, Washington, and Wyoming.

13. Connecticut, Delaware, Hawaii, Illinois, Louisiana, Michigan, Minnesota, Montana, New Mexico, North Dakota, Ohio, Oklahoma, Rhode Island, South Carolina, Tennessee, Washington, and Wisconsin.

14. California, Connecticut, Delaware, and North Dakota.

15. Arizona, Delaware, Florida, Illinois, Kentucky, Ohio, Oklahoma, Texas, Utah, West Virginia, Wisconsin, and Wyoming.

16. Alaska, Arizona, Delaware, Idaho, Indiana, Iowa, Massachusetts, Minnesota, Nevada, New Hampshire, New Jersey, New Mexico, North Carolina, North Dakota, Oregon, Rhode Island, South Carolina, South Dakota, Tennessee, Vermont, Washington, West Virginia, Wisconsin, and Wyoming.

17. California, Connecticut, Delaware, Idaho, Iowa, Maine, Michigan, Montana, Rhode Island, South Carolina, Tennessee, Texas, and Wisconsin.

18. Alaska, Arizona, California, Connecticut, Florida, Georgia, Hawaii, Idaho, Illinois, Iowa, Kansas, Kentucky, Louisiana, Maryland, Massachusetts, Minnesota, Missouri, Montana, Nevada, New Mexico, North Carolina, North Dakota, Ohio, Oklahoma, Pennsylvania, Rhode Island, South Carolina, South Dakota, Tennessee, Texas, Vermont, Washington, and Wisconsin.

19. In a state with an affirmative defense provision, a parent or agent of the parent can be charged and prosecuted, but the act of leaving the baby safely at a safe haven can be a defense to such charges. The states with an affirmative defense provision include Alabama, Arkansas, Colorado, Delaware, Indiana, Maine, Michigan, Mississippi, Missouri, New Jersey, New York, Oregon, Utah, Virginia, West Virginia, and Wyoming.

20. California, Delaware, Idaho, Illinois, Kentucky, Louisiana, Montana, New Hampshire, Oklahoma, South Carolina, Texas, Utah, and Wyoming.

21. Illinois, Iowa, Missouri, Utah, and Wyoming.

22. California, Connecticut, Delaware, Florida, Hawaii, Idaho, Illinois, Iowa, Kentucky, Louisiana, Michigan, Montana, Nevada, New Mexico, North Dakota, Ohio, Oklahoma, Tennessee, Wisconsin, and Wyoming.

23. Hawaii, Missouri, Montana, South Dakota, and Tennessee.

24. Alaska, Delaware, Florida, Idaho, Illinois, Kentucky, Michigan, Missouri, Montana, Nevada, Rhode Island, South Carolina, South Dakota, Tennessee, Utah, and Wisconsin.

Chapter 28

Sex Offender Registries and Community Notice Programs

Registration and Community Notification

Within the past few years, the nation has witnessed an unprecedented proliferation of sex offender–specific legislation designed to enhance community safety through increasing accountability and tightening restrictions for the individuals who have committed sex offenses. States have proposed and enacted a number of measures, including the use of electronic monitoring devices, residency restrictions, lifetime supervision, increased penalties and sanctions, and civil commitment for violent and predatory sex offenders. However, the most longstanding and far-reaching trends involving sex offender–specific legislation are the use of registration and community notification. Broadly speaking, registration requires convicted sex offenders to provide identifying information to law enforcement agencies, where it is entered into a central registry as a means of tracking these offenders. Community notification, on the other hand, is the process by which members of the public obtain information about registered sex offenders, either by accessing sex offender registries themselves or through the active dissemination of information by local law enforcement or other state officials.

From: *The Comprehensive Assessment Protocol: A Systemwide Review of Adult and Juvenile Sex Offender Management Strategies*, July 2007. Prepared by the Center for Sex Offender Management, a program of the U.S. Department of Justice, Office of Justice Programs, Bureau of Justice Assistance. The complete document, including references, is available online beginning at http://www.csom.org/pubs/cap/6/6_0.htm.

The widespread adoption of registration and notification laws has been driven primarily by a series of federal proposals that have been ratified during the past decade. While not intended to be an exhaustive review, the key provisions of these laws are highlighted briefly below:

- Enacted in 1994, The Jacob Wetterling Crimes Against Children and Sexually Violent Offender Registration Act essentially required all states to create and maintain registry systems that included specific identifying information about sex offenders who target children and those who commit violent sex crimes. It included provisions pertaining to collecting registry information from sex offenders upon release from incarceration, updating registry information when sex offenders change residences, and conducting routine address verifications.

- When Megan's Law was passed in 1996, all states were mandated to establish provisions that allow for the release of information about registered sex offenders when necessary for public protection. Although it did not require states to actively notify communities about sex offenders, it did require public access to registry information in order to allow for heightened awareness of sex offenders living in their communities.

- The Pam Lychner Sex Offender Tracking and Identification Act of 1996 required a national database to be established at the Federal Bureau of Investigation. This database, known as the National Sex Offender Registry (NSOR), was designed to ensure registration and address verification for sex offenders residing in states whose registration systems were not yet deemed as minimally sufficient.

- In 1998, The Jacob Wetterling Improvements Act expanded the class of registerable sex offenders to those who had been convicted in federal and military courts. It also required sex offenders who relocate to another state to register in that state, and required sex offenders to also register in the state in which they work or attend school, if different from their permanent residence. Furthermore, through this amendment, states were mandated to participate in the National Sex Offender Registry program.

- The Campus Sex Crimes Prevention Act was enacted in 2000 and required individuals who are attending, employed by, or working at institutions of higher education (that is, colleges or universities) to notify those institutions of their registration status, who in turn must forward the information for inclusion in the state's sex offender registration database.

- Most recently, the Adam Walsh Child Protection and Safety Act of 2006 (the Adam Walsh Act) established a more standardized and expanded registration process to be implemented nationwide, including the posting of specific information on states' websites as a means of notification. It also requires states to submit an expanded set of data about each sex offender in their jurisdiction to the National Sex Offender Registry and allows law enforcement officials access to the more detailed information. Among multiple other expectations, the Act creates a tiered classification of sex offenders with minimum registration periods, expands registration requirements to include certain juvenile sex offenders, requires that sex offenders register in person, and makes failure to register a felony crime.

Taken together, these and other policies enacted both at the state and federal levels have had, and will continue to have, a significant influence on adult and juvenile sex offender management efforts throughout the country. As interested jurisdictions strive toward establishing evidence-based policies and practices and consider their approaches to registration and notification, it will be important to explore the ways in which these legal policies have been implemented within the context of contemporary research and practice. For example, because assessment-driven case management leads to better outcomes, particularly when the intensity of interventions and strategies is commensurate with the assessed level of risk, jurisdictions should consider the implications for the ways in which registration and notification policies are developed and implemented. Finally, as discussed later in this chapter, the contemporary research and literature about adult and juvenile sex offenders can be instructive for jurisdictions that are considering how to address registration and notification most effectively.

Sex Offender Registration

The overarching goal of creating centralized registries of convicted sex offenders is to enhance public safety through multiple processes. For example, because these registries contain identifying information and offense summary data about sex offenders residing in a particular jurisdiction, the investigation of sex crimes can be facilitated and enhanced. Law enforcement officials and other criminal justice agents can utilize registry data to narrow the focus of investigations, compare forensic evidence, and identify potential suspects with similar crime patterns. In addition, registries are designed to make sex offenders more visible to community members who, when they access or receive information about registered sex offenders living in their communities, may take increased protective steps. Sex offender registration is also believed to play a role in deterrence, as sex offenders are acutely aware of the increased visibility and scrutiny by the criminal justice system and the public at large. Finally, for individuals who have either not engaged in sex offending behaviors, or who have thus far gone undetected, the idea of being placed on a public registry may also have a deterrent effect.

In order to meet these and other goals, jurisdictions must ensure that the following elements are in place:

• Policies and procedures are clear and understood

• Registry information is current and accurate

• Ongoing registration efforts are coordinated and collaborative

Clear Policies and Procedures

Unlike the considerable latitude that agencies and entities have with respect to implementing core sex offender management strategies such as treatment and supervision, the approach to sex offender registration is firmly established by statutes at the federal and state levels. Therefore, the key to effective implementation and utilization of sex offender registries is ensuring that the associated policies are clear, comprehensive in scope, and well understood by those with a role and a stake in the process. This requires that staff are well-trained in the specific statutory requirements, agency policies, and specific procedures regarding the registration process, and that quality assurance or other monitoring practices are in place to ensure adherence to these procedures.

Of primary importance is the intended applicability of sex offender registration policies. Some state statutes expressly indicate that registration is intended only for adult sex offenders, while other laws explicitly include juveniles adjudicated within the juvenile courts, waived to adult courts, or both. Still other statutes are silent on the applicability of registration to juveniles. In addition, the specific types of crimes that qualify for registration must be defined, whether limited only to sex offenses as defined within criminal codes or including other crimes that may have an underlying sexual component or similar motivation (for example, kidnapping, forcible confinement, aggravated assault, abuse of a child). It is also important that policies outline the respective responsibilities of the various agencies or individuals that have a role in sex offender registration.

Policies must also specify the type of information that is to be collected for sex offender registries. This varies to some degree across states, but typically includes names and aliases of sex offenders, dates and types of convictions, last known addresses, law enforcement identification numbers, photographs, and fingerprints. Some states also include employment information, vehicle registration, and blood samples for DNA analysis. The recent enactment of the Adam Walsh Act is likely to promote increased consistency with respect to collecting registry data throughout the country. Similarly, the implementation of the National Sex Offender Registry, which provides law enforcement officials with greater access to cross-state registration information, may increase the consistency of sex offender registry data.

Ideally, registration statutes and agency policies specifically outline expected protocols for ensuring that incarcerated sex offenders are informed of the applicable registration requirements prior to their release or that allow the registration process to be initiated prior to release. In these instances, procedures must take into account documentation and record-keeping, including documentation that the offender was notified of and understood the registration requirements. For sex offenders who are placed directly under supervision with no period of incarceration, policies should outline the process by which they are required to register, and the role that court officers or community supervision officers will have in ensuring that offenders comply with registration following sentencing or disposition.

Also important to explicate in statutes is the duration of registration requirements (for example, 10 years, lifetime). This may vary based on whether an adult or juvenile is the subject of the registration process, the crimes of conviction, or tiered classification systems. For example, for states implementing the provisions of the Adam Walsh Act, minimum registration requirements are prescribed based upon a three-tiered system, with registration durations ranging from 15 years to life. In jurisdictions that use a tiered system for registration, it may be beneficial for procedures to specify the inclusion of an empirically validated sex offender–specific actuarial risk assessment tool to provide an informed foundation for risk management decisions. When the duration of registration responsibilities is finite (either because of statutory limitations on duration, or because a court issues an order for relief from registration), policies and procedures should outline the process for inactivating records and/or removing the names from public registries.

Current and Accurate Registry Information

Collecting registry information at the point of initial registration requires a significant amount of staff time and resources, but it may not be the most significant challenge facing jurisdictions with respect to sex offender registration.

Rather, maintaining accurate and up-to-date registry information is perhaps the most difficult aspect. Most statutes clarify offenders' requirements for notifying relevant law enforcement or criminal justice agencies of any address changes, and many policies require sex offenders to present themselves to local law enforcement agencies at routine intervals (for example, annually) in order to verify that all information is current and to update the offender's photograph. Within the Adam Walsh Act, for example, provisions mandate sex offenders to appear in person for routine registration verification purposes (that is, every three months, six months, or year) based on their tier classification. However, because these expectations are dependent upon the offenders themselves, the assurance of accurate and current registry information is not guaranteed. Therefore, many jurisdictions have implemented requirements for law enforcement and other agencies to take active steps to update and verify registry information on an ongoing basis (for example, some states now require law enforcement agencies to conduct routine in-person address verifications by going door-to-door), which often requires significant fieldwork, manpower, and resources.

With the growing number of sex offenders entering the criminal justice system, verifying and updating addresses and other registry information is likely to become even more time, staff, and resource intensive. Because accurate information is vital to the integrity of registries, a formal verification process must be established and should include the following:

- Types of information that must be updated or verified

- Agency or agencies responsible for these verifications

- Specific timeframes and frequencies expected for verifications

- Methods by which verification must occur

- Requirements for forwarding updates or changes in registration information to the designated state law enforcement agency, and on to the national registry

- Penalties for offenders' failure to verify or update registry information

Coordinated and Collaborative Efforts

It is common for multiple agencies to be involved with the sex offender registration process, particularly as offenders move through various stages of the criminal or juvenile justice process. As such, sex offender registration has the potential to be most effective in those jurisdictions where collaboration and coordination exist among the sentencing courts, corrections departments, state and local law enforcement, and community supervision agencies. Strong working relationships can bring these agencies together to ensure that complete registry information is collected, duplication of effort is minimized, and capacity for initial registration and ongoing verification processes is enhanced. The law enforcement officers who are charged with the responsibility for registration will ideally work in concert with others in the community (for example, supervision officers) who are active in the monitoring of those sex offenders under supervision.

Formalized partnerships between law enforcement and supervision and corrections agencies may provide an ideal means of managing the initial and ongoing registration process. For example, jurisdictions may wish to explore collaborations between law enforcement and corrections agencies to allow institutional caseworkers to initiate or facilitate the registration process with incarcerated sex offenders prior to release from the institution. Similarly, because supervision officers are generally expected to conduct home visits and other field contacts with sex offenders, they can verify addresses of sex offenders under supervision and communicate those verifications formally to law enforcement officials. And through partnerships with volunteer programs, law enforcement agencies can receive administrative assistance with registration processes (for example, organizing and filing paperwork associated with registration, updating databases), distributing community notification materials, developing and disseminating educational materials, and conducting address verifications (that is, through auxiliary officers). Depending upon agencies' statutory mandates pertaining to registration and verification processes, efforts to implement these and other types of collaborative approaches may require attention at the policy level.

Community Notification

All states are authorized to release information to the public about registered sex offenders and must have in place procedures that allow for the public to access that information when deemed necessary. In addition, states are now expected to make some of the sex offender registry information available to the public through their state registry websites and through the National Sex Offender Registry. However, outside of the public access requirements, states continue to have a level of discretion regarding their approaches to releasing information to the public or actively notifying the public about registered sex offenders. Not surprisingly, then, these processes vary from state to state.

Some states limit their information-sharing about registered sex offenders to a "passive" notification approach, which involves the posting of information on the state registry website. Interested parties are able to access and review the information about registered sex offenders living in their area or in other parts of the state, and through the National Sex Offender Registry citizens have the ability to search a national database. At the same time, other states have implemented an "active" notification approach, whereby they take specific steps within the community to disseminate information about certain sex offenders. This may include conducting community meetings in jurisdictions in which a high risk sex offender may be returning, posting fliers in neighborhoods, advertising information in local newspapers, or even going door-to-door to inform local citizens about specific sex offenders who will be residing in those areas. Active notification most often occurs when a sex offender is released from incarceration and returns to a community, although it may also take place when a sex offender moves into a community or neighborhood after residing elsewhere.

As noted previously, with the exception of the requirements for passive notification systems through public access to web-based and other sex offender registries, states continue to have flexibility around the approaches they use for notification with one exception: the provisions of the Adam Walsh Act are much more prescribed, and include active notification to specific parties, such as schools, public housing agencies, volunteer programs where minors or other vulnerable parties may be present, social services agencies responsible for child welfare, and others.

Applicability of Notification

In addition to the variations in community notification practices between jurisdictions (that, passive versus active), states also vary with respect to the specific sex offenders (for example, all sex offenders, adults only, sexually violent predators, sex offenders with child victims) to whom notification applies. Indeed, recognizing that sex offenders are a heterogeneous group with varying levels of risk for recidivism, it may be worthwhile to establish different processes (for example, ranging from passive notification to broad, active notification) that are based on tiered levels of risk. To illustrate, when a sex offender is classified as high risk, active and broad notification may be conducted, including the use of community notification meetings that are open to the public. Conversely, for a sex offender in a lower risk category, information dissemination may be restricted only to those individuals or organizations with increased vulnerability to specific offenders or classes of offenders, leaving law enforcement officials with discretion about who should receive such information.

Risk classification protocols should outline the specific processes and tools used to establish any tier classifications for community notification purposes, so that practices are consistent throughout the state. To ensure that these risk classifications are well-informed, jurisdictions may wish to include an empirically validated, sex offender–specific risk assessment tool as part of the classification protocol. Because offender risk can increase or decrease over time, jurisdictions that employ tier-based community notification practices may wish to include specific provisions for reclassification or reassignment within the system. This should include the circumstances under which reclassification should be considered, the process by which changes in risk will be assessed, specific criteria that will be used for reassigning sex offenders to tiers, and any modifications to community notification practices that may result from reclassification.

Community Education to Enhance Notification

Very little research has been conducted on community notification, making it difficult to determine the relative effectiveness of different approaches to notification. However, the process of community notification in and of itself has the potential to create unintended consequences for sex offenders and their families (for example, loss of employment, housing, and social supports) that may exacerbate existing difficulties with community reintegration. These collateral consequences are noteworthy in that some of them are associated with recidivism among sex offenders. Therefore, when planning for community notification, multidisciplinary teams should develop collaboratively the policies, practices, and strategies that may facilitate community notification in a manner that reduces the potential for unintended consequences for offenders, family members, victims, other affected individuals, and communities at large. For example, approaching family members, victims, landlords, and employers before conducting a notification allows these individuals time to prepare for the disclosure.

Some jurisdictions have also developed protocols for conducting community meetings in a manner that reduces the potential for these collateral consequences. When thoughtfully implemented by trained professionals, community notification meetings can provide useful information to the public about the prevention of sexual assault and can help communities understand the nature of offending. Moreover, community notification and education meetings can enhance public confidence in the agencies established to serve and protect their communities. Based on this literature, and to reduce the likelihood of negative impact of notification, community meetings should be designed to serve these functions:

- Inform communities about the benefits and limitations of community notification

- Dispel common myths and misperceptions about sex offenders while providing education about effective treatment and supervision strategies

- Educate the public about the incidence and prevalence of sexual victimization, including the data that suggests that stranger attacks are not as commonplace as believed

- Ensure that community members understand the implications of further stigmatizing and ostracizing offenders

- Encourage community assistance with offender reintegration and subsequently, promote offender success

Victim advocates can play an important role in the development of a successful community notification program. For example, states that use review committees to assess an offender's risk of reoffense often enlist the help of victim advocates. Victim advocates can also be helpful in strategizing with corrections and law enforcement officials regarding who should be notified and how, as well as assisting in the notification itself. Moreover, victim advocates can ensure that policies and procedures protect the identities of victims during the notification process.

Some states that conduct community meetings use victim advocates to help educate audiences about the nature of sex crimes and teach parents how to protect themselves and their children from sex offenders. Victim advocacy groups, such as the National Alliance to End Sexual Violence, the National Center for Missing and Exploited Children, the National Center for Victims of Crime, the National Sexual Violence Resource Center, as well as many state-based and local sexual assault advocacy programs, develop and provide educational materials that raise awareness about taking protective measures against sexual assault that may prove helpful in these endeavors.

Special Considerations for Juvenile Sex Offenders

Although the initial establishment of sex offender registration and community notification policies primarily targeted adult sex offenders, many states have since enacted legislation to include juvenile sex offenders. The application of these types of legal policies paralleled the trend with treatment and supervision strategies, whereby adult models of treatment and adult-oriented approaches to supervision were simply applied to juvenile sex offenders.

As professionals' understanding of juvenile sex offenders began to expand, controversies about their existing "adult-like" clinical and legal management arose, primarily because of concerns about the negative impact that labeling could have on peer relationships, social isolation, and a sense of identity. In addition, because many victims of juvenile sex offenders are family members, the identities of victims may be identifiable through community notification.

Nonetheless, a "treat juveniles like adults" philosophy remains even today and is perhaps most notable in the legal policy arena. This speaks to the importance of collaboration between researchers in the field of juvenile sex offender management and key policymakers, in order to ensure that they have the benefit of specialized information about juvenile sex offenders as a means of informing policy development.

For jurisdictions that opt to require registration and notification for juvenile sex offenders, it may be worthwhile for stakeholders to consider the agency within which juveniles' information will be maintained, the range of parties that will have access to this information, and the potential for termination of registration requirements. Some states maintain juvenile sex offender registries within the juvenile court or juvenile supervision agency rather than with the local law enforcement agency. This allows for collecting and maintaining registry information, while also allowing for increased protections and safeguards. Rather than being maintained on the statewide registry used for adults, information is provided about these youth only to a limited range of parties on a "need to know" basis. Similarly, recognizing the importance of developmental considerations for juvenile sex offenders and the promising treatment outcome data, some states have enacted registration provisions for juveniles that allow for the termination of registration requirements once registrants reach adulthood (that is, ranging from 18–21 years of age). Where such provisions do not exist, states may wish to consider policies that afford juvenile sex offenders the ability to petition the courts for relief from registration requirements after a demonstrated period of community adjustment and stability. Some states exempt juveniles from community notification practices altogether, or have limited notification practices only to those juveniles who have been determined to pose a high risk to the community.

Sex offender management experts and legal scholars alike emphasize the importance of taking into account the ever-growing body of research about juvenile sex offenders when crafting policies such as registration and notification. Most salient are the key developmental differences between adults and juveniles, low rates of sexual recidivism among juvenile sex offenders, evidence which suggests that these youth are not likely to continue offending sexually as adults, the effectiveness of community-based treatment, and concerns about collateral consequences.

Research on the Impact of Registration and Notification

Creating evidence-based policies in the sex offender management arena requires an understanding about what is currently known about sex offenders, victims, and the impact of sex offender management strategies. For the core components of an integrated and comprehensive approach to managing sex offenders (for example, treatment, supervision), there is evidence—albeit to greater and lesser degrees—that some strategies seem to "work" to enhance public safety and to facilitate positive offender outcomes. Unfortunately, empirical analyses of sex offender-specific policy analyses are very limited, and remain a critical need in the overall sex offender management field. Thus far, only a handful of studies have begun to address the impact of registration and community notification on sex offender management. Below is a summary of the limited research studies and the questions that they were designed to answer:

- **Does registration reduce sexual recidivism?** Researchers in the state of Iowa compared sex offenders involved in the criminal justice system prior to the enactment of the state's registration statute with sex offenders who were involved in the system after the registration statute was enacted. No significant differences were revealed for sexual recidivism (that is, reconviction) after a more than four year follow-up period.

- **Does community notification reduce sexual recidivism?** Tracking high risk sex offenders in the state of Washington, researchers compared the sexual recidivism rates of sex offenders "pre-enactment" and "post-enactment" of the community notification legislation. After a 4.5 year follow-up, the sexual recidivism rates (that is, re-arrests) for the two groups did not differ significantly.

- **Does community notification reduce sexual recidivism?**
  Researchers in the state of Washington compared the five year sexual recidivism rates (that is, reconvictions) of sex offenders released from prisons pre-enactment, post-enactment, and post-amendment of the registration and notification statutes. After a five year follow-up, the sexual recidivism rate for the pre-enactment group was 7%, the rate for the post-enactment group was 4%, and the rate for the post-amendment group was 2%. Although these differences were statistically significant, the researchers noted that other confounding variables (for example, increased state incarceration rates, decreased crime rate within the state and nationally) may have influenced the findings.

- **Do sex offenders who fail to register recidivate sexually at higher rates?** With the growing rate of failure to register convictions in the state of Washington, researchers explored the relationship between failing to comply with registration requirements and sexual recidivism. When comparing the failure-to-register group to the registration-compliant group over a five year follow-up period, the sexual recidivism rates (that is, reconvictions) were 4.3% and 2.8%, respectively. The differences were not statistically significant.

The primary goal of registration and community notification—to promote community safety by increasing the visibility of convicted sex offenders in the community—is laudable. Indeed, enhancing community safety is the thread that connects all stakeholders involved in the management of adult and juvenile sex offenders. Unfortunately, very limited research has been conducted to identify the extent to which registration and notification approaches are achieving that goal.

Summary

As emphasized throughout this protocol, the key to ensuring community safety, whether via treatment or supervision interventions, reentry practices, or sex offender-specific legislation, is to make well-informed decisions based on the best available research. Therefore, policymakers and agency administrators are well-advised to conduct cost-benefit analyses of their current registration and notification strategies. Ideally, this would be operationalized through specific requirements and dedicated funding for outcome evaluations that investigate the short-and long-term impact of these policies, both in terms of effects on recidivism and impact on key stakeholders (for example, law enforcement, citizens, victims, sex offenders, and families).

Chapter 29

Reporting Child Abuse

Reporting Child Abuse and Neglect

If you suspect abuse, reporting it can protect the child and get help for the family. Each state identifies mandatory reporters (groups of people who are required to report suspicions of child abuse or neglect). However, any concerned person can and should report suspected child abuse. A report is not an accusation; it is an expression of concern and a request for an investigation or evaluation of the child's situation. If you suspect a child is in a dangerous situation, take immediate action. Your suspicion of child abuse or neglect is enough to make a report. You are not required to provide proof. Investigators in your community will make the determination of whether abuse or neglect has occurred. Almost every state has a law to protect people who make good-faith reports of child abuse from prosecution or liability.

How do I report child abuse or neglect?

If you suspect a child is being harmed, contact your State Child Abuse Hotline, local child protective services (CPS), or law enforcement agency so professionals can assess the situation. For more information about

This chapter includes excerpts from "Factsheet: Reporting Child Abuse and Neglect," 2006, and "Penalties for Failure to Report and False Reporting of Child Abuse and Neglect: Summary of State Laws," December 2009, both produced by Child Welfare Information Gateway (www.childwelfare.gov), U.S. Department of Health and Human Services.

where and how to file a report, call Childhelp, National Child Abuse Hotline (800-4-A-CHILD).

When calling to report child abuse, you will be asked for specific information, which may include these details:

- The child's name and location

- The suspected perpetrator's name and relationship to the child (if known)

- A description of what you have seen or heard regarding the abuse or neglect

- The names of any other people having knowledge of the abuse

- Your name and phone number

The names of reporters are not given out to families reported for child abuse or neglect; however, sometimes by the nature of the information reported, your identity may become evident to the family. You may request to make your report anonymously, but your report may be considered more credible and can be more helpful to CPS if you give your name.

What will happen when I make a report?

Your report of possible child maltreatment will first be screened by hotline staff or a CPS worker. If the worker feels there is enough credible information to indicate that maltreatment may have occurred or is at risk of occurring, your report will be referred to staff who will conduct an investigation. Investigators respond within a particular time period (anywhere from a few hours to a few days), depending on the potential severity of the situation. They may speak with the child, the parents, and other people in contact with the child (such as doctors, teachers, or childcare providers). Their purpose is to determine if abuse or neglect has occurred and if it may happen again.

If the investigator finds that no abuse or neglect occurred, or what happened does not meet the state's definition of abuse or neglect, the case will be closed and the family may or may not be referred elsewhere for services. If the investigator feels the children are at risk of harm, the family may be referred to services to reduce the risk of future maltreatment. These may include mental health care, medical care, parenting skills classes, employment assistance, and concrete support such as financial or housing assistance. In rare cases where the child's safety cannot be ensured, the child may be removed from the home.

Penalties for Failure to Report

Many cases of child abuse and neglect are not reported, even when mandated by law. Therefore, nearly every state and U.S. territory imposes penalties, often in the form of a fine or imprisonment, on mandatory reporters who fail to report suspected child abuse or neglect as required by law.[1]

Approximately 47 states, the District of Columbia, American Samoa, Guam, the Northern Mariana Islands, and the Virgin Islands impose penalties on mandatory reporters who knowingly or willfully fail to make a report when they suspect that a child is being abused or neglected.[2] Failure to report is classified as a misdemeanor in 39 states and American Samoa, Guam, and the Virgin Islands.[3] In Arizona, Florida, and Minnesota, misdemeanors are upgraded to felonies for failure to report more serious situations, while in Illinois and Guam, second or subsequent violations are classified as felonies.

Twenty states and the District of Columbia, Guam, the Northern Mariana Islands, and the Virgin Islands specify in the reporting laws the penalties for failure to report.[4] Upon conviction, a mandated reporter who fails to report can face jail terms ranging from 10 days to five years or fines ranging from $100 to $5,000. In seven states and American Samoa, in addition to any criminal penalties, the reporter may be civilly liable for any damages caused by the failure to report.[5]

Penalties for False Reporting

Approximately 28 states carry penalties in their civil child protection laws for any person who willfully or intentionally makes a report of child abuse or neglect that the reporter knows to be false.[6] In New York, Ohio, and the Virgin Islands, making false reports of child maltreatment is made illegal in criminal sections of state code.

Twenty states and the Virgin Islands classify false reporting as a misdemeanor or similar charge.[7] In Florida, Tennessee, and Texas, false reporting is a felony, while in Arkansas, Illinois, Indiana, Missouri, and Virginia, second or subsequent offenses are upgraded to felonies. In Michigan, false reporting can be either a misdemeanor or a felony, depending on the seriousness of the alleged abuse in the report. No criminal penalties are imposed in California, Maine, Montana, Minnesota, and Nebraska; however, immunity from civil or criminal action that is provided to reporters of abuse or neglect is not extended to those who make a false report.

Eleven states and the Virgin Islands specify the penalties for making a false report.[8] Upon conviction, the reporter can face jail terms ranging from 30 days to five years or fines ranging from $200 to $5,000. Florida imposes the most severe penalties: In addition to a court sentence of five years and $5,000, the Department of Children and Family Services may fine the reporter up to $10,000. In six states the reporter may be civilly liable for any damages caused by the report.[9]

To access the statutes for a specific state or territory, visit the State Statutes Search (http://www.childwelfare.gov/systemwide/laws_policies/state/).

Notes

1. See Child Welfare Information Gateway's *Mandatory Reporters of Child Abuse and Neglect* (http://www.childwelfare.gov/systemwide/laws_policies/statutes/manda.cfm).

2. The word *approximately* is used to stress the fact that the states frequently amend their laws. This information is current through December 2009. Maryland, North Carolina, Wyoming, and Puerto Rico currently do not have statutes imposing penalties for failure to report.

3. The states that do not use the misdemeanor classification for failure to report include Connecticut, Delaware, Massachusetts, Mississippi, New Jersey, Vermont, Virginia, and Wisconsin.

4. Alabama, California, Connecticut, Delaware, Florida, Louisiana, Maine, Massachusetts, Michigan, Minnesota, Mississippi, New Mexico, Rhode Island, South Carolina, Tennessee, Vermont, Virginia, Washington, West Virginia, and Wisconsin.

5. Arkansas, Colorado, Iowa, Michigan, Montana, New York, and Rhode Island.

6. Arizona, Arkansas, California, Colorado, Connecticut, Florida, Idaho, Illinois, Indiana, Iowa, Kansas, Kentucky, Louisiana, Maine, Massachusetts, Michigan, Minnesota, Missouri, Montana, Nebraska, Oklahoma, Rhode Island, South Carolina, Tennessee, Texas, Virginia, Washington, and Wyoming.

7. Arizona, Arkansas, Colorado, Illinois (disorderly conduct), Indiana, Iowa, Kansas, Kentucky, Louisiana, Michigan, Missouri, New York, North Dakota, Ohio, Oklahoma, Rhode Island, South Carolina, Virginia, Washington, and Wyoming.

8. Connecticut, Florida, Louisiana, Massachusetts, Michigan, Oklahoma, Rhode Island, South Carolina, Texas, Washington, and Wyoming.

9. California, Colorado, Idaho, Indiana, Minnesota, and North Dakota.

Chapter 30

Professionals Who Are Required to Report Child Abuse And Neglect

Mandatory Reporters of Child Abuse and Neglect

All states, the District of Columbia, American Samoa, Guam, the Northern Mariana Islands, Puerto Rico, and the U.S. Virgin Islands have statutes identifying persons who are required to report child maltreatment under specific circumstances.

Professionals Required to Report

Approximately 48 states, the District of Columbia, American Samoa, Guam, the Northern Mariana Islands, Puerto Rico, and the Virgin Islands designate professions whose members are mandated by law to report child maltreatment.[1] Individuals designated as mandatory reporters typically have frequent contact with children. Such individuals may include the following:

This chapter includes excerpts from the following three documents produced by Child Welfare Information Gateway (www.childwelfare.gov), U.S. Department of Health and Human Services: "Mandatory Reporters of Child Abuse and Neglect: Summary of State Laws," April 2010; "Clergy as Mandatory Reporters of Child Abuse and Neglect: Summary of State Laws," April 2010; "Penalties for Failure to Report and False Reporting of Child Abuse and Neglect: Summary of State Laws," December 2009. These publications were produced by Child Welfare Information Gateway. While every attempt has been made to be as complete as possible, additional information on these topics may be in other sections of a state's code as well as agency regulations, case law, and informal practices and procedures. This chapter concludes with "Sources of Child Maltreatment Reports," which is excerpted from *Child Maltreatment 2010*, produced by the Children's Bureau, Administration for Children and Families (www.acf.hhs.gov), 2011.

- Social workers

- Teachers and other school personnel

- Physicians and other health-care workers

- Mental health professionals

- Child care providers

- Medical examiners or coroners

- Law enforcement officers

Some other professions frequently mandated across the states include commercial film or photograph processors (in 11 states, Guam, and Puerto Rico), substance abuse counselors (in 14 states), and probation or parole officers (in 17 states).[2] Seven states and the District of Columbia include domestic violence workers on the list of mandated reporters, while seven states and the District of Columbia include animal control or humane officers.[3] Court-appointed special advocates are mandatory reporters in nine states.[4] Members of the clergy now are required to report in 26 states.[5]

Reporting by Other Persons

In approximately 18 states and Puerto Rico, any person who suspects child abuse or neglect is required to report. Of these 18 states, 16 states and Puerto Rico specify certain professionals who must report but also require all persons to report suspected abuse or neglect, regardless of profession.[6] New Jersey and Wyoming require all persons to report without specifying any professions. In all other states, territories, and the District of Columbia, any person is permitted to report. These voluntary reporters of abuse are often referred to as "permissive reporters."

Standards for Making a Report

The circumstances under which a mandatory reporter must make a report vary from state to state. Typically, a report must be made when the reporter, in his or her official capacity, suspects or has reasons to believe that a child has been abused or neglected. Another standard frequently used is when the reporter has knowledge of, or observes a child being subjected to, conditions that would reasonably result in harm to the child. Permissive reporters follow the same standards when electing to make a report.

Privileged Communications

Mandatory reporting statutes also may specify when a communication is privileged. "Privileged communications" is the statutory recognition of the right to maintain confidential communications between professionals and their clients, patients, or congregants. To enable states to provide protection to maltreated children, the reporting laws in most states and territories restrict this privilege for mandated reporters. All but three states and Puerto Rico currently address the issue of privileged communications within their reporting laws, either affirming the privilege or denying it (that is, not allowing privilege to be grounds for failing to report).[7] Here are some examples:

- The physician-patient and husband-wife privileges are the most common to be denied by states.

- The attorney-client privilege is most commonly affirmed.

- The clergy-penitent privilege is also widely affirmed, although that privilege usually is limited to confessional communications and, in some states, denied altogether.[8]

Inclusion of the Reporter's Name in the Report

Most states maintain toll-free telephone numbers for receiving reports of abuse or neglect.[9] Reports may be made anonymously to most of these reporting numbers, but states find it helpful to their investigations to know the identity of reporters. Approximately 18 states, the District of Columbia, American Samoa, Guam, and the Virgin Islands currently require mandatory reporters to provide their names and contact information, either at the time of the initial oral report or as part of a written report.[10] The laws in Connecticut, Delaware, and Washington allow child protection workers to request the name of the reporter. In Wyoming, the reporter does not have to provide his or her identity as part of the written report, but if the person takes and submits photographs or x-rays of the child, his or her name must be provided.

Disclosure of the Reporter's Identity

All jurisdictions have provisions in statute to maintain the confidentiality of abuse and neglect records. The identity of the reporter is specifically protected from disclosure to the alleged perpetrator in 39 states, the District of Columbia, Puerto Rico, American Samoa, Guam, Puerto Rico, and the Northern Mariana Islands.[11] This protection is maintained even when other information from the report may be disclosed.

395

Release of the reporter's identity is allowed in some jurisdictions under specific circumstances or to specific departments or officials. For example, disclosure of the reporter's identity can be ordered by the court when there is a compelling reason to disclose (in California, Mississippi, Tennessee, Texas, and Guam) or upon a finding that the reporter knowingly made a false report (in Alabama, Arkansas, Connecticut, Kentucky, Louisiana, Minnesota, South Dakota, Vermont, and Virginia). In some jurisdictions (California, Florida, Minnesota, Tennessee, Texas, Vermont, the District of Columbia, and Guam), the reporter can waive confidentiality and give consent to the release of his or her name.

To find statute information for a particular state, go to http://www .childwelfare.gov/systemwide/laws_policies/state/index.cfm.

Notes

1. The word *approximately* is used to stress the fact that states frequently amend their laws. This information is current only through April 2010. At that time, New Jersey and Wyoming were the only two states that did not enumerate specific professional groups as mandated reporters but required all persons to report.

2. Film processors are mandated reporters in Alaska, California, Colorado, Georgia, Illinois, Iowa, Louisiana, Maine, Missouri, Oklahoma, and South Carolina. Substance abuse counselors are required to report in Alaska, California, Connecticut, Illinois, Iowa, Kansas, Massachusetts, Nevada, New York, North Dakota, Oregon, South Carolina, South Dakota, and Wisconsin. Probation or parole officers are mandated reporters in Arkansas, California, Colorado, Connecticut, Hawaii, Illinois, Louisiana, Massachusetts, Minnesota, Missouri, Nevada, North Dakota, South Dakota, Texas, Vermont, Virginia, and Washington.

3. Domestic violence workers are mandated reporters in Alaska, Arizona, Arkansas, Connecticut, Illinois, Maine, and South Dakota. Humane officers are mandated reporters in California, Colorado, Illinois, Maine, Ohio, Virginia, and West Virginia.

4. Arkansas, California, Louisiana, Maine, Montana, Oregon, Virginia, Washington, and Wisconsin.

5. Alabama, Arizona, Arkansas, California, Colorado, Connecticut, Illinois, Louisiana, Maine, Massachusetts, Michigan, Minnesota, Mississippi, Missouri, Montana, Nevada, New Hampshire, New Mexico, North Dakota, Ohio, Oregon, Pennsylvania, South

Carolina, Vermont, West Virginia, and Wisconsin. For more information, see Child Welfare Information Gateway's Clergy as Mandatory Reporters of Child Abuse and Neglect at www .childwelfare.gov/systemwide/laws_policies/statutes/ clergymandated.cfm.

6.   Delaware, Florida, Idaho, Indiana, Kentucky, Maryland, Mississippi, Nebraska, New Hampshire, New Mexico, North Carolina, Oklahoma, Rhode Island, Tennessee, Texas, and Utah.

7.   Connecticut, Mississippi, and New Jersey do not currently address the issue of privileged communications within their reporting laws. The issue of privilege may be addressed elsewhere in the statutes of these states, such as rules of evidence.

8.   New Hampshire, North Carolina, Oklahoma, Rhode Island, Texas, and West Virginia disallow the use of the clergy-penitent privilege as grounds for failing to report suspected child abuse or neglect. For a more complete discussion of the requirement for clergy to report child abuse and neglect, see the Information Gateway's Clergy as Mandatory Reporters of Child Abuse and Neglect at www.childwelfare.gov/systemwide/laws_policies/ statutes/clergymandated.cfm.

9.   For state-specific information about these hotlines, see Information Gateway's State Child Abuse Reporting Numbers at www .childwelfare.gov/pubs/reslist/rl_dsp.cfm?rs_id=5&rate _chno=W-00082.

10.   California, Colorado, Florida, Illinois, Indiana, Iowa, Louisiana, Maine, Massachusetts, Minnesota, Mississippi, Missouri, Nebraska, New Mexico, New York, North Carolina, Pennsylvania, and Vermont have this requirement.

11.   The statutes in Alaska, Arizona, Delaware, Idaho, Maryland, Massachusetts, New Hampshire, Oklahoma, Rhode Island, West Virginia, Wyoming, and the Virgin Islands do not specifically protect reporter identity but do provide for confidentiality of records in general.

Clergy as Mandatory Reporters of Child Abuse and Neglect

Every state, the District of Columbia, American Samoa, Guam, the Northern Mariana Islands, Puerto Rico, and the U.S. Virgin Islands have statutes that identify persons who are required to report child maltreatment under specific circumstances.[1] *Approximately* 26 states currently include members of the clergy among those professionals specifically mandated by law to report known or suspected instances of child abuse or neglect.[2] In approximately 18 states and Puerto Rico, any person who suspects child abuse or neglect is required to report.[3] This inclusive language appears to include clergy but may be interpreted otherwise.

Privileged Communications

As a doctrine of some faiths, clergy must maintain the confidentiality of pastoral communications. Mandatory reporting statutes in some states specify the circumstances under which a communication is "privileged" or allowed to remain confidential. Privileged communications may be exempt from the requirement to report suspected abuse or neglect. The privilege of maintaining this confidentiality under state law must be provided by statute. Most states do provide the privilege, typically in rules of evidence or civil procedure.[4] If the issue of privilege is not addressed in the reporting laws, it does not mean that privilege is not granted; it may be granted in other parts of state statutes.

This privilege, however, is not absolute. While clergy-penitent privilege is frequently recognized within the reporting laws, it is typically interpreted narrowly in the context of child abuse or neglect. The circumstances under which it is allowed vary from state to state, and in some states it is denied altogether. For example, among the states that list clergy as mandated reporters, New Hampshire and West Virginia deny the clergy-penitent privilege in cases of child abuse or neglect. Four of the states that enumerate "any person" as a mandated reporter (North Carolina, Oklahoma, Rhode Island, and Texas) also deny clergy-penitent privilege in child abuse cases.

In states where neither clergy members nor "any person" are enumerated as mandated reporters, it is less clear whether clergy are included as mandated reporters within other broad categories of professionals who work with children. For example, in Virginia and Washington, clergy are not enumerated as mandated reporters, but the clergy-penitent privilege is affirmed within the reporting laws.

Many states and territories include Christian Science practitioners or religious healers among professionals who are mandated to report suspected child maltreatment. In most instances, they appear to be regarded as a type of health-care provider. Only nine states (Arizona, Arkansas, Louisiana, Massachusetts, Missouri, Montana, Nevada, South Carolina, and Vermont) explicitly include Christian Science practitioners

Table 30.1. State-by-State Status of Clergy as Mandatory Reporters

Clergy status	Privilege granted but limited to pastoral communications	Privilege denied in cases of suspected child abuse or neglect	Privilege not addressed in the reporting laws
Clergy enumerated as mandated reporters	Alabama, Arizona, Arkansas, California, Colorado, Illinois, Louisiana, Maine, Massachusetts, Michigan, Minnesota, Missouri, Montana, Nevada, New Mexico, North Dakota, Ohio, Oregon, Pennsylvania, South Carolina, Vermont, Wisconsin	New Hampshire, West Virginia	Connecticut, Mississippi
Clergy not enumerated as mandated reporters but may be included with "any person" designation	Delaware, Florida, Idaho, Kentucky, Maryland, Utah, Wyoming	North Carolina, Oklahoma, Rhode Island, Texas	Indiana, Nebraska, New Jersey, Tennessee, Puerto Rico
Neither clergy nor "any person" enumerated as mandated reporters	Virginia, Washington[5]	Not applicable	Alaska, American Samoa, District of Columbia, Georgia, Guam, Hawaii, Iowa, Kansas, New York, Northern Mariana Islands, South Dakota, Virgin Islands

among classes of clergy required to report. In those states the clergy-penitent privilege is also extended to those practitioners by statute.

The Table 30.1 summarizes how states have or have not addressed the issue of clergy as mandated reporters (either specifically or as part of a broad category) and/or clergy-penitent privilege (either limiting or denying the privilege) within their reporting laws. To access the statutes for a specific state or territory, visit the State Statutes Search portion of the Child Welfare Information Gateway website at www.childwelfare.gov.

Notes

1. For more information on mandated reporters, see Child Welfare Information Gateway's Mandatory Reporters of Child Abuse and Neglect (https://www.childwelfare.gov/systemwide/laws _policies/statutes/manda.pdf).

2. The word *approximately* is used to stress the fact that states frequently amend their laws. This information is current only through April 2010; states that include clergy as mandated re-porters are Alabama, Arizona, Arkansas, California, Colorado, Connecticut, Illinois, Louisiana, Maine, Massachusetts, Michigan, Minnesota, Mississippi, Missouri, Montana, Nevada, New Hampshire, New Mexico, North Dakota, Ohio, Oregon, Pennsylvania, South Carolina, Vermont, West Virginia, and Wisconsin.

3. Delaware, Florida, Idaho, Indiana, Kentucky, Maryland, Mississippi, Nebraska, New Hampshire, New Jersey, New Mexico, North Carolina, Oklahoma, Rhode Island, Tennessee, Texas, Utah, and Wyoming. Three of these states (Mississippi, New Hampshire, and New Mexico) also enumerate clergy as mandated reporters.

4. The issue of clergy-penitent privilege also may be addressed in case law, which this text does not cover.

5. Clergy are not mandated reporters in Washington, but if they elect to report, their report and any testimony are provided statutory immunity from liability.

Penalties for Failure to Report and False Reporting of Child Abuse and Neglect

Many cases of child abuse and neglect are not reported, even when mandated by law. Therefore, nearly every state and U.S. territory imposes penalties, often in the form of a fine or imprisonment, on mandatory reporters who fail to report suspected child abuse or neglect as required by law. In addition, to prevent malicious or intentional reporting of cases that are not founded, many states and the U.S. Virgin Islands impose penalties against any person who files a report known to be false.

Sources of Child Maltreatment Reports

For 2010, three-fifths of reports of alleged child abuse and neglect were made by professionals. The term professional means that the person had contact with the alleged child maltreatment victim as part of the report source's job. This term includes teachers, police officers, lawyers, and social services staff. "Other" and unknown report sources submitted 13.7 percent of reports. An "other" report source includes any state code that does not fit into one of the National Child Abuse and Neglect Data System (NCANDS) codes. The remaining reports were made by nonprofessionals, including friends, neighbors, and relatives:

- The three largest percentages of report sources were from such professionals as teachers (16.4%), law enforcement and legal personnel (16.7%), and social services staff (11.5%).

- Anonymous sources (9.0%), other relatives (7.0%), parents (6.8%), and friends and neighbors (4.4%), accounted for nearly all of the nonprofessional reporters.

Chapter 31

The Role of Educators in Preventing and Responding to Child Abuse and Neglect

Forms of Child Abuse and Neglect

Every form of maltreatment (for example, physical abuse, neglect, sexual abuse, and emotional maltreatment) is inflicted on school-age children. In addition, many children who live in homes where domestic violence occurs are not only in danger of a misdirected blow, but probably suffer emotional consequences from witnessing this disturbing behavior. Knowledgeable educators can pick up indicators of possible maltreatment by observing children's behavior at school, recognizing physical signs, and noticing family dynamics during routine interactions with parents.

Educators are in an excellent position to notice behavioral indicators. As trained observers, they are sensitive to the range of behaviors exhibited by children at various developmental stages, and they are quick to notice behaviors that fall outside this range. Teachers also can talk with a child's previous teacher to note any major changes in his or her behavior. Abused and neglected children sometimes get the reputation for being "bad kids" or extremely difficult to control or understand. Research suggests that challenging behavior is often a cry for help that concerned adults need to learn to decode.

Excerpted from "The Role of Educators in Preventing and Responding to Child Abuse and Neglect," Office on Child Abuse and Neglect, Children's Bureau, U.S. Department of Health and Human Services, 2003. The entire text of this manual is available from the Child Welfare Information Gateway, https://www.childwelfare .gov. Reviewed by David A. Cooke, MD, FACP, January 2013.

In the past, lists of physical and behavioral indicators have been provided as guidelines to help educators recognize maltreatment, and Table 31.1 lists several of the key indicators. Recognition of child maltreatment, however, is not based always upon the detection of one or two clues, but rather on the recognition of a cluster of indicators that make up a composite or pattern. It also is very important to remember that some indicators, both physical and behavioral, may be indications of something other than abuse. This chapter is dedicated to recognizing composites that might be seen specifically by educators and that warrant the consideration of maltreatment as a cause.

Table 31.1. Behavioral Clues That May Indicate Child Abuse

Although there are many other potential indicators, the abused child may demonstrate these characteristics:

- Be aggressive, oppositional, or defiant
- Cower or demonstrate fear of adults
- Act out, displaying aggressive or disruptive behavior
- Be destructive to self or others
- Come to school too early or not want to leave school—indicating a possible fear of going home
- Show fearlessness or extreme risk taking
- Be described as "accident prone"
- Cheat, steal, or lie (may be related to too high expectations at home)
- Be a low achiever (to learn, children must convert aggressive energy into learning; children in conflict may not be able to do so)
- Be unable to form good peer relationships
- Wear clothing that covers the body and that may be inappropriate in warmer months (be aware that this may be a cultural issue as well)
- Show regressive or less mature behavior
- Dislike or shrink from physical contact (may not tolerate physical praise such as a pat on the back)

General Indicators of Abuse and Neglect

There are some indicators that serve as general signs that a child may be experiencing abuse or neglect rather than signaling the presence of one particular type of maltreatment. These general indicators include academic as well as emotional or psychological clues. It is important to remember that these also can be signs of other problems such as substance abuse, a reaction to divorce, or the witnessing of domestic violence, so it is crucial to follow each school's protocol in reporting suspected abuse.

Academic Clues

Academic performance may be a clue to the presence of child abuse and neglect. This is particularly true when there are sudden or extreme changes in performance. Previously good students who suddenly seem disinterested in school or who are no longer prepared for class may be maltreated. Students who suddenly refuse to change for gym class may be concealing evidence of beatings. There can be numerous clues suggesting neglect. Some of these factors may affect academic performance, such as children whose broken glasses have not been replaced.

Studies have revealed a relationship between child maltreatment and certain learning problems. For example, Cornell University's Family Life Development Center matched maltreated children with 530 children who had not suffered abuse or neglect and evaluated the school performance of each child based upon grades, grade repetition, achievement test scores, and other school adjustment issues (for example, truancies, suspensions, and infractions of disciplinary codes). Results indicated that maltreatment has a significant negative influence on children's performance in school. The maltreated children scored lower in test scores, especially in reading, and earned fewer As and Bs and more Fs than children who were not mistreated. In addition, children who have been maltreated show discipline problems at school, poor achievement, increased absences and dropout rates, and greater likelihood of repeating grades.

A similar study in Georgia using a smaller population (21 physically abused children, 47 neglected children) and a nonmatched control group compared test scores, grades, and teacher and parent interviews to examine the academic, social, and adaptive behavior of school-age children. Significant differences between the maltreated children and those in the control groups were found. Abused and neglected children were more likely to demonstrate disturbed behaviors (for example, aggression, hyperactivity, anxiety, depression). Maltreated children had lower self-concepts and felt unpopular in school. In addition, maltreated children scored significantly lower in language, math, and reading scores in the Iowa and Georgia Criterion Reference Test. Teachers felt these children were learning at below-average levels and were more likely to repeat a grade.

Research also indicates that a child who is physically disabled or developmentally delayed is at a statistically greater risk of child abuse and neglect. In some instances, the disabled child may be viewed as a disappointment, a burden, or proof of the parents' "failure." Educators should be sensitive to the particular stresses that having a disabled child can produce in some families. Children whose physical needs and problems are ignored also may experience learning difficulties. Children who are always hungry, who cannot see the blackboard because they need glasses, or who cannot hear the teacher because they need hearing aids, cannot learn well, and this inability to learn will be reflected in academic achievement.

Academic difficulties may have a variety of causes, and the presence of an academic problem does not prove that child abuse or neglect exists. The possibility of child abuse or neglect, however, must be considered along with other possible causes when the problem is assessed.

Emotional and Psychological Clues

Educators typically are sensitive to children who are "different" (for example, physically or mentally challenged). That sensitivity should be extended to abused and neglected children, who also may appear to be different.

Educators should be alert to children who are hostile and angry, those that effectively alienate all who come in contact with them, or children who may be passive, withdrawn, and uncommunicative. These represent extreme ranges in the expected behaviors and attitudes of abused and neglected children. Additionally, sudden changes in a child's emotional or psychological well-being may serve as clues to child abuse and neglect. The previously gregarious child who becomes uncommunicative and withdrawn might be concealing maltreatment.

Familial Clues

The educator often has several opportunities to observe family dynamics. Normal interactions with the parents may indicate how they feel about the child. There may be an increased risk of child abuse and neglect if the parents consistently demonstrate these characteristics:

- Blame or belittle the child

- See the child as very different from his or her siblings (in a negative way)

- See the child as "bad," "evil," or a "monster"

- Find nothing good or attractive in the child
- Seem unconcerned about the child
- Fail to keep appointments or refuse to discuss problems the child may be having in school
- Behave in a bizarre or an irrational manner

There are instances when the educator knows a child's family is in marital crisis, experiencing economic or emotional turmoil, or has other significant stressors .Such information may be relevant and helpful to CPS when maltreatment is suspected and a report made.

Conversations with Families and Children

In all states, educators are mandated reporters for child maltreatment cases. It is important to understand that, legally speaking, educators only need reasonable suspicion rather than hard evidence or proof to report alleged child abuse. It may be tempting to call the parents and see what they have to say, but such action can pose several serious problems, such as increasing the risk of further abuse to the child or interfering with the initial CPS investigation. Many schools have protocols detailing how suspected maltreatment is to be reported to CPS. These protocols delineate what information the educator will need to provide when reporting, or whether teachers, administrators, and other school personnel should refer all suspicions to the school's social worker or Child Protection Team who will then make the report to CPS.

Talking with the Child

It is the educator's role to report any suspicions of child maltreatment. There are times when CPS may request more information in order to meet statutory guidelines for accepting a report. In these instances or when a child discloses maltreatment to an educator, it is important to remember these points:

- CPS or law enforcement has the responsibility to assess and investigate.
- It is critical that the educator not lead the child.
- The child may be afraid to tell the whole truth because of fear of being further hurt by the abuser if he or she tells; a belief that the abuser may go to jail; fear that the child may be removed from the

home; feelings of loyalty and attachment to the parent, no matter how bad the situation might be.

- The child may feel that the abuse or neglect is normal.

Unfortunately, it can be very easy to fall into the role of confidant to an abused child who has begged that no one be told.

If CPS needs more information before accepting a report and requests that the educator talk with the child or if the child self-discloses, it is important to remember these things:

- The educator should not appear shocked as a strong reaction may affect the child's comfort level.

- If self-disclosing, praise the child for revealing what has happened to him or her. It is not up to the educator to determine if the child is telling the truth.

- When talking with a child concerning a possible inflicted injury or condition of neglect, the educator should refrain from asking leading questions.

- Let the child tell his or her story without probing for information that the child is unwilling to give.

- The child should be made as comfortable as possible under the circumstances.

- The child should be put at ease, and the educator should sit near the child, not behind a desk or table.

- The educator who talks with the child should be the designated person to handle such matters (for example, the school social worker).

- Children often feel or are told that they are to blame for their own maltreatment and for bringing "trouble" to the family; therefore, it is important to reassure children that they are not at fault.

- If maltreatment is suspected, the educator must always remember that he or she is a mandated reporter, and this should be explained to the child in an age-appropriate way.

- The child may be afraid that either he or she will be taken from the home or the parent may be arrested. If such a fear is expressed, the educator should acknowledge not knowing what will occur.

- Children may be fearful of others learning about their maltreatment issues. The educator should assure the child that the information would not be shared with classmates or others who have no need to know. It is vital, however, that the educator also acknowledge that in order to provide help to the child, it may be necessary to discuss these issues with other school personnel, law enforcement, or CPS. It is important that the educator abides by the promise to protect the child's right to confidentiality.

It also is important to realize how difficult it is for most children to discuss abuse, because of emotional elements or a limited ability to express themselves. When talking with the child, use language that a child will understand. When describing an incident of abuse, if the child uses a term with which the educator is not familiar (for example, a word for a part of the body), the educator should ask for clarification or have the child point to the body part. The educator should not disparage the child's choice of language or supply terms; rather, the educator should use the child's terms to put the child at ease and to avoid confusion. Educators can actually do more harm by probing for answers or supplying children with terms or information. Several major child sexual abuse cases have been dismissed in court because it was felt that the initial interviewers had biased the children. Additionally, it is important for the educator to not display feelings of anger, disgust, or disapproval toward the parents or the child for any action disclosed.

If the child wishes to show his or her injuries to the educator, he or she should be allowed to do so. The educator should never insist on seeing the child's injuries. At no time should the child be asked or forced to remove clothing. It may be important to have the school nurse present should a child decide to remove his or her clothes.

If further action is to be taken, the child should be told what will happen and when. The educator should assure the child of support and assistance throughout the process and should follow through on the assurances. It is important that the onus or responsibility not be placed on the child, nor should the child be asked to conceal from the parents that the conversation has taken place or that further action is contemplated.

The educator should be especially sensitive to the safety of the child following the disclosure. Ask the child if he or she feels safe returning home and observe how this question is answered. While CPS must be involved in any situation of suspected maltreatment, it is particularly important to involve CPS or law enforcement immediately in situations where the child's imminent safety is a concern. If a CPS caseworker needs to interview the child at school, the school should provide a private place for the interview. In addition, ensure that the interview location does not alert peers and other classmates to the presence of a CPS caseworker. The child's right to confidentiality must be respected.

If it is necessary for the CPS caseworker to remove the child from school for a medical examination, the school may request a written release from the caseworker, or this may be an established element of a memorandum of understanding (MOU) between the school and CPS. This varies by locale and it is important to know the practice and requirements of a particular school.

Talking with the Parents

Some educators may feel that it is important to contact parents to inform them that the school has made a report of suspected child abuse and neglect, because they feel that contact will help maintain the parents' relationship with the school and keep the door open for further communication. It is very rarely appropriate, however, for educators to communicate directly with parents regarding alleged child maltreatment. CPS caseworkers and law enforcement personnel are trained and primarily responsible for contacting and discussing these concerns with parents. The following issues may arise if educators seek to talk with parents before reporting:

- The danger to the child may increase, particularly if the child disclosed the maltreatment.

- The parent may try to have the child recant upon learning that the child has told someone about the abuse.

- The parent may flee or withdraw the child from school.

- The risk for suicide increases for both the victim and the perpetrator immediately after a report is made in sexual abuse cases, especially in cases of incest. It is crucial that such cases be handled swiftly by experts.

There may be instances when a parent contacts a school regarding a report made to CPS. Many school systems have one point of contact to handle CPS reports, such as the school social worker, nurse, or principal. The educator should listen to parents and refer them to that point of contact. In talking with the parents, the educator should respond in a professional, direct, and honest manner without displaying anger, shock, or an insinuation of guilt. It is critical to remember that the educator should not reveal any information pertinent to the report made to CPS or law enforcement. Parents also should be informed about the limitations to confidentiality of the present discussion. Further threats or revelations of abuse typically require the educator to reveal what was discussed to a third party (for example, CPS).

Occasionally, an angry parent will come to school demanding to know why someone is "telling me how to raise my children." The parent may feel betrayed or that someone has "gone behind their back" because the school did not communicate with him or her directly. Even though CPS caseworkers are legally mandated not to reveal the name of the referral source, the parent often suspects the source of the report. If an angry parent appears at school, the educator should attempt to diffuse the situation by remaining calm and maintaining a professional demeanor. The educator should be mindful of his or her own safety, as well as the safety of others, if the parent is threatening or violent. School protocol should delineate who needs to be contacted in such situations. An angry parent usually will calm down to a reasonable degree if he or she feels listened to and is treated with respect.

Child Abuse within the School

It is extremely disturbing for most educators to consider that a fellow colleague might be abusing children. In the event that this does occur, however, children need special protection. A common response when a fellow educator is suspected of abuse, especially if that person is popular or a long-time employee, is to deny or ignore it. Sometimes the abuser is transferred to another school. Even with a suspension or reprimand, the violation is likely to recur in the absence of intervention and monitoring.

If a child reports that he or she is being sexually, physically, or even emotionally abused by school personnel, the educator should remember that it takes courage for an abused child to talk to someone. The educator must consider facts and consistencies. Older children may invent stories, but they usually contain obvious inconsistencies. The educator should follow school policy and procedures, which usually involve contacting CPS. CPS personnel then interview the child or refer the allegations to law enforcement (depending on the state's laws) to determine if the child knows anyone else to whom this has happened. If so, the CPS investigator should talk with any other victims. Protocols usually require immediate notification of the school administrator. The situation should not be discussed among other school staff. The accused has a reputation and the right to know of the accusation, but it is the investigator (who may be a CPS caseworker or law enforcement) who should talk with the accused colleague. Not doing so often leads to a witch-hunt atmosphere and is not beneficial to students or faculty. It also is inappropriate to ask the children to tell their stories initially in front of the accused. There is a significant difference in power and resources between teachers and students.

411

It is important to remember that schools are mandated reporters whether the abuser is an outsider or a school employee. Under state child abuse and neglect reporting statutes, educators have the same liabilities for failing to report suspected incidents perpetrated by colleagues as for incidents resulting from interfamilial abuse or neglect. If allegations are made and there is suspicion of abuse, CPS or law enforcement must become involved.

Reporting Child Abuse and Neglect

In addition to trying to help families in which maltreatment is suspected, the involvement of educators in reporting child abuse and neglect is guided by federal standards and regulations and mandated by state and local laws, which identify what is required of the educator and how that obligation is to be fulfilled. Schools are frequently concerned with creating protocols to enable them to address maltreatment issues more efficiently. Established protocols help address concerns over quality control, fear of lawsuits, and the protection of staff in reporting cases, as well as ensure that there are effective steps for helping children.

Federal Legislation

The Keeping Children and Families Safe Act of 2003 (P.L. 108-36) included the reauthorization of the Child Abuse Prevention and Treatment Act (CAPTA) in its Title I, Sec. 111. CAPTA provides minimum standards for defining child physical abuse and neglect and sexual abuse that states must incorporate into their statutory definitions in order to receive federal funds. Under this Act, child maltreatment is defined as any recent act or failure to act on the part of a parent or caretaker that results in death, serious physical or emotional harm, sexual abuse, or exploitation; and/or an act or failure to act that presents an imminent risk of serious harm.

A "child" under this definition generally means a person who is under the age of 18 or who is not an emancipated minor. In cases of child sexual abuse, a "child" is one who has not attained the age of 18 or the age specified by the child protection law of the state in which the child resides, whichever is younger. While CAPTA provides specific definitions for sexual abuse and for special cases related to withholding or failing to provide medically indicated treatment, it does not provide such definitions for other types of maltreatment—physical abuse, neglect, or psychological maltreatment. Each state has statutes providing that information.

Also at the federal level, the Federal Family Educational Rights and Privacy Act (FERPA) of 1974 (P.L. 93-380), provides standards and regulations that are relevant to educators for reporting child abuse and neglect. While amended numerous times since it was first authorized, FERPA still governs the release of information from school records.

In a small number of cases, it may be necessary to consult school records to determine if a report of suspected child abuse and neglect should be made. Usually, parental consent is required before releasing information contained in school records. However, there are exceptions that can apply in cases of suspected child abuse and neglect.

State Law

All states, the District of Columbia, and U.S. territories have reporting statutes for child abuse and neglect. These statutes outline who must report, to whom the abuse or neglect must be reported, and the form and content of the report. Given the diversity of statutes, educators should be familiar with or obtain a copy of the law in their state.

Who reports: Most states specifically require educators to report suspected child maltreatment unless educators are grouped under the category of "anyone." Some states specifically define what is meant by an "educator" (for example, teachers, principals, administrators, school nurses, school social workers, and guidance counselors) in any school, whether public or private, day or residential. Those professionals mandated to report vary from state to state. Educators should check their state reporting statute to determine who has been designated as a mandated reporter. They also should be familiar with their school system's policy and procedures regarding child abuse and neglect reporting. Additionally, it should be noted that when schools have a Child Protection Team, an educator's report to the team may or may not free him or her from further obligation, and a child protective services (CPS) caseworker may still contact him or her. The Child Protection Team representative would make the actual report to CPS. This regulation also should be researched within the educator's own state.

What to report: States specify what can be defined as child maltreatment in their particular jurisdiction, often specifically defining nonaccidental physical abuse and neglect, sexual abuse, and emotional (or psychological) maltreatment. Many of the definitions for sexual abuse include the production of child pornography or compelling children to view sexually explicit materials or acts. Some states require that domestic violence within a child's family be reported to CPS, as it may adversely affect the child. Every school should have or know how to access the definitions for abuse and neglect in their jurisdiction.

While states require the reporting of suspected abuse, no state requires that the reporter have conclusive proof that the abuse or neglect occurred before reporting. The law clearly specifies that reports must be made when the educator "suspects" or "has reasonable cause to believe" that there is abuse. In any case, the intent is clear—incidents are to be reported as soon as they are noticed. Waiting for conclusive proof may involve further risk to the child.

When to report: Again, state statutes differ as to when a report must be made. While early reporting is vital, educators may find it useful to keep notes on behaviors, bruises, or other potentially relevant information regarding the child. These informal, personally kept notes may be invaluable not only in filing a report, but in providing information to CPS. Notes should be taken even after the report is made in order to provide updates for CPS investigators. It is important to realize, however, that personal notes also can be subpoenaed if the case goes to court.

State and local statutes, as well as school system policies, vary regarding whether oral or written reports are necessary. Some require only an oral report, while others ask the reporter to follow up with a written report within a specific period of time. Secured internet reporting to CPS also is allowed in some states. Some states and school districts identify special reporting requirements.

Where to report: Every school should have identified, current, and accessible contact information for the appropriate agency for reporting suspected child maltreatment. State law specifies the agency that will receive reports of suspected child abuse and neglect. Usually this agency is a state's department of social services, human resources, family and children's services, CPS, or department of children and youth services. Other agencies mandated to receive reports may include law enforcement, the health department, the county or district attorney's office, and the juvenile or district court.

The local department of social services or other receiving agency may maintain a special child abuse and neglect unit, usually CPS. If there is no special unit, the local department itself will have CPS responsibility. The CPS unit receives and investigates all reports of suspected child maltreatment (that meet the state's statutory definitions) and may be involved in treatment and rehabilitation of affected families, by either performing such services or referring families to other agencies.

It is important to understand who receives reports of suspected child abuse and neglect in a particular jurisdiction. Requirements of confidentiality should be observed so that reports are made only to authorized persons. The state reporting statute will provide this information. An attorney should be consulted if questions arise.

How to report: Educators should follow local school system policies and procedures for reporting suspected abuse. These build upon state statutes, which vary regarding the form and content of reports of suspected maltreatment. All states require that an oral or written report (or both) be made to the agency or agencies responsible for child abuse and neglect. When two reports are required, the oral report is usually required immediately, with the written report often following within 24 to 48 hours. Some state statutes will specify the type of information to submit in a report of suspected child maltreatment. Usually this includes the following details:

- Child's name, age, gender, and address

- Parent's name and address

- Nature and extent of the injury or condition observed

- Prior injuries and when observed

- Actions taken by the reporter (for example, talking with the child)

- Where the act occurred

- Reporter's name, location, and contact information (sometimes not required, but extremely valuable to CPS staff).

In some states, additional information is required. This may include any previous injury observed by the reporter to the child or to a sibling; any information that would aid in establishing the cause of the injury; information that would aid in identifying the person responsible for the injury; if a previous report has been made to CPS; and other information about the child and family that will help CPS in their assessment of the risk of maltreatment to the child.

To assist citizens making oral reports of suspected child abuse and neglect, some states maintain a toll-free, 24-hour telephone hotline just for receiving reports of suspected maltreatment. Anyone may use hotlines to report an incident of suspected child abuse and neglect anywhere in their state.

To facilitate written reports, most states and some local school districts provide a reporting form. Schools should keep a supply of these forms for more efficient reporting. An educator would not be excused for failing to report a suspected case of maltreatment because a reporting form was unavailable. The reporter may submit a report using any form, so long as the required information is provided.

Difficulties That May Be Encountered when Reporting

A report of child maltreatment is not an accusation; rather, it is a request to determine if abuse or neglect has taken place and, if so, to begin the helping process. The reporting process, however, does not always proceed smoothly. Difficulties may be encountered that serve as barriers to reporting and discourage the educator from making future reports.

Personal feelings: One of the biggest obstacles to reporting may be the feelings of the potential reporter. Some individuals would prefer not to get involved. As one educator put it: "Although I realize that a child abuse report is not an accusation, I really hated to be the one to do it. What if the parents become angry with me? What if they pull their child out of my classroom? What if they see me as a troublemaker? I also wonder if I would be in any personal danger. Some of the abuse seems awfully violent. Will the parents come after me?"

These are typical concerns of educators and should be addressed. Parents who are subjects of a child abuse report typically feel angry. Anger is a natural response when threatened. If the parents angrily confront the reporter, however, a sensitive presentation with the desire to help may actually turn the parents into allies. These parents certainly have the right to pull their child out of a particular classroom, but only a small percentage actually do so, especially when the school makes clear its intention to help rather than punish.

When cultural values conflict with the laws of the state, this is problematic, but the laws remain the same. Where culturally based behaviors could be seen as abusive, it is usually the practice of CPS to try to educate the parents about the laws and to work with them. Some educators question their right to intervene in such instances. One educator described a family who had recently come to this country: "In their country hitting the children severely is accepted practice," she said. "What right do I have to tell them to change their cultural values?"

One of the most difficult situations for educators is discovering that abuse or neglect is being perpetrated by someone they know well. It may be extremely difficult for an educator to face the fact that the child of a colleague or a neighbor is being maltreated, or that a respected member of the community is sexually abusing a child. This is a natural feeling, but it must be overcome. Even if an educator knows the abusive family well, making a report is still necessary. All children are protected by law and, no matter what the circumstances, the educator remains a mandated reporter.

While the report may help protect the child, the process of reporting suspected child maltreatment is often a stressful experience. Confidentiality issues limit those with whom the educator can discuss the situation. Many educators may benefit from identifying support mechanisms and coping strategies while going through the process. Some schools have Child Protection Teams that aid the process of reporting and provide support to the reporter. Other schools may have developed their own support strategies.

Problems internal to the school: On occasion, school personnel indicate that school administrators create obstacles to reporting. They may fail to make an official report of suspected maltreatment once a situation has been brought to their attention or make it difficult for other school personnel to report. This may be done for the same reasons discussed above or because the administrator does not want to "make waves." Such actions may be more than obstructive; they may be illegal.

Administrators who refuse to report or who make it difficult to report cause several problems for other adults on their staff. Not only does the educator feel unsupported and even undermined, but educators whose administrators do not report may be held liable for the unreported maltreatment. Thus, the educator is put in a position of being vulnerable to legal sanction or having to bypass the administrator. In some instances, central administrative staff may provide no backup to educators, thus undercutting the reporter who has acted in the best interests of the child and complied with the law. Suddenly reporters find their motives questioned. Superintendents or principals who fail to provide inservice training to staff to inform them of their legal obligations also maybe an obstacle to reporting. Educators who do not know the signs and implications of child maltreatment or who are unaware of their legal responsibilities will be at a disadvantage and possibly, unwittingly, a disservice to children in need of assistance.

While some states allow anonymous reporting, the educator would not be protected, as there would be no proof that he or she had ever reported. It is difficult for the educator to know what to do or how to react to an unresponsive or obstructive administrator. The best answer is that it depends on the individual circumstances and available options. For instance, educators in certain locales may be able to develop a relationship with a CPS caseworker or with mental health, law enforcement, or other child welfare professionals who can help facilitate making a report. In other situations, there may be other school personnel, such as the school social worker or someone else in the school's administration, who may be willing to seek alternative avenues for reporting the situation.

Previous experiences reporting: Educators who have had a negative or difficult experience when reporting suspected maltreatment might be reluctant to become involved again. Such educators may feel that a previous case was not handled appropriately or to their satisfaction. These concerns are real and sometimes valid, but a previous bad experience does not mean that the next case will not be handled well. CPS agencies throughout the country are continually working to upgrade their services. In many communities, they are becoming steadily more responsive and highly skilled. After experiencing an unsatisfactory response with the CPS agency, however, the reporter should not hesitate to request that an agency supervisor intervene in the handling of the case. Exemptions are not granted to mandated reporters who have previously had a negative experience. In addition, while reporting does not guarantee that the situation will improve, not reporting virtually guarantees that the child will continue to be at risk if the abuse or neglect exists.

Belief that nothing will be done: Sometimes potential reporters believe that nothing will be done if they report, so they choose not to. Such reasoning often is faulty. If an incident of suspected child maltreatment is reported, some action will occur. At the very least, a record of the report will be made, the educator's legal obligation will be fulfilled, and the investigative process will begin. If the incident is not reported, however, it is likely that nothing will be done. Maltreated children cannot be protected unless they are first identified, and the key to identification is reporting. While not all calls result in an investigation, educators may not know what information was previously or subsequently reported about the child or the family. The cumulative effect of all the reports may allow CPS to substantiate a case and to provide help and intervention.

Some educators find it frustrating that CPS will not let them know whether the case is being investigated. Confidentiality laws and policies often make followup impossible. Educators may offer to keep in touch with CPS during the treatment phase, however, to help the children as much as possible. Some state laws will allow release of information from CPS to other professionals when the individual is a member of a multidisciplinary team.

Providing Support after the Report: What Schools Can Offer

Reporting suspected cases of maltreatment is just the beginning of the child protection process. Treatment, rehabilitation, strengthening the family, and preventing future abuse still lie ahead. Traditionally, the roles of the school and the educator in dealing with child maltreatment have ended with reporting, but this is changing. Increasingly, educators are providing assistance and support to child protective services (CPS) staff by sharing relevant information about families and children after they have been reported; providing services to the child, parents, and the family; and participating on multidisciplinary teams. Schools also are actively involved in community efforts to reduce the incidence of child maltreatment.

Chapter 32

Legal Interventions in Suspected Child Abuse Cases

Chapter Contents

Section 32.1

How the Child Welfare System Works

From: Child Welfare Information Gateway. (2012). *How the child welfare system works*. Washington, DC: U.S. Department of Health and Human Services, Children's Bureau. The complete text and other resources can be found online through the Child Welfare Information Gateway at http://www.childwelfare.gov.

The child welfare system is a group of services designed to promote the well-being of children by ensuring safety, achieving permanency, and strengthening families to care for their children successfully. While the primary responsibility for child welfare services rests with the states, the federal Government plays a major role in supporting states in the delivery of services through funding of programs and legislative initiatives.

The primary responsibility for implementing federal child and family legislative mandates rests with the Children's Bureau, within the Administration on Children, Youth and Families, Administration for Children and Families, U.S. Department of Health and Human Services (HHS). The Children's Bureau works with state and local agencies to develop programs that focus on preventing the abuse of children in troubled families, protecting children from abuse, and finding permanent families for children who cannot safely return to their parents.

The Child Abuse Prevention Act

The Child Abuse Prevention and Treatment Act (CAPTA), originally passed in 1974, brought national attention to the need to protect vulnerable children in the United States. CAPTA provides federal funding to states in support of prevention, assessment, investigation, prosecution, and treatment activities as well as grants to public agencies and nonprofit organizations for demonstration programs and projects. Additionally, CAPTA identifies the federal role in supporting research, evaluation, technical assistance, and data collection activities. CAPTA also sets forth a minimum definition of child abuse and neglect. Since it was signed into law, CAPTA has been amended several times. It was most recently amended and reauthorized on December 20, 2010, by the CAPTA Reauthorization Act of 2010 (P.L. 111-320).

Encountering the Child Welfare System

Most families first become involved with their local child welfare system because of a report of suspected child abuse or neglect (sometimes called "child maltreatment"). Child maltreatment is defined by CAPTA as serious harm (neglect, physical abuse, sexual abuse, and emotional abuse or neglect) caused to children by parents or primary caregivers, such as extended family members or babysitters. (Each state has its own laws. Visit the Child Welfare Information Gateway online at http://www.childwelfare.gov for information about specific state laws.)

Child maltreatment also can include harm that a caregiver allows to happen or does not prevent from happening to a child. In general, child welfare agencies do not intervene in cases of harm to children caused by acquaintances or strangers. These cases are the responsibility of law enforcement. While some states authorize child protective services agencies to respond to all reports of alleged child maltreatment, other states authorize law enforcement to respond to certain types of maltreatment, such as sexual or physical abuse.

The child welfare system is not a single entity. Many organizations in each community work together to strengthen families and keep children safe. Public agencies, such as departments of social services or child and family services, often contract and collaborate with private child welfare agencies and community-based organizations to provide services to families, such as in-home family preservation services, foster care, residential treatment, mental health care, substance abuse treatment, parenting skills classes, domestic violence services, employment assistance, and financial or housing assistance.

Child welfare systems are complex, and their specific procedures vary widely by state. The purpose of this text is to give a brief overview of the purposes and functions of child welfare from a national perspective. Child welfare systems typically provide these services:

- Receive and investigate reports of possible child abuse and neglect

- Provide services to families that need assistance in the protection and care of their children

- Arrange for children to live with kin or with foster families when they are not safe at home

- Arrange for reunification, adoption, or other permanent family connections for children leaving foster care

When Possible Abuse or Neglect Is Reported

Any concerned person can report suspicions of child abuse or neglect. Most reports are made by "mandatory reporters"—people who are required by state law to report suspicions of child abuse and neglect. As of April 2010, statutes in approximately 18 states and Puerto Rico require any person who suspects child abuse or neglect to report it. (The word approximately is used to stress the fact that states frequently amend their laws.) These reports are generally received by child protective services (CPS) workers and are either "screened in" or "screened out." A report is screened in when there is sufficient information to suggest an investigation is warranted. A report may be screened out if there is not enough information on which to follow up or if the situation reported does not meet the state's legal definition of abuse or neglect. In these instances, the worker may refer the person reporting the incident to other community services or law enforcement for additional help.

During federal fiscal year (FFY) 2010, an estimated 3.3 million referrals, which included approximately 5.9 million children, were made to CPS agencies. Three-fifths (60.7 percent) of the reports were screened in for further investigation, and 39.3 percent were screened out.

After a Report Is "Screened In"

CPS caseworkers, often called investigators, respond within a particular time period, which may be anywhere from a few hours to a few days, depending on the type of maltreatment alleged, the potential severity of the situation, and requirements under state law. They may speak with the parents and other people in contact with the child, such as doctors, teachers, or child care providers. They also may speak with the child, alone or in the presence of caregivers, depending on the child's age and level of risk. Children who are believed to be in immediate danger may be moved to a shelter, a foster home, or a relative's home during the investigation and while court proceedings are pending. An investigator's primary purpose is to determine whether the child is safe, whether abuse or neglect has occurred, and whether there is a risk of it occurring again.

Some jurisdictions now employ an alternative, or differential, response system. In these jurisdictions, when the risk to the children involved is considered low, the CPS caseworker may focus on assessing family strengths, resources, and difficulties and identifying supports and services needed, rather than on gathering evidence to confirm the occurrence of abuse or neglect.

At the end of an investigation, CPS caseworkers typically make one of two findings—unsubstantiated (unfounded) or substantiated (founded). These terms vary from state to state. Typically, a finding of unsubstantiated means there is insufficient evidence for the worker to conclude that a child was abused or neglected, or what happened does not meet the legal definition of child abuse or neglect. A finding of substantiated typically means that an incident of child abuse or neglect, as defined by state law, is believed to have occurred. Some states have additional categories, such as "unable to determine," that suggest there was not enough evidence to either confirm or refute that abuse or neglect occurred.

The agency will initiate a court action if it determines that the authority of the juvenile court (through a child protection or dependency proceeding) is necessary to keep the child safe. To protect the child, the court can issue temporary orders placing the child in shelter care during the investigation, ordering services, or ordering certain individuals to have no contact with the child. At an adjudicatory hearing, the court hears evidence and decides whether maltreatment occurred and whether the child should be under the continuing jurisdiction of the court. The court then enters a disposition, either at that hearing or at a separate hearing, which may result in the court ordering a parent to comply with services necessary to alleviate the abuse or neglect. Orders can also contain provisions regarding visitation between the parent and the child, agency obligations to provide the parent with services, and services needed by the child.

In FFY 2010, an estimated 695,000 children were found to be victims of maltreatment. This number refers to unique victims. The unique count of child victims counts a child only once, regardless of the number of times he or she was found to be victim during the reporting year. The duplicate count of child victims counts a child each time he or she was found to be a victim. The number of nationally estimated duplicate victims was 754,000 for FFY 2010.

Substantiated Cases

If a child has been abused or neglected, the course of action depends on state policy, the severity of the maltreatment, an assessment of the child's immediate safety, the risk of continued or future maltreatment, the services available to address the family's needs, and whether the child was removed from the home and a court action to protect the child was initiated. The following general options are available:

- **No or low risk:** The family's case may be closed with no services if the maltreatment was a one-time incident, the child is considered to be safe, there is no or low risk of future incidents, and any services the family needs will not be provided through the child welfare agency but through other community-based resources and service systems.

- **Low to moderate risk:** Referrals may be made to community-based or voluntary in-home child welfare services if the CPS worker believes the family would benefit from these services and the child's present and future safety would be enhanced. This may happen even when no abuse or neglect is found, if the family needs and is willing to participate in services.

- **Moderate to high risk:** The family may again be offered voluntary in-home services to address safety concerns and help reduce the risks. If these are refused, the agency may seek intervention by the juvenile dependency court. Once there is a judicial determination that abuse or neglect occurred, juvenile dependency court may require the family to cooperate with in-home services if it is believed that the child can remain safely at home while the family addresses the issues contributing to the risk of future maltreatment. If the child has been seriously harmed, is considered to be at high risk of serious harm, or the child's safety is threatened, the court may order the child's removal from the home or affirm the agency's prior removal of the child. The child may be placed with a relative or in foster care.

Nationally, it is estimated that 216,000 children, including more than 130,000 victims and almost 86,000 nonvictims (duplicate count), were removed from their homes in 2010 as a result of a child abuse investigation or assessment.

People Who Abuse or Neglect Children

People who are found to have abused or neglected a child are generally offered support and treatment services or are required by a juvenile dependency court to participate in services that will help keep their children safe. In more severe cases or fatalities, police are called on to investigate and may file charges in criminal court against the perpetrators of child maltreatment. In many states, certain types of abuse, such as sexual abuse and serious physical abuse, are routinely referred to law enforcement.

Whether or not criminal charges are filed, the perpetrator's name may be placed on a state child maltreatment registry if abuse or neglect is confirmed. A registry is a central database that collects information about maltreated children and individuals who are found to have abused or neglected those children. These registries are usually confidential and used for internal child protective purposes only. However, they may be used in background checks for certain professions that involve working with children to protect children from contact with individuals who may mistreat them.

Children Who Enter Foster Care

Most children in foster care are placed with relatives or foster families, but some may be placed in group homes. While a child is in foster care, he or she attends school and should receive medical care and other services as needed. The child's family also receives services to support their efforts to reduce the risk of future maltreatment and to help them, in most cases, be reunited with their child. Visits between parents and their children and between siblings are encouraged and supported, following a visitation plan.

Every child in foster care should have a permanency plan. Families typically participate in developing a permanency plan for the child and a service plan for the family, and these plans guide the agency's work. Reunification with parents, except in unusual and extreme circumstances, is the permanency plan for most children. In some cases, when prospects for reunification appear less likely, a concurrent permanency plan is developed. If the efforts toward reunification are not successful, the plan may be changed to another permanent arrangement, such as adoption or transfer of custody to a relative.

Under the Adoption and Safe Families Act, while reasonable efforts to preserve and reunify families are still required, state agencies are required to seek termination of the parent-child relationship when a child has been in foster care for 15 of the most recent 22 months. This requirement does not, at the state's option, apply if a child is cared for by a relative, if the termination is not in the best interests of the child, or if the state has not provided adequate services for the family.

Federal law requires the court to hold a permanency hearing, which determines the permanent plan for the child, within 12 months after the child enters foster care and every 12 months thereafter. Many courts review each case more frequently to ensure that the agency is actively pursuing permanency for the child.

Whether or not they are adopted, older youth in foster care should receive support in developing some form of permanent family connection, in addition to transitional or Independent Living services, to assist them in being self-sufficient when they leave foster care between the ages of 18 and 21.

In FFY 2010, 128,913 children leaving foster care (51 percent) were returned to their parents or primary caregivers. The median length of stay in foster care for these children was 13.5 months. The average age of a child exiting foster care was 9.6 years old.

Summary

The goal of the child welfare system is to promote the safety, permanency, and wellbeing of children and families. Even among children who enter foster care, most will leave it to return safely to the care of their own families, or go to live with relatives or an adoptive family.

For more detailed information about the child welfare system, please refer to the resources listed below. For more information about the child welfare system in your state or local jurisdiction, contact your local public child welfare agency.

References

Child Welfare Information Gateway. (2011). *About CAPTA: A legislative history*. Retrieved from http://www.childwelfare.gov/pubs/factsheets/about.pdf

U.S. Department of Health and Human Services. (2011a). *The AFCARS report: Preliminary FY 2010 estimates as of June 2011 (18)*. Retrieved from http://www.acf.hhs.gov/programs/cb/stats_research/afcars/tar/report18.htm

U.S. Department of Health and Human Services. (2011b). *Child maltreatment 2010*. Retrieved from http://www.acf.hhs.gov/programs/cb/pubs/cm10

Additional Resources

Badeau, S., and Gesiriech, S. (2003). *A child's journey through the child welfare system*. Washington, DC: The Pew Commission on Children in Foster Care. Retrieved from http://www.pewtrusts.org/our_work_report_detail.aspx?id=48990

Child Welfare Information Gateway. (2011). *Understanding child welfare and the courts*. Washington, DC: U.S. Department of Health and Human Services, Children's Bureau.

Goldman, J., and Salus, M. (2003). *A coordinated response to child abuse and neglect: The foundation for practice* (The User Manual Series). Washington, DC: U.S. Department of Health and Human Services. Retrieved from http://www.childwelfare.gov/pubs/usermanuals/foundation/index.cfm

McCarthy, J., Marshall, A., Collins, J., Arganza, G., Deserly, K., and Milon, J. (2003). *A family's guide to the child welfare system*. Washington, DC: National Technical Assistance Partnership for Child and Family Mental Health at Georgetown University Center for Child and Human Development. Retrieved from http://gucchd.georgetown.edu/72140.html

Section 32.2

Court Appointed Special Advocates for Children

The National CASA [Court Appointed Special Advocates] Association is a network of 946 programs that are recruiting, training, and supporting volunteers to represent the best interests of abused and neglected children in the courtroom and other settings.

How do CASA volunteers help children?

CASA volunteers are appointed by judges to watch over and advocate for abused and neglected children, to make sure they don't get lost in the overburdened legal and social service system or languish in inappropriate group or foster homes. Volunteers stay with each case until it is closed and the child is placed in a safe, permanent home. For many abused children, their CASA volunteer will be the one constant adult presence in their lives.

Independent research has demonstrated that children with a CASA volunteer are substantially less likely to spend time in long-term foster care and less likely to reenter care.

Who are CASA volunteers?

Last year, more than 77,000 CASA and guardian ad litem (GAL) volunteers helped 234,000 abused and neglected children find safe, permanent homes. CASA volunteers are everyday citizens who have undergone screening and training with their local CASA/GAL program.

Who are the children CASA volunteers help?

Judges appoint CASA volunteers to represent the best interests of children who have been removed from their homes due to abuse or neglect. Each year, more than 600,000 children experience foster care in this country. Because there are not enough CASA volunteers to represent all of the children in care, judges typically assign CASA volunteers to their most difficult cases.

How did the CASA movement begin?

In 1977, a Seattle juvenile court judge concerned about making drastic decisions with insufficient information conceived the idea of citizen volunteers speaking up for the best interests of abused and neglected children in the courtroom. From that first program has grown a network of more than 946 CASA and guardian ad litem programs that are recruiting, training and supporting volunteers in 49 states.

How do I find a CASA program in my area?

To find a CASA program near you and inquire about becoming a volunteer, visit the CASA website at www.casaforchildren.org and click on the "State and Local Programs Tab." Enter your zip code in the "Find a CASA Program" box or click on "Advanced Search" to search with other options.

How is National CASA funded?

The primary source of National CASA's funding is the federal government, through the Office of Juvenile Justice and Delinquency Prevention (OJJDP). Additional support comes from Jewelers for Children, individuals, and other private funders.

Chapter 33

Therapy Options for Children Impacted by Abuse

Chapter Contents

Section 33.1

Cognitive Behavioral Therapy for Physical Abuse

Excerpted from: Child Welfare Information Gateway. (2007). Abuse-focused cognitive behavioral therapy for child physical abuse. Washington, DC: U.S. Department of Health and Human Services. The full text of this document, including references, is available online at http://www.childwelfare.gov/pubs/cognitive/cognitive.pdf. Reviewed by David A. Cooke, MD, FACP, January 2013.

Children who have experienced physical abuse are at risk for developing significant psychiatric, behavioral, and adjustment difficulties. During the past three decades, research has documented the efficacy of several behavioral and cognitive-behavioral methods, many of which have been incorporated in abuse-focused cognitive behavioral therapy (AF-CBT). AF-CBT has been found to improve functioning in school-aged children, their parents (caregivers), and their families. AF-CBT is an evidence-supported intervention that targets individual child and parent characteristics related to the abusive experience, and the family context in which coercion or aggression occurs. This approach emphasizes training in interpersonal skills designed to enhance self-control and reduce violent behavior.

This report is intended to build a better understanding of the characteristics and benefits of AF-CBT. It was written primarily to help child welfare caseworkers and other professionals who work with at-risk families make more informed decisions about when to refer children and their parents and caregivers to AF-CBT programs. This information also may help parents, foster parents, and other caregivers understand what they and their children can gain from AF-CBT and what to expect during treatment. In addition, it may be useful to others with an interest in implementing or participating in effective strategies for the treatment of child physical abuse.

What Makes AF-CBT Unique

The families in which physical child abuse occurs have often experienced stressful life events that may lead parents to maintain negative perceptions or attributions of their children, heightened anger or hostility, coercive family interactions, and harsh or punitive parenting practices. As a result, abused children from these families may experience aggression, behavioral problems, trauma-related emotional symptoms, poor social and relationship skills, and cognitive impairment.

AF-CBT addresses both the risk factors and the consequences of physical abuse in a comprehensive manner. This approach draws from a variety of therapeutic approaches and implements procedures that have been successful in improving positive family relations and reducing family conflict in diverse populations of parents, children, and families.

Reflects a Comprehensive Treatment Strategy

The diversity of family circumstances and individual problems associated with physical abuse points to the need for a comprehensive treatment strategy that targets both the contributors to abusive behavior and children's subsequent behavioral and emotional adjustment. Treatment approaches that focus on several aspects of the problem (for example, a caretaker's parenting skills, a child's anger, family coercion) may have a greater likelihood of reducing re-abuse and more fully remediating any mental health problems. Therefore, AF-CBT adopts a comprehensive treatment strategy that addresses the complexity of the issues more completely.

Integrates Several Therapeutic Approaches

AF-CBT combines elements drawn from several therapeutic approaches:

- Cognitive therapy, which aims to change behavior by addressing a person's thoughts or perceptions, particularly those thinking patterns that create distorted views

- Behavioral and learning therapy, which focuses on modifying habitual responses (for example, anger, fear) to identified situations or stimuli

- Family therapy, which examines patterns of interactions among family members to identify and alleviate problems

- Developmental victimology, which describes processes involved in the onset and maintenance of abusive behavior, and how the specific sequelae of the abusive experience may vary for children at different developmental stages and across the lifespan

433

AF-CBT pulls together many techniques currently used by practitioners, such as behavior and anger management, problem solving, social skills training, and cognitive restructuring. The advantage of this program is that all of these techniques, relevant handouts, training examples, and outcome measures are integrated in a structured approach that practitioners and supervisors can easily access and use.

Treats Children and Parents Simultaneously

During AF-CBT, school-aged children and parents (or caretakers) participate in separate but coordinated therapy sessions, often using somewhat parallel treatment materials. In addition, children and parents attend joint sessions together at various times throughout treatment. This approach seeks to address individual and parent-child issues in an integrated fashion.

Discourages Aggressive or Violent Behavior

The AF-CBT approach is designed to promote appropriate and prosocial behavior, while discouraging coercive, aggressive, or violent behavior. Consistent with cognitive-behavioral approaches, AF-CBT includes procedures that target three related ways in which people respond to different circumstances:

- Cognition (thinking)

- Affect (feeling)

- Behavior (doing)

AF-CBT includes training in various psychological skills in each of these channels that are designed to promote self-control and to enhance interpersonal effectiveness.

Tailors Treatment to Meet Specific Needs and Circumstances

Child maltreatment research has documented a variety of risk factors and consequences of physical abuse, and this variability requires treatment that can be adapted for different needs. So, for example, the treatment needs of a suicidal teen abused by an alcoholic father may differ from those of a child reported to be aggressive at school and hostile toward a mother who is also a victim of violence.

AF-CBT begins with a multisource assessment to identify the nature of the problems the child is experiencing, specific parental and family difficulties that may be contributing to the risk of abuse, and the child's and family's strengths that may help influence change. Tailoring the treatment to the family's specific strengths and challenges is key to efficient outcomes.

Key Components

AF-CBT is a short-term treatment typically provided over the course of 12 to 24 hours during three to six months (although treatment may last as long as determined necessary). Treatment generally is provided in an outpatient or in-home setting, but it may be used in residential settings (for example, group home, residential treatment facility) or other placement settings (such as foster care) when the parent or caregiver is in regular contact with the child. Treatment includes separate individual sessions with the child and parent. Joint sessions with the child and parent also are held. Where relevant, family interventions may be applied before, during, or after the individual services. Following a brief outline of treatment goals, the key components in each treatment area are listed below.

Goals

Generally, the goals of AF-CBT treatment are to achieve the following:

- Reduce parental anger and use of force
- Promote alternative (nonaggressive) discipline approaches
- Minimize risks for additional abusive incidents
- Enhance the child's coping skills and overall adjustment
- Encourage prosocial problem-solving and communication in the family

Treatment for School-Aged Children

The school-aged child-directed therapy elements include the following:

- Identifying the child's exposure to and views of family hostility, coercion, and violence
- Understanding the child's perceptions of the circumstances and consequences of the physical abuse
- Educating the child on topics related to child welfare and safety, child abuse laws, and common reactions to abuse

- Discussing healthy vs. unhealthy coping
- Training in techniques to identify, express, and manage emotions appropriately (for example, anxiety management, anger control)
- Training in interpersonal skills to enhance social competence
- Developing social support plans

The treatment program for children incorporates the use of specific skills, role-playing exercises, performance feedback, and home practice exercises.

Treatment for Parents (or Caregivers)

Parent-directed therapy elements include the following:

- Identifying views on violence, physical punishment, and sources of stress
- Understanding the role of parental and family stressors that may contribute to conflict
- Examining the role of expectations related to child development and general attributions that may promote coercive interactions
- Identifying and managing reactions to abuse-specific triggers, heightened anger, anxiety, and depression to promote self-control
- Training in effective discipline strategies (for example, time out, attention reinforcement) as alternates to the use of physical force

The treatment program for parents incorporates the use of specific skills, role-playing exercises, performance feedback, and home practice exercises.

Treatment for Families (or the Parent and Child)

Parent-child or family therapy elements include the following:

- Conducting a family assessment using multiple methods and identifying family treatment goals
- Discussing a no-violence agreement
- Clarifying attributions of responsibility for the abuse and developing safety plans, as needed

- Training in communication skills to encourage constructive interactions

- Training in nonaggressive problem-solving skills with home practice applications

- Involving community and social systems, as needed

Target Population

AF-CBT is most appropriate for use with physically abusive or coercive parents and their school-aged children.

Appropriate Populations for Use of AF-CBT

The following groups are appropriate candidates for this program:

- Parents of physically abused children who need to improve their child behavior management skills, lack knowledge of alternatives to punitive forms of child discipline, and/or need guidance in creating more positive interaction with their child

- Physically abused children who exhibit externalizing behavior problems, including aggressive behavior and poor social competence. Often these characteristics are found in families with heightened levels of conflict and coercion.

Limitations for Use of AF-CBT

Parents with psychiatric disorders that may significantly impair their general functioning or their ability to learn new skills (for example, substance use disorders, major depression) may benefit from alternative or adjunctive interventions designed to address these problems. In addition, children or parents with very limited intellectual functioning, or very young children, may require more simplified services or translations of some of the more complicated treatment concepts. Children with psychiatric disorders such as attention-deficit disorder (ADD) or major depression may benefit from additional interventions. Traumatized children, especially sexually abused children, may respond better to trauma-focused therapy. (For more information, see the Child Welfare Information Gateway issue brief, *Trauma-Focused Cognitive Behavioral Therapy: Addressing the Mental Health of Sexually Abused Children*, available online at https://www.childwelfare.gov/pubs/trauma/trauma.pdf.)

Summary of AF-CBT Outcomes

Parent Outcomes

- Achievement of individual treatment goals related to the use of more effective discipline methods
- Decreased parental reports of overall psychological distress
- Lowered parent-reported child abuse potential (risk)
- Reduction in parent-reported drug use

Child Outcomes

- Reduction in parent-reported severity of children's behavior problems (externalizing behavior)
- Reduction in parent-reported severity of child-to-parent aggression

Family Outcomes

- Greater child-reported family cohesion
- Reduced child-reported and parent-reported family conflict

Child Welfare Outcome

- Low rate of abuse recidivism

What to Look for in a Therapist

Caseworkers should become knowledgeable about commonly used treatments before recommending a treatment provider to families. Parents or caregivers should receive as much information as possible on the treatment options available to them. If AF-CBT appears to be an appropriate treatment model for a family, the caseworker should look for a provider who has received adequate training, supervision, and consultation in the AF-CBT model. If feasible, both the caseworker and the family should have an opportunity to interview potential AF-CBT therapists prior to beginning treatment.

AF-CBT Training

Mental health professionals with at least some advanced training in psychotherapy skills and methods and experience working with physically abusive caregivers and their children are eligible for training in AF-CBT. Training generally involves at least two days of initial instruction involving a review of background materials, discussion of key procedures (for example, session guide), and presentation of case examples/tapes. Additional learning experiences are recommended, including ongoing follow-up consultation and supervision (by phone) on the implementation of AF-CBT with a small caseload (for three to six months) and booster training and advanced case review. The duration of this experience may vary by level of experience and case difficulty.

Questions to Ask Treatment Providers

In addition to appropriate training and thorough knowledge of the AF-CBT model, it is important to select a treatment provider who is sensitive to the particular needs of the child, caregiver, and family. Caseworkers recommending an AF-CBT therapist should ask the treatment provider to explain the course of treatment, the role of each family member in treatment, and how the family's specific cultural considerations will be addressed. The child, caregiver, and family should feel comfortable with and have confidence in the therapist.

Some specific questions to ask regarding AFCBT include the following:

- Will the child and parent each receive individualized therapy using corresponding (coordinated) treatment protocols?

- Will social learning principles be used to address the thoughts, emotions, and behaviors of the child and parent?

- Is there a focus on enhancing the parent-child relationship and improving parental discipline practices?

- Is the practitioner sensitive to the cultural background of the child and family?

- Is there a standard assessment process used to gather baseline information on the functioning of the child and family and to monitor their progress in treatment over time?

- Is this the most appropriate treatment for this child and family?

Conclusion

AF-CBT is an evidence-supported treatment intervention for parents and school-aged children in families where physical abuse has occurred. AF-CBT uses an integrated approach to address beliefs about abuse and violence and improve skills to enhance emotional control and reduce violent behavior. Improvements resulting from the use of AF-CBT include reductions in the risk of child abuse, fewer abuse-related behavior problems in children, and improvements in family cohesion. Increased awareness of this treatment option among those making referrals, coupled with increased availability, may create opportunities for helping to strengthen families and reduce the risks for and consequences of child physical abuse.

Section 33.2

Play Therapy for Victims of Child Abuse

Play is the child's language and toys are the child's words.

Why play?

In recent years a growing number of noted mental health professionals have observed that play is as important to human happiness and wellbeing as love and work. Some of the greatest thinkers of all time, including Aristotle and Plato, have reflected on why play is so fundamental in our lives. The following are some of the many benefits of play that have been described by play theorists.

Play is a fun, enjoyable activity that elevates our spirits and brightens our outlook on life. It expands self-expression, self-knowledge, self-actualization and self-efficacy. Play relieves feelings of stress and boredom, connects us to people in a positive way, stimulates creative thinking and exploration, regulates our emotions, and boosts our ego. In addition, play allows us to practice skills and roles needed for survival. Learning and development are best fostered through play.

Why play in therapy?

Play therapy is a structured, theoretically based approach to therapy that builds on the normal communicative and learning processes of children. The curative powers inherent in play are used in many ways. Therapists strategically utilize play therapy to help children express what is troubling them when they do not have the verbal language to express their thoughts and feelings. In play therapy, toys are like the child's words and play is the child's language. Through play, therapists may help children learn more adaptive behaviors when there are emotional or social skills deficits. The positive relationship that develops between therapist and child during play therapy sessions provides a corrective emotional experience necessary for healing. Play therapy may also be used to promote cognitive development and provide insight about and resolution of inner conflicts or dysfunctional thinking in the child.

What is play therapy?

Initially developed in the turn of the 20th century, today play therapy refers to a large number of treatment methods, all applying the therapeutic benefits of play. Play therapy differs from regular play in that the therapist helps children to address and resolve their own problems. Play therapy builds on the natural way that children learn about themselves and their relationships in the world around them. Through play therapy, children learn to communicate with others, express feelings, modify behavior, develop problem-solving skills, and learn a variety of ways of relating to others. Play provides a safe psychological distance from their problems and allows expression of thoughts and feelings appropriate to their development.

The Association for Play Therapy (APT) defines play therapy as "the systematic use of a theoretical model to establish an interpersonal process wherein trained play therapists use the therapeutic powers of play to help clients prevent or resolve psychosocial difficulties and achieve optimal growth and development."

How does play therapy work?

Children are referred for play therapy to resolve their problems. Often, children have used up their own problem solving tools, and they misbehave, may act out at home, with friends, and at school. Play therapy allows trained mental health practitioners who specialize in play therapy, to assess and understand children's play. Further, play therapy is utilized to help children cope with difficult emotions and find solutions to problems. By confronting problems in the clinical play therapy setting, children find healthier solutions. Play therapy allows children to change the way they think about, feel toward, and resolve their concerns. Even the most troubling problems can be confronted in play therapy and lasting resolutions can be discovered, rehearsed, mastered and adapted into lifelong strategies.

Who benefits from play therapy?

Although everyone benefits, play therapy is especially appropriate for children ages three through 12 years old. Teenagers and adults have also benefited from play techniques and recreational processes. To that end, use of play therapy with adults within mental health, agency, and other healthcare contexts is increasing. In recent years, play therapy interventions have also been applied to infants and toddlers.

How will play therapy benefit a child?

Play therapy is implemented as a treatment of choice in mental health, school, agency, developmental, hospital, residential, and recreational settings, with clients of all ages.

Play therapy treatment plans have been utilized as the primary intervention or as an adjunctive therapy for multiple mental health conditions and concerns (for example, anger management, grief and loss, divorce and family dissolution, and crisis and trauma) and for modification of behavioral disorders (for example, anxiety, depression, attention deficit hyperactivity (ADHD), autism or pervasive developmental, academic and social developmental, physical and learning disabilities, and conduct disorders).

Research supports the effectiveness of play therapy with children experiencing a wide variety of social, emotional, behavioral, and learning problems, including: children whose problems are related to life stressors, such as divorce, death, relocation, hospitalization, chronic illness, assimilate stressful experiences, physical and sexual abuse, domestic violence, and natural disasters. Play therapy helps children:

- Become more responsible for behaviors and develop more successful strategies.

- Develop new and creative solutions to problems.

- Develop respect and acceptance of self and others.

- Learn to experience and express emotion.

- Cultivate empathy and respect for thoughts and feelings of others.

- Learn new social skills and relational skills with family.

- Develop self-efficacy and thus a better assuredness about their abilities.

How long does play therapy take?

Each play therapy session varies in length but usually last about 30 to 50 minutes. Sessions are usually held weekly. Research suggests that it takes an average of 20 play therapy sessions to resolve the problems of the typical child referred for treatment. Of course, some children may improve much faster while more serious or ongoing problems may take longer to resolve.

How may my family be involved in play therapy?

Families play an important role in children's healing processes. The interaction between children's problems and their families is always complex. Sometimes children develop problems as a way of signaling that there is something wrong in the family. Other times the entire family becomes distressed because the child's problems are so disruptive. In all cases, children and families heal faster when they work together.

The play therapist will make some decisions about how and when to involve some or all members of the family in the play therapy. At a minimum, the therapist will want to communicate regularly with the child's caretakers to develop a plan for resolving problems as they are identified and to monitor the progress of the treatment. Other options might include involving a) the parents or caretakers directly in the treatment in what is called filial play therapy and b) the whole family in family play therapy. Whatever the level the family members choose to be involved, they are an essential part of the child's healing.

Who practices play therapy?

The practice of play therapy requires extensive specialized education, training, and experience. A play therapist is a licensed (or certified) mental health professional who has earned a Master's or Doctorate degree in a mental health field with considerable general clinical experience and supervision.

With advanced, specialized training, experience, and supervision, mental health professionals may also earn the Registered Play Therapist (RPT) or Registered Play Therapist-Supervisor (RPT-S) credentials conferred by the Association for Play Therapy (APT). The Registered

Play Therapist (RPT) or Registered Play Therapist-Supervisor (RPT-S) credentials can be viewed online at http://www.a4pt.org/ps.credentials. cfm?ID=1637.

Chapter 34

Therapy Options for Adult Survivors of Childhood Abuse

Research tells us that nobody is "magically" resilient. Everyone needs a network of supportive people around them in order to enjoy psychological and emotional health. Many adult survivors of child abuse lack that network: they may not be able to rely on their families, and they may find it difficult to establish and maintain friendships and relationships.

Many health professionals acknowledge the impact of child abuse in their everyday work with adult clients in a range of contexts, from general practice, to mental health services, to alcohol and drug services, and beyond. Nonetheless, Australia has yet to develop a trauma-informed public health system that provides adequate care to adult survivors of child abuse. Australia's mental health system is underfunded, with far fewer dedicated beds and services than comparable Western countries. In Australia, patients with psychoses and/or otherwise "acute needs" are prioritized over patients with complex, chronic mental health problems, such as those that adult survivors of child abuse can display.

This text provides a comprehensive overview of your options for care and support. Please contact us [Adults Surviving Childhood Abuse; www .asca.org.au] to discuss any questions or concerns you may have and we will try and help you as best we can. ASCA is currently actively seeking funding to expand services for adult survivors of child abuse through the formation of therapeutic alliances, and education, and training.

What Would Be the Benefit of Disclosing My Story?

- At times, there are big hurdles and sometimes you don't feel like dredging up any more... You get tired of the gut churning feelings, but the pain is just below the surface at all times anyway and facing it has really helped it to lose its powerful hold over me. Sometimes it is hard to talk about things. I just allow the emotions and pain to come up and I try to ride with it. Then when I feel comfortable enough I speak of why I am feeling the way I am... —Study participant in van Loon, A. M., and Kralik, D. Reclaiming Myself after Child Sexual Abuse. SA: RDNS Research Unit, 2005a.

There are some professionals who feel there is nothing to be gained by going back over past experiences, nor delving into them. Others believe that telling your story relieves the burden of you carrying your abuse history around, as though it is the sum total of who you are. Your abuse is not your whole story. Talking externalizes those past experiences and disentangles the issues they invoke from who you are, making it possible to separate yourself from the abuse experiences (van Loon & Kralik, 2005a). In relation to exploring the past, some survivors conclude that they do not need to dig too deep because the process of exploring may become re-traumatizing. Some survivors explain that it is important to acknowledge that the abuse happened and speak about the aspects of the abuse story that relate to the impacts of the abuse, rather than the details of what happened (van Loon, A. M., and Kralik, D. Promoting Capacity with Homeless Women Survivors of Child Sexual Abuse Misusing Alcohol, Drugs or Gambling. SA: RDNS Research Unit, 2005b).

It is important only to share your story when and if you feel ready to do so, and only within a safe environment, with a person you can trust. If you don't want to talk about your abuse experiences, you may not be ready to do, in which case it might be preferable not to.

Many survivors feel that they have few people to whom they can talk, or from whom they can seek and receive support. However, it is important not to try to recover from your abuse in a vacuum. Learning to trust others and to turn to them for support is a crucial step in recovery. Doing so challenges one of the basic notions arising from a history of abuse: namely, that people are dangerous. Trust your own feelings. Choose people who are interested in you and who can engage with your situation.

Professional help can be of tremendous value to survivors attempting to overcome the negative impacts of their abuse. Recovery usually proceeds more quickly and more safely if you are working with a skilled professional. In a relationship with an ethical and clinically appropriate therapist, the client experiences safety, respect for boundaries, sensitivity to needs, and validation of both the abuse that occurred and the role of recovery in creating a happy and meaningful life.

Disclosing your experiences will rob the abuse of its potency. Even though the effects of abuse cannot be completely erased, they can certainly be diminished and coped with in a healthier way.

Shopping for a Therapist

ASCA is currently expanding its referral database to help you identify suitably qualified therapists in your area. It is recommended that you choose a therapist who holds a recognized qualification in counseling, psychology, or a similarly skilled area. In addition, particular experience and expertise in working with survivors of childhood abuse is vital. Make sure you feel safe in the consulting rooms of the health care professional you choose and that they are sensitive and encouraging. Your chosen therapist would ideally answer any questions you have about their experience, models of working, professional memberships, and qualifications. So, feel free to ask.

Once you have entered into a therapeutic relationship with a professional, if you feel yourself being pushed too hard, or you are uncomfortable with suggested therapeutic methods, try to discuss your concerns with your therapist. If the therapist's suggestions aren't compatible with your feelings or beliefs about your abuse, then try to discuss this as well. You should be comfortable with the pace of your therapy and be able to discuss your progress openly with your therapist. If you are not comfortable after discussing your concerns consider choosing a different therapist.

Even though you may need support to reclaim your capacity to make decisions, a good therapist will allow you to keep control of your life and encourage you to join in decisions about your care. You may want your therapist to make a decision for you while you are in a state of crisis, and doing so may be necessary at times, but it is still important that you are offered that choice (van Loon and Kralik, 2005a).

Choosing a therapist can be intimidating, confusing, and time-consuming. It is often advisable to 'shop around' before you make your choice.

447

The following advice might help you:

- Seek personal recommendations from other survivors.

- Seek recommendations from ASCA.

- Prepare a list of questions to ask the therapist you have chosen, for example, What is his/her experience in working with survivors (particularly with issues that are relevant to you)?

- What approach(es) does he/she use in therapy?

- How much will it cost?

- Is there any possibility of a concession rate?

- What are the options for payment?

- How available is he/she?

- What form do the sessions take?

- How long are the sessions?

- What are the rules about canceling a session?

- Is there any facility for contact between sessions?

- What are the arrangements for holidays?

- What is the process followed when therapy finishes?

- Will you be given the option of returning?

- Will you be involved in the decision-making process?

- Beware of therapists who stress a particular approach or technique, or who are dogmatic about issues such as forgiveness, confrontation, etc.

- Beware of therapists who give hugs, shake hands too readily, or sit too close without invitation. If you do feel uncomfortable when interviewing a therapist, trust your instincts.

- Beware if your therapist seems overly interested in your sexual history and questions you in detail, especially when the questioning appears irrelevant.

- Beware if your therapist avoids sensitive issues and talks in generalities. Is your therapist able to handle the feelings and content that you bring to therapy?

Ask yourself the following:

- Do I feel intimidated by this therapist?
- Does he/she listen to me?
- Do I believe that I can disagree with him/her?

The therapist you choose should be a good listener, who is both empathetic and non-judgmental. Your therapist needs to be a trusted partner in your process.

Psychotherapy

Psychotherapy is the umbrella term for a set of healing techniques practised by accredited psychologists, psychiatrists, and psychoanalysts. There are many different forms of psychotherapy, and they are often combined within a therapeutic program that is developed between a therapist and their client.

Psychotherapy is now accessible through Medicare, and so you are able to access free, or discounted, psychotherapeutic services once you have been given a referral through your local doctor. A therapeutic alliance with a well-trained and sensitive psychotherapist is an important resource for adult survivors of child abuse.

Ideally, a psychotherapist working with an adult survivor of child abuse should have a basic understanding of abuse and trauma, or else be open to further education and training on the matter. Unfortunately, abuse and trauma remains a specialized area of psychotherapy, and many psychologists complete their training without a basic understanding of the dynamics of trauma, and how to work effectively with adult survivors of child abuse.

Research has found that the strongest predictor of good outcomes in psychotherapy is not the type of therapy that is being practiced, but rather the ability of the psychotherapist to establish a strong rapport with their clients. It is natural to, at times, for uncomfortable during psychotherapy, however, it is crucial that you feel comfortable and safe with your psychotherapist, and that they are working with you to build on your strengths, and providing you with new tools to cope with day-to-day life.

Counseling

Counseling is a broader term than "psychotherapy" and refers to any professional guidance in resolving personal conflicts and emotional problems. There are many different counseling approaches, and they often draw on psychological theory and techniques. Many counselors have

449

related qualifications and accreditations. However, counseling remains a largely unregulated field of care at this time. It is a good idea to check the qualifications and expertise of any counselor before establishing an ongoing professional relationship with them.

Sexual Assault Services

Sexual assault services exist in all states and territories of Australia. While their main focus is on recent sexual assault victims, adult survivors of child abuse comprise approximately a quarter of clients seen by these services. In 60% of these cases, the time between the assault and presentation at the service was more than 10 years.

Sexual assault services are excellent resources for adult survivors of child abuse. Many such services provide phone counseling, one-on-one counseling, online counseling, as well as group programs and referral options for adult survivors of child sexual abuse. It is worth noting, however, that these services are chronically underfunded, and are often forced to prioritize services to recent victims of sexual assault.

Complementary Therapy

Complementary therapies, or alternative therapies, refer to a range of practices and techniques outside of those usually practiced by accredited psychotherapists and counselors. Complementary therapies have become increasingly popular in many different areas of health over the last thirty years, and mental health is no exception. Examples of complementary therapies in mental health include practices based on yoga, Reiki, and other meditative traditions, as well as techniques that incorporate dance, massage, or other physical activities.

When investigating complementary therapies, it is important to note that practitioners are not necessarily bound by the same standards of conduct and care as psychotherapists and other accredited mental health care professionals. Psychotherapeutic techniques are regularly evaluated and tested for their effectiveness, whereas complementary therapies are often not. It is often preferable to maintain a therapeutic relationship with a qualified and experienced mental health professional whilst exploring complementary and alternative therapies.

Part Six

Parenting Issues and Child Abuse Risks

Chapter 35

Family Matters and Child Abuse Risk

Chapter Contents

Section 35.1

Risk Factors for Potential Abuse by Parents

Excerpted from "Preventing Child Abuse and Neglect with Parent Training: Evidence," by Richard P. Barth, The Future of Children, Fall 2009, pp 95–118. From *The Future of Children*, a collaboration of The Woodrow Wilson School of Public and International Affairs at Princeton University and the Brookings Institution. To view the complete text of this document including references, visit www.princeton.edu/futureofchildren.

What Parental Behaviors May Lead to Child Abuse and Neglect?

A description of the prevalence of the co-occurring risk factors among parents who abuse and neglect their children sets the stage for a discussion of parenting education elements that may mitigate the untoward effects of these co-occurring problems.

Substance Abuse

Substance abuse by a child's parent or guardian is commonly considered to be responsible for a substantial proportion of child maltreatment reported to the child welfare services. Studies examining the prevalence of substance abuse among caregivers who have maltreated their children have found rates ranging from 19 percent to 79 percent or higher. One widely quoted estimate of the prevalence of substance abuse among caregivers involved in child welfare is 40 to 80 percent. An epidemiological study published in the *American Journal of Public Health* in 1994 found 40 percent of parents who had physically abused their child and 56 percent who had neglected their child met lifetime criteria for an alcohol or drug disorder.

Substance abuse has its greatest impact on neglect. In the 1994 study noted above, respondents with a drug or alcohol problem were 4.2 times as likely as those without such a problem to have neglected their children. In another study conducted during the 1990s, child welfare workers were asked to identify adults in their caseloads with either suspected or known alcohol or illicit drug abuse problems. In 29 percent of the cases, a family member abused alcohol; in 18 percent, at least one adult abused illicit drugs. These findings approximate those of the more recent National Survey of Child and Adolescent Well-Being (NSCAW) that 20 percent of children in an investigation for abuse and neglect had a mother who, by either the child welfare worker's or mother's account, was involved with drugs or alcohol; that figure rises to 42 percent for children who are placed into foster care. These studies have clearly established a positive relationship between a caregiver's substance abuse and child maltreatment among children in out-of-home care and among children in the general population. Among children whose abuse was so serious that they entered foster care, the rate of substance abuse was about three times higher. Thus, substance abuse by parents of victims of child abuse may not be as common in the general child welfare services-involved population as often believed, but substance abuse appears to be a significant contributor to maltreatment.

The mechanism by which substance abuse is responsible for child maltreatment is not as evident (outside of the direct relationship created by the mandated reporting of children who have been tested to have been born drug-exposed). Stephen Magura and Alexandre Laudet argue that in-utero exposure to cocaine and other drugs can lead to congenital deficits that may make a child more difficult to care for and, therefore, more prone to being maltreated. Parenting skills can also suffer among substance-abusing parents, who may be insufficiently responsive to their infants. Caregivers who abuse substances also may place a higher priority on their drug use than on caring for their children, which can lead them to neglect their children's needs for such things as food, clothing, hygiene, and medical care. Findings from the NSCAW indicate that substance abuse was much more highly associated with "neglect, failure to provide basic necessities" than with "neglect, failure to supervise" or any type of abuse. Finally, violence may be more likely to erupt in homes where stimulant drugs and alcohol are used. The interplay between substance abuse and child maltreatment within family dynamics and across children's developmental periods is gradually becoming clearer. Dana Smith and several colleagues showed that prenatal maternal alcohol and substance abuse and postnatal paternal alcohol and substance abuse are most highly associated with child maltreatment. Mothers most often maltreat infants or very young children; fathers involved with alcohol and other substances are more likely to maltreat non-infants. These findings can help in developing parent education programs aimed at preventing child abuse.

Parental Mental Illness

Relatively little has been written about the effect of serious and persistent parental mental illness on child abuse, although many studies show that substantial proportions of mentally ill mothers are living away from their children. Much of the discussion about the effect of maternal mental illness on child abuse focuses on the poverty and homelessness of mothers who are mentally ill, as well as on the behavior problems of their children—all issues that are correlated with involvement with child welfare services. Jennifer Culhane and her colleagues followed a five-year birth cohort among women who had ever been homeless and found an elevated rate of involvement with child welfare services and a nearly seven-times-higher rate of having children placed into foster care. More direct evidence on the relationship between maternal mental illness and child abuse in the general population, however, is strikingly scarce, especially given the 23 percent rate of self-reported major depression in the previous twelve months among mothers involved with child welfare services, as shown in NSCAW.

The relationship between maternal depression and parenting has been better explored and offers guidance regarding the design of parent education programs to prevent child abuse and neglect. Penny Jameson and several colleagues show that depressed mothers have difficulty maintaining interactions with their children and that toddlers tend to match the negative behavior rates of their depressed mothers (but not of their non-depressed mothers). Along similar lines, Casey Hoffman, Keith Crnic, and Jason Baker have shown that maternal depression interferes with parenting and is linked with the development of emotional regulation and behavior problems in children—thus making subsequent parenting even more difficult. Sang Kahng and several colleagues tested the relationship between changes in psychiatric symptoms and changes in parenting and concluded that as symptoms of mental illness lessened, a mother's parental stress decreased and her nurturance increased. Contextual factors—on the positive side, more education and social support; on the negative side, a history of substance abuse and increased daily stress—predict both symptoms and parenting. Taking these contextual factors into account helps to weaken the relationship between psychiatric symptoms and poor parenting. Nicole Shay and John Knutson concur that maternal depression is a risk factor for child abuse and neglect, though they find that it is not so much depression as the irritability that accompanies depression that causes mothers to be physically abusive.

Considerable evidence has also accumulated over many years that as parenting improves, symptoms of maternal depression may lift. Long-term analyses of maternal depression and child problem behavior show that completing parent management training is effective, overall, in improving parenting and reducing conduct problems. Significantly, mothers who improve their parenting skills over a period of a year also show significant reductions in depression during that same interval. And the lifting of depression contributes significantly to improved parenting and child conduct over the next eighteen months.

Domestic Violence

Many families involved with child welfare services must also cope with domestic violence. According to the NSCAW, the lifetime and past-year self-reported rates of intimate partner violence against mothers were 44.8 percent and 29.0 percent, respectively. Caregiver major depression was also strongly associated with violence against women. In a pair of analyses based on NSCAW, Cecilia Casaneueva and colleagues showed that about one-third of parents with low parenting skills had experienced domestic violence. Such violence was also associated with harsher parenting: children over the age of eighteen months were more likely to be spanked if their parents were facing domestic violence. But parents who had once experienced domestic violence, but had been able to put it behind them, did not show elevated rates of impaired or violent parenting. The parenting of women currently suffering interpersonal partner violence is significantly worse than that of women who have faced it in the past, suggesting that the context of the violence is creating the problems in parenting and child conduct problems and that its cessation may be a more important contributor to child outcomes than parent instruction.

Child Behavior Problems

Many studies have shown that children who are involved with child welfare services have high rates of behavioral problems. Indeed, during the 1970s, child welfare services were specifically targeted at two types of children—those without extraordinary behavior problems who needed protection from parental abuse and those with extraordinary behavior problems whose parents often needed the assistance of treatment or placement services. Although the Adoption Assistance and Child Welfare Act of 1980 and subsequent child welfare legislation made federal funding for child welfare services contingent on parental incapacity or abuse, many children continue to enter care because of behavior problems. (They are often reclassified as abused or neglected or abandoned to meet the requirements of funding). Whatever the reason for their involvement with child welfare services —whether difficult child behavior or some measure of parental incapacity—the share of children involved with these services who have behavior problems is substantial. NSCAW indicates that, at least according to parental reports using the Child Behavior Checklist, 42 percent of children between the ages of three and fourteen score high enough to warrant clinical treatment for their problem behaviors. The high rates of behavior problems reported by parents of these children may, however, exaggerate the actual rates. Anna Lau and several colleagues show that physically abusive parents rate the "externalizing" misbehavior (that is, delinquent or aggressive behavior) of their children far more negatively than do independent raters—a difference that does not exist for non-abusive parents. This pattern is consistent with a commonly noted sign of physical abuse—the description by the parent of the child as "bad." Indeed, according to a study by Michael Hurlburt and several colleagues, "The tendency to overreact to child misbehavior, and to overstate behavior problems, may represent a key dispositional risk factor that predicts child physical abuse."

Barbara Burns and several colleagues found that only a small proportion of children with behavior problems receives treatment and, in all likelihood, a still smaller proportion receives evidence-based services. Therefore, because parents believe that their children's behavior is poor and few practitioners are providing evidence-based methods to help them, the risk of abuse is elevated.

Section 35.2

Domestic Violence and Child Abuse

From "Domestic Violence and the Child Welfare System," Child Welfare Information Gateway (www.childwelfare.gov), a service of the Children's Bureau, Administration for Children and Families, U.S. Department of Health and Human Services, 2009. The complete text of this document, including references, is available online at http://www.childwelfare.gov/pubs/factsheets/domesticviolence.cfm.

Domestic violence is a devastating social problem that impacts every segment of the population. While system responses are primarily targeted toward adult victims of abuse, increased attention is now being focused on the children who witness domestic violence. Studies estimate that 10 to 20 percent of children are at risk for exposure to domestic violence. These findings translate into approximately 3.3 to 10 million children who witness the abuse of a parent or adult caregiver each year. Research also indicates children exposed to domestic violence are at an increased risk of being abused or neglected. A majority of studies reveal there are adult and child victims in 30 to 60 percent of families experiencing domestic violence.

Impact of Domestic Violence on Children

Children who live with domestic violence face increased risks: the risk of exposure to traumatic events, the risk of neglect, the risk of being directly abused, and the risk of losing one or both of their parents. All of these may lead to negative outcomes for children and may affect their well-being, safety, and stability. Childhood problems associated with exposure to domestic violence fall into three primary categories:

- **Behavioral, social, and emotional problems:** Higher levels of aggression, anger, hostility, oppositional behavior, and disobedience; fear, anxiety, withdrawal, and depression; poor peer, sibling, and social relationships; and low self-esteem.

- **Cognitive and attitudinal problems:** Lower cognitive functioning, poor school performance, lack of conflict resolution skills, limited problem solving skills, pro-violence attitudes, and belief in rigid gender stereotypes and male privilege.

- **Long-term problems:** Higher levels of adult depression and trauma symptoms and increased tolerance for and use of violence in adult relationships.

Children's risk levels and reactions to domestic violence exist on a continuum where some children demonstrate enormous resiliency while others show signs of significant maladaptive adjustment. Protective factors, such as social competence, intelligence, high self-esteem, outgoing temperament, strong sibling and peer relationships, and a supportive relationship with an adult, can help protect children from the adverse effects of exposure to domestic violence.

Comprehensive assessment regarding the protective factors of children and the effects of domestic violence can inform decision-making regarding the types of services and interventions needed for children living with violence. Additional assessment factors that influence the impact of domestic violence on children include the following:

- **Nature of the violence:** Children who witness frequent and severe forms of violence or fail to observe their caretakers resolving conflict may undergo more distress than children who witness fewer incidences of physical violence and experience positive interactions between their caregivers.

- **Coping strategies and skills:** Children with poor coping skills are more likely to experience problems than children with strong coping skills and supportive social networks.

- **Age of the child:** Younger children appear to exhibit higher levels of emotional and psychological distress than older children. Age-related differences might result from older children's more fully developed cognitive abilities to understand the violence and select various coping strategies to alleviate upsetting symptoms.

- **Elapsed time since exposure:** Children often have heightened levels of anxiety and fear immediately after a violent event. Fewer observable effects are seen in children as more time passes after the violent event.

- **Gender:** In general, boys exhibit more "externalized behaviors" (for example, aggression or acting out) while girls exhibit more "internalized" behaviors" (for example, withdrawal or depression).

460

- **Presence of child physical or sexual abuse:** Children who witness domestic violence and are physically abused are at risk for increased levels of emotional and psychological maladjustment than children who only witness violence and are not abused.

Implications on Practice

Since children respond differently to domestic violence, professionals are cautioned against assuming that witnessing domestic violence constitutes child maltreatment or child protective services intervention. Some states are considering legislation that broadens the definition of child neglect to include children who witness domestic violence. Expanding the legal definition of child maltreatment, however, may not always be the most effective method to address the needs of these children. Communities can better serve families by allocating resources that build partnerships between service providers, child protective services, and the array of informal and formal systems that offer a continuum of services based upon the level of risk present.

Increased awareness regarding the co-occurrence of domestic violence and child abuse compelled child welfare and domestic violence programs to re-evaluate their services and interventions with families experiencing both forms of violence. Although adult and child victims often are found in the same families, child welfare and domestic violence programs historically responded separately to victims. The divergent responses are largely due to differences in each system's development, philosophy, mandate, policies, and practices. For example, some child welfare advocates have charged domestic violence service providers with discounting the safety needs of children by focusing solely on the adult victim. Conversely, some domestic violence advocates accuse child protective services caseworkers of "revictimizing" adult victims by blaming them for the violence, removing their children and charging them with "failure to protect." Despite these differences, child welfare advocates and service providers share areas of common ground that can bridge the gap between them, including these concerns:

- Ending violence against adults and children

- Ensuring children's safety

- Protecting adult victims so their children are not harmed by the violence

- Promoting parents' strengths

461

- Deferring child protection services intervention, if possible, and referring adult victims and children to community based services

A number of national, state, and local initiatives are demonstrating that a collective ownership and intolerance for abuse against adults and children can form the foundation of a solid, coordinated, and comprehensive approach to ending child abuse and domestic violence. These are some examples of promising practice approaches:

- Co-locating domestic violence advocates in child welfare offices for case consultation and supportive services

- Developing cross-system protocols and partnerships to ensure coordinated services and responses to families

- Instituting family court models that address overlapping domestic violence and child abuse cases

- Cross training domestic violence and child welfare advocates

- Creating domestic violence units in child welfare agencies

- The Temporary Assistance for Needy Families Program provides funding, services, exceptions from work requirements, and other waivers, under the Family Violence Option, for families experiencing domestic violence.

Institutional and societal changes can only begin when an expansive network of service providers integrate their expertise, resources, and services to eliminate domestic violence in their communities. Thus, child welfare and domestic violence service providers can collaborate to achieve a shared goal of freeing victims from violence and working to prevent future violence.

Section 35.3

Postpartum Depression

"Depression During and After Pregnancy Fact Sheet," Office on Women's Health (www.womehshealth.gov), March 6, 2009.

What is depression?

Depression is more than just feeling "blue" or "down in the dumps" for a few days. It's a serious illness that involves the brain. With depression, sad, anxious, or "empty" feelings don't go away and interfere with day-to-day life and routines. These feelings can be mild to severe. The good news is that most people with depression get better with treatment.

How common is depression during and after pregnancy?

Depression is a common problem during and after pregnancy. About 13 percent of pregnant women and new mothers have depression.

How do I know if I have depression?

When you are pregnant or after you have a baby, you may be depressed and not know it. Some normal changes during and after pregnancy can cause symptoms similar to those of depression. But if you have any of the following symptoms of depression for more than two weeks, call your doctor:

- Feeling restless or moody
- Feeling sad, hopeless, and overwhelmed
- Crying a lot
- Having no energy or motivation
- Eating too little or too much
- Sleeping too little or too much
- Having trouble focusing or making decisions
- Having memory problems

- Feeling worthless and guilty

- Losing interest or pleasure in activities you used to enjoy

- Withdrawing from friends and family

- Having headaches, aches and pains, or stomach problems that don't go away

Your doctor can figure out if your symptoms are caused by depression or something else.

What causes depression? What about postpartum depression?

There is no single cause. Rather, depression likely results from a combination of factors:

- Depression is a mental illness that tends to run in families. Women with a family history of depression are more likely to have depression.

- Changes in brain chemistry or structure are believed to play a big role in depression.

- Stressful life events, such as death of a loved one, caring for an aging family member, abuse, and poverty, can trigger depression.

- Hormonal factors unique to women may contribute to depression in some women. We know that hormones directly affect the brain chemistry that controls emotions and mood. We also know that women are at greater risk of depression at certain times in their lives, such as puberty, during and after pregnancy, and during perimenopause. Some women also have depressive symptoms right before their period.

Depression after childbirth is called postpartum depression. Hormonal changes may trigger symptoms of postpartum depression. When you are pregnant, levels of the female hormones estrogen and progesterone increase greatly. In the first 24 hours after childbirth, hormone levels quickly return to normal. Researchers think the big change in hormone levels may lead to depression. This is much like the way smaller hormone changes can affect a woman's moods before she gets her period.

Levels of thyroid hormones may also drop after giving birth. The thyroid is a small gland in the neck that helps regulate how your body uses and stores energy from food. Low levels of thyroid hormones can cause symptoms of depression. A simple blood test can tell if this condition is causing your symptoms. If so, your doctor can prescribe thyroid medicine.

Other factors may play a role in postpartum depression. You may feel these effects:

- Tired after delivery
- Tired from a lack of sleep or broken sleep
- Overwhelmed with a new baby
- Doubts about your ability to be a good mother
- Stress from changes in work and home routines
- An unrealistic need to be a perfect mom
- Loss of who you were before having the baby
- Less attractive
- A lack of free time

Are some women more at risk for depression during and after pregnancy?

Certain factors may increase your risk of depression during and after pregnancy:

- A personal history of depression or another mental illness
- A family history of depression or another mental illness
- A lack of support from family and friends
- Anxiety or negative feelings about the pregnancy
- Problems with a previous pregnancy or birth
- Marriage or money problems
- Stressful life events
- Young age
- Substance abuse

Women who are depressed during pregnancy have a greater risk of depression after giving birth. If you take medicine for depression, stopping your medicine when you become pregnant can cause your depression to come back. Do not stop any prescribed medicines without first talking to your doctor. Not using medicine that you need may be harmful to you or your baby.

What is the difference between "baby blues," postpartum depression, and postpartum psychosis?

Many women have the baby blues in the days after childbirth. If you have the baby blues, you may experience these effects:

- Have mood swings
- Feel sad, anxious, or overwhelmed
- Have crying spells
- Lose your appetite
- Have trouble sleeping

The baby blues most often go away within a few days or a week. The symptoms are not severe and do not need treatment.

The symptoms of postpartum depression last longer and are more severe. Postpartum depression can begin anytime within the first year after childbirth. If you have postpartum depression, you may have any of the symptoms of depression listed above. Symptoms may also include thoughts of hurting the baby, thoughts of hurting yourself, or not having any interest in the baby. Postpartum depression needs to be treated by a doctor.

Postpartum psychosis is rare. It occurs in about one to four out of every 1,000 births. It usually begins in the first two weeks after childbirth. Women who have bipolar disorder or another mental health problem called schizoaffective disorder have a higher risk for postpartum psychosis. Symptoms may include the following:

- Seeing things that aren't there
- Feeling confused
- Having rapid mood swings
- Trying to hurt yourself or your baby

What should I do if I have symptoms of depression during or after pregnancy?

Call your doctor if you experience these symptoms:

- Your baby blues don't go away after two weeks

- Symptoms of depression get more and more intense
- Symptoms of depression begin any time after delivery, even many months later
- It is hard for you to perform tasks at work or at home
- You cannot care for yourself or your baby
- You have thoughts of harming yourself or your baby

Your doctor can ask you questions to test for depression. Your doctor can also refer you to a mental health professional who specializes in treating depression.

Some women don't tell anyone about their symptoms. They feel embarrassed, ashamed, or guilty about feeling depressed when they are supposed to be happy. They worry they will be viewed as unfit parents.

Any woman may become depressed during pregnancy or after having a baby. It doesn't mean you are a bad or "not together" mom. You and your baby don't have to suffer. There is help.

Here are some other helpful tips:

- Rest as much as you can. Sleep when the baby is sleeping.
- Don't try to do too much or try to be perfect.
- Ask your partner, family, and friends for help.
- Make time to go out, visit friends, or spend time alone with your partner.
- Discuss your feelings with your partner, family, and friends.
- Talk with other mothers so you can learn from their experiences.
- Join a support group. Ask your doctor about groups in your area.
- Don't make any major life changes during pregnancy or right after giving birth. Major changes can cause unneeded stress. Sometimes big changes can't be avoided. When that happens, try to arrange support and help in your new situation ahead of time.

How is depression treated?

The two common types of treatment for depression are talk therapy and medicine:

- **Talk therapy:** This involves talking to a therapist, psychologist, or social worker to learn to change how depression makes you think, feel, and act.

- **Medicine:** Your doctor can prescribe an antidepressant medicine. These medicines can help relieve symptoms of depression.

These treatment methods can be used alone or together. If you are depressed, your depression can affect your baby. Getting treatment is important for you and your baby. Talk with your doctor about the benefits and risks of taking medicine to treat depression when you are pregnant or breastfeeding.

What can happen if depression is not treated?

Untreated depression can hurt you and your baby. Some women with depression have a hard time caring for themselves during pregnancy. They may experience these effects:

- Eat poorly

- Not gain enough weight

- Have trouble sleeping

- Miss prenatal visits

- Not follow medical instructions

- Use harmful substances, like tobacco, alcohol, or illegal drugs

Depression during pregnancy can raise the risk of problems during pregnancy or delivery, having a low-birth-weight baby, or premature birth. Untreated postpartum depression can affect your ability to parent. You may lack energy, have trouble focusing, feel moody, or not be able to meet your child's needs. As a result, you may feel guilty and lose confidence in yourself as a mother. These feelings can make your depression worse.

Researchers believe postpartum depression in a mother can affect her baby. It can cause the baby to have delays in language development, problems with mother-child bonding, behavior problems, or increased crying. It helps if your partner or another caregiver can help meet the baby's needs while you are depressed.

All children deserve the chance to have a healthy mom. And all moms deserve the chance to enjoy their life and their children. If you are feeling depressed during pregnancy or after having a baby, don't suffer alone. Please tell a loved one and call your doctor right away.

Section 35.4

Returning War Veterans and Family Matters

Trauma and Family Safety

As tours of duty in Iraq and Afghanistan place more soldiers and their families under greater strain, many are concerned about the adequacy of mental health services available to the millions of men and women in uniform, especially those in the Reserves and National Guard (currently 30–40% of those deployed).

A series of domestic homicides at Fort Bragg in 2002 helped to focus a spotlight on the problem, in particular because some of the perpetrators had recently returned from tours of duty in Afghanistan. Since then, numerous incidents and reports indicate that domestic violence remains a serious problem in the military, especially after service members return from war. CBS' *60 Minutes* reported that rates of marital aggression are considerably higher in the military than in civilian life, as much as three to five times greater ("The War At Home," Jan. 17, 1999). Confronted with this mounting problem of domestic violence in the military, Congress created The Defense Task Force on Domestic Violence and the Joint Task Force for Sexual Assault Prevention and Response.

Also, among veterans of the wars in Iraq and Afghanistan who received care from the Department of Veterans Affairs (VA) between 2001 and 2005, nearly-one third were diagnosed with mental health and/or psychosocial problems and one-fifth were diagnosed with a substance use disorder.[1] Victims of trauma are at a much higher risk for co-occurring mental health and substance abuse disorders, violence victimization and perpetration, self-injury, and a host of other coping mechanisms which themselves have devastating human, social, and economic costs.

In March, 2007, the White House formed the President's Commission on Care for America's Returning Wounded Warriors. The commission has recommended fundamental changes to the military health care system, including aggressive steps to prevent and treat post-traumatic stress disorder (PTSD) and traumatic brain injury (TBI)—two key injuries in the current conflicts. In its report issued July 31, 2007, the commission stated: "A sizeable fraction of service members returning from Iraq and Afghanistan suffer from PTSD. Best estimates are that PTSD of varying degrees of severity affects 12 to 20 percent of returnees from Iraq and 6 to 11 percent of returnees from Afghanistan. To date, 52,375 returnees have been seen in the Veterans Administration for PTSD symptoms." What is also known is that many service members never seek out mental health services when they are struggling because of the many stigma barriers and the impact that diagnosis can have (on career, security clearance, the perception that peers will question their reliability in future situations of combat and reduce trust in those relationships, the perception family members will have in seeing this as a weakness rather than an injury, and more). These silent wounds impact more than just the veteran—they affect the soldier's parents, spouses, children, and friendships.

The following is some research that looks at how the impact of combat trauma can play a role in responses that can put the family in a situation that is not safe—and one that is often seen as domestic violence. It is only when we understand the role that trauma plays in this dynamic that we can begin to consider preventive measures and the trauma-informed care that will promote healing with our returning veterans.

Veterans

Both veterans of the current conflicts in Afghanistan and Iraq who are still active in the military and those who have separated from military service and may be utilizing VA services are included in our view of veterans.

Veterans and Combat Stress

- The traumatic impact of the repeat and prolonged nature of war is significant.

- Repeat deployments increase stress and strain on veterans and their families exponentially. [2]

- Adrenalin levels are much higher than normal, which is partly why returning veterans partake in thrill seeking and risk taking behaviors.

470

- The condition of combat creates strong startle responses and trauma triggers that can be not only divisive with family members after return, but they can be potentially dangerous.

- Trauma and PTSD-related symptoms like flashbacks and nightmares can cause a veteran to react quickly with intense response, and this can create a safety concern for family members.

- The war and military condition create a sense of wanting immediate response and results (perhaps stemming from anxiety and/or hypervigilance), which means that many soldiers do not stick with services and recovery programs they have sought out.

Reports on Veterans, Substance Abuse and Mental Health[3]

- "Nearly 20 percent of military service members who have returned from Iraq and Afghanistan—300,000 in all—report symptoms of post-traumatic stress disorder or major depression, yet only slightly more than half have sought treatment."

- "Since October 2001, about 1.6 million U.S. troops have deployed to the wars in Iraq and Afghanistan, with many exposed to prolonged periods of combat-related stress or traumatic events. Early evidence suggests that the psychological toll of the deployments may be disproportionately high compared with physical injuries."

- Just 53 percent of service members with PTSD or depression sought help from a provider over the past year, and of those who sought care, roughly half got minimally adequate treatment.

- If PTSD and depression go untreated or are under treated, there is a cascading set of consequences. Drug use, suicide, marital problems, and unemployment are some of the consequences.

- National Guard and Reserve combat troops in Iraq and Afghanistan are more likely to develop drinking problems than active-duty soldiers.[4]

- Veterans "use" alcohol, drugs, and cigarettes more often than nonveterans.[5] Veterans also often use substances to self-medicate the psychological wounds that go unaddressed.

- Evidence based practices (EBP) indicate that substance abuse and mental health treatment (especially PTSD) must be done concurrently. Treatment of co-occurring disorders is widely accepted, although not always practiced, and has the most successful treatment outcomes for those in recovery. All too often the focus is on addressing the symptom (for example, self-medicating with alcohol or drugs) rather than the root of what happened to the veteran which is combat trauma.

Veterans and Family Relationships

- Start to distance from the family before deployment. The time away and new routines and norms at home require time for the returning parent to feel a part of the family unit again.

- Tend to "bark" orders, as they would in a military unit, after returning home.

Spouses of Veterans

Spouses/Partners

- Start to distance from their partner before deployment.

- Sometimes experience a resentment that they have to provide all of the financial and parenting support to the family while the veteran is away.

- Assume all parenting responsibilities that sometimes continue even after their partner returns from war.

- Avoiding groups, crowds, and family events may feel more comfortable to the returning veteran, but that kind of emotional withdrawal further isolates the family.

- May struggle with anger from the returning veteran which, while it may be a means of coping, lessens communication, distances loved ones, and creates greater loneliness. Because of the anger, spouses may see their partner as unpredictable, hostile, and frightening.[6]

- May be aware that a solider changes while away at war, but do not understand how these changes may impact their relationship with their spouse or their family dynamic

- If domestic violence was experienced prior to deployment, spouses may see an increase in violence and intensity after returning from a tour.

Reports on Domestic Violence

- "There is increasing recognition that active duty military (ADM) women, like their civilian counterparts, are at risk for domestic violence defined as physical and/or sexual assault or threats between sexually intimate partners."[7]

Children of Veterans

Children

- There are 1.1 million children with a parent that is an OEF/OIF [Operation Enduring Freedom/Operation Iraqi Freedom] veteran.
- Start to distance with a deploying parent before departure. Getting close again after the return home takes time.
- Are used to the home parent caring for and disciplining them. When the veteran parent returns and steps back into their role, it may be met with resistance.
- May wonder what they did to cause their parent to be quiet or withdrawn, when the emotional distance may be the result of combat trauma.

Reports on Child Abuse

- A report commissioned by the Army determined that during deployment, rates jump, outstripping civilian abuse rates: neglect (increases four-fold), maltreatment (increases three-fold), and physical abuse (increases two-fold).[8]
- Maltreatment of children in families of enlisted soldiers was 42 percent higher if a parent was deployed and away from home than when they were home.[9]

Parents of Veterans

Parents

- Feel a strong responsibility and continue to care for and help their son or daughter.
- Sometimes take the experience of dissociation and isolation (common following the traumatic impact of war) of their son or daughter as something personal, and struggle to remain close and connected.
- Can experience added stress from verbal abuse, substance abuse, and anxiety-creating changes like seeing their veteran son or daughter sleeping with a loaded gun.

- Are impacted economically when their veteran son or daughter becomes dependant needing emotional and/or physical care, living expenses, and housing.

- Depending on their own physical, emotional, and economic history and situation, the parent may not be adequately equipped to address the needs of their adult son or daughter.

- Are unlikely to reach out for help if they experience a stressful, abusive, or violent situation with their adult son or daughter because they do not want to create added problems for him or her, because of stigma and family secrecy on these issues, and because parents sometimes see the animosity or stress as their own failure as a parent.

Reports on Parents

- "An estimated 10,000 recent veterans of these conflicts now depend on their parents for their care. Working unheralded, these parents have quit jobs, shelved retirement plans, and relocated so they can be with their injured sons and daughters. Many have become warriors themselves, fighting to make sure this new wave of injured veterans gets the medical care and rehabilitation it needs." [10]

Editor's Note

It is being increasingly recognized that a significant number of veterans of the Iraq and Afghanistan wars sustained traumatic brain injuries (TBI) during their deployments, frequently from roadside bomb explosions. A history of TBI has been shown to sharply increase the risk of subsequent psychiatric disorders, including PTSD and substance abuse. It is possible that this is a significant factor in the high rates of mental health problems seen among veterans of these conflicts.

Notes

1. National Survey on Drug Use and Health. 2005. SAMHSA [Substance Abuse and Mental Health Services Administration].

2. Combat Duty in Iraq and Afghanistan, Mental Health Problems, and Barriers to Care. July 1, 2004. *The New England Journal of Medicine.*

3. *Invisible Wounds of War Project*. 2008. The Rand Corporation: http://www.rand.org/multi/military/veterans/

4. "After combat, soldiers turning to alcohol - Guard and Reserve combat troops at higher risk than active-duty soldiers." August 12, 2008. The Associated Press.

5. National Survey on Drug Use and Health. 2005. SAMHSA.

6. "Trauma and the Military Family: Responses, Resources, and Opportunities for Growth." January/February 2008. *Social Work Today*. Sherman, M.D. http://www.socialworktoday.com/archive/janfeb2008p36.shtml

7. "Domestic Violence in the Military: Women's Policy Preferences and Beliefs Concerning Routine Screening and Mandatory Reporting." August 2006. *Military Medicine*. Carlson, G., Campbell, J., Garza, M., and O'Campo, P. http://findarticles.com/p/articles/mi_qa3912/is_200608/ai_n17183184/pg_1?tag=artBody;col1

8. "Child Maltreatment in Enlisted Soldiers' Families During Combat-Related Deployments." August 1, 2007. *Journal of the American Medical Association (JAMA)*. Gibbs, D., Martin, S, Kupper, L. Johnson, R. Issue 298, pages 528–535.

9. "Military Deployment Stress Tied to Child-Abuse Increase." September 7, 2007. Levin, A. *Psychiatr News*. Volume 42, Number 17, page 8.

10. "When Wounded Vets Come Home." July & August 2008. *AARP The Magazine*. Yeoman, B. http://www.aarpmagazine.org/family/when_wounded_vets_come_home.html

Chapter 36

Parental Substance Abuse and Child Abuse Risks

Chapter Contents

Section 36.1

Connection between Substance Abuse and Child Abuse

"Parental Substance Use and the Child Welfare System,"
Child Welfare Information Gateway (www.childwelfare.gov),
U.S. Department of Health and Human Resources, 2009.

Parental substance use continues to be a serious issue in the child welfare system. Maltreated children of parents with substance use disorders often remain in the child welfare system longer and experience poorer outcomes than other children. Addressing the multiple needs of these children and families is challenging.

This section provides a brief overview of some of the issues confronting families affected by parental substance use who enter the child welfare system, and it examines some of the service barriers as well as the innovative approaches child welfare agencies have developed to best meet the needs of these children and families.

Statistics and Costs

It is estimated that nine percent of children in this country (six million) live with at least one parent who abuses alcohol or other drugs. Studies indicate that between one-third and two-thirds of child maltreatment cases involve substance use to some degree.

It is difficult to determine the numbers of child welfare cases that involve substance-using parents. One article notes that not all child welfare agencies systematically record information on parental substance use disorders, and many substance abuse treatment programs do not routinely ask patients if they have children. The article goes on to summarize available data from a number of national studies, estimating that 22,440 children receiving in-home services for maltreatment and 128,640 to 211,720 children in out-of-home care had a parent with a substance use disorder in 2004. In that same year, approximately 295,000 parents receiving treatment for substance use had one or more children removed by child protective services.

Expenditures related to substance use are significant, because maltreated children of parents with a substance use disorder may experience more severe problems and remain in the foster care system longer than maltreated children from other families. One study estimates that of the more than $24 billion states spend annually to address different aspects of substance use, $5.3 billion (slightly more than 20 percent) goes to child welfare costs related to substance abuse.

Impact of Parental Substance Use on Parenting

Parents with substance use disorders may not be able to function effectively in a parental role. This can be due to problems such as these:

- Impairments (both physical and mental) caused by alcohol or other drugs

- Domestic violence, which may be a result of substance use

- Expenditure of often limited household resources on purchasing alcohol or other drugs

- Frequent arrests, incarceration, and court dates

- Time spent seeking out, manufacturing, or using alcohol or other drugs

- Estrangement from primary family and related support

Families in which one or both parents have substance use disorders, and particularly families with an addicted parent, often experience a number of other problems that affect parenting, including mental illness, unemployment, high levels of stress, and impaired family functioning, all of which can put children at risk for maltreatment. The basic needs of children, including nutrition, supervision, and nurturing, may go unmet due to parental substance use, resulting in neglect. Depending on the extent of the substance use and other circumstances (for example, the presence of another caregiver), dysfunctional parenting can also include physical and other kinds of abuse.

Impact on Child Outcomes

The impact of parental substance use disorders on a child can begin before the child is born. While the full effects of prenatal drug exposure depend on a number of factors, alcohol or drug use during pregnancy has been associated with infant mortality, premature birth, miscarriage, low birth weight, and a variety of behavioral and cognitive problems in the child. A 2007 study of children in foster care found that prenatal maternal alcohol use predicted child maltreatment, and combined prenatal maternal alcohol and drug use predicted foster care transitions.

Fetal alcohol spectrum disorders (FASD) are among the most well-known consequences, affecting an estimated 40,000 infants born each year. Children with FASD may experience mental, physical, behavioral, and learning disabilities. Children with the most severe disorders may suffer from fetal alcohol syndrome, alcohol-related neurodevelopmental disorder, or alcohol-related birth defects.

Research has demonstrated that children of parents with substance use disorders are more likely to experience abuse (physical, sexual, or emotional) or neglect than children in other households. As infants, they may suffer from attachment difficulties that develop because of inconsistent care and nurturing, which may interfere with their emotional development. As growing children, they may experience chaotic households that lack structure, positive role models, and adequate opportunities for socialization.

In addition, children of parents who use or abuse substances have an increased chance of experiencing a variety of other negative outcomes:

- Maltreated children of parents with substance use disorders are more likely to have poorer physical, intellectual, social, and emotional outcomes.

- They are at greater risk of developing substance use problems themselves.

- They are more likely to be placed in foster care and to remain there longer than maltreated children of parents without substance use problems.

Methamphetamine

Over the last decade, there has been an increase in the manufacture and use of methamphetamine. From 1995 to 2005, the percentage of substance abuse treatment admissions for primary abuse of methamphetamine/amphetamine more than doubled from four percent to nine percent.

Parental use of methamphetamine has many of the same effects on children as other kinds of drug use. Prenatal exposure can produce birth defects and low birth weight and may lead to developmental disorders. Parents who use methamphetamine may suffer physical and psychological effects that lead to abuse and neglect of their children. In addition, some methamphetamine users also are producers of the drug, which can be manufactured using common household products. These home "labs" put children in additional danger from exposure to the drugs and the conditions under which they are manufactured and distributed.

Surveys conducted by the National Association of Counties indicate that methamphetamine has increased the burden of child welfare agencies in many areas of the country. In addition to increasing caseloads in some areas, the unique dangers of methamphetamine labs have prompted many jurisdictions to develop specific protocols for meeting the needs of children who may have been exposed to the drug.

Other Substances

While methamphetamine continues to garner much attention, other drugs actually account for the bulk of substance use disorders. The Substance Abuse and Mental Health Service Administration (SAMHSA) reports the following statistics:

- Marijuana was the most commonly used illicit drug in 2006, accounting for 72.8 percent of illicit drug use.

- In 2006, there were 2.4 million cocaine users, a figure that remained the same from 2005 but was an increase from 2002 (at 2.0 million).

- The number of heroin users increased from 136,000 in 2005 to 338,000 in 2006, and the corresponding prevalence rate increased from 0.06 to 0.14 percent.

- The most widely used substance continues to be alcohol. In 2006, heavy drinking was reported by 6.9 percent of the population (17 million people), while binge drinking was reported by 23 percent (57 million people).

Service Delivery Issues

Child welfare agencies face a number of difficulties in serving children and families affected by parental substance use disorders:

- Inadequate funds for services and/or dependence on client insurance coverage

- Insufficient service availability or scope of services to meet existing needs

- Lack of training for child welfare workers on substance use issues

- Lack of coordination between the child welfare system and other services and systems, including hospitals that may screen for drug exposure, the criminal justice system, and the courts

- Conflicts in the time required for sufficient progress in substance abuse recovery to develop adequate parenting potential, legislative requirements regarding child permanency, and the developmental needs of children

Agencies are faced with timeframes imposed by the Adoption and Safe Families Act of 1997 (ASFA) that may not coincide with substance abuse treatment. Although ASFA requires that an agency file a petition for termination of parental rights if a child has been in foster care for 15 of the past 22 months, unless it is not in the best interest of the child, many states cannot adhere to this timeframe due to problems with accessing substance abuse services in a timely manner. This results in delayed permanency decisions for children in the foster care system. For example, despite a federal mandate that pregnant and parenting women receive priority for accessing substance abuse treatment services, states report it is often difficult for these parents to access an open treatment slot quickly. Once a slot is available, treatment itself may take many months, and achieving sufficient stability to care for their children may take parents even longer. In addition, relapse is often part of the recovery process for parents undergoing treatment, especially in the early phases, so it is especially important that parents access treatment quickly. Custodial parents who require residential treatment may face an additional barrier since many of these programs do not allow children to live in the facility.

Promising Practices

There is a growing movement toward collaboration among the child welfare, substance abuse, courts, and other systems that provide services for children and families affected by substance use by their parents. Communication, understanding, and active collaboration among service systems are vital to ensuring that child welfare-involved parents in need of substance abuse treatment are accurately identified and receive appropriate treatment in a timely manner.

These are some examples of effective approaches:

Prevention and Treatment

- Focusing on early identification of at-risk families in substance abuse treatment programs so that prevention services can be provided to ensure children's safety and well-being in the home

- Providing coaching or mentoring to parents for their treatment, recovery, and parenting

- Offering shared family care in which a family experiencing parental substance use and resulting child maltreatment is placed with a host family for support and mentoring

- Giving mothers involved in the child welfare system priority access to substance abuse treatment slots

- Providing inpatient treatment for mothers in facilities where they can have their children with them

- Motivating parents to enter and complete treatment by offering such incentives as support groups or housing

Systems Changes

- Stationing addiction counselors in child welfare offices or forming ongoing teams of child welfare and substance abuse workers

- Developing or modifying dependency drug courts to ensure treatment access and therapeutic monitoring of compliance with court orders

- Developing cross-system partnerships to ensure coordinated services (for example, formal linkages between child welfare and other community agencies to address each family's needs)

- Providing wraparound services that streamline the recovery and reunification processes

- Conducting cross-system training

- Recruiting and training a diverse workforce and including training in cultural competence

- Exploring various funding streams to support these efforts (for example, using state or local funds to maximize child welfare funding for substance abuse-related services or using Temporary Assistance to Needy Families [TANF] funds to support substance abuse treatment for families also involved with the child welfare system)

The Children's Bureau has funded a number of discretionary grants to promote demonstration projects with a goal of improved outcomes for children growing up in families in which one or more parents has a substance use problem. These grants have included the following:

- Family Support Services for Grandparents and Other Relatives Providing Care for Children and Substance Abusing and HIV-Positive Women (awarded in 2001 with six grantees)

- Family Support Services for Grandparents and Other Relatives Providing Caregiving for Children of Substance Abusing and/or HIV-Positive Women (awarded in 2004 with four grantees)

- Model Development or Replication to Implement the CAPTA Requirement to Identify and Serve Substance Exposed Newborns (awarded in 2005, with four grantees)

- Targeted Grants to Increase the Well-Being of, and to Improve the Permanency Outcomes for, Children Affected by Methamphetamine or Other Substance Abuse (awarded in 2007, with 53 grantees under four program options)

Replication or adaptation of any of the above approaches requires a careful assessment of state or local capacity, including needs and strengths of families served, as well as a careful assessment of the evaluation findings to ensure funds are targeted toward effective programs. Agencies also should focus on the specific needs of the families they serve when selecting among these (and other) approaches.

Section 36.2

Substance Abuse during Pregnancy

From "Chapter 3: Protecting Children in Families Affected by Substance Use Disorders," *How Parental Substance Use Disorders Affect Children*, prepared by the Office on Child Abuse and Neglect, Children's Bureau, and ICF International; available from Child Welfare Information Gateway (www .childwelfare.gov), U.S. Department on Health and Human Services, 2009.

The lives of millions of children are touched by substance use disorders (SUDs). The 2007 National Survey on Drug Use and Health reports that 8.3 million children live with at least one parent who abused or was dependent on alcohol or an illicit drug during the past year. This includes 13.9 percent of children aged two years or younger, 13.6 percent of children aged 3 to 5 years, 12.0 percent of children aged 6 to 11 years, and 9.9 percent of youths aged 12 to 17 years. These children are at increased risk for abuse or neglect, as well as physical, academic, social, and emotional problems.

A predictable, consistent environment, coupled with positive caregiver relationships, is critical for normal emotional development of children. Parental substance abuse and dependence have a negative impact on the physical and emotional well-being of children and can cause home environments to become chaotic and unpredictable, leading to child maltreatment. The children's physical and emotional needs often take a back seat to their parents' activities related to obtaining, using, or recovering from the use of drugs and alcohol.

This section discusses how prenatal and postnatal substance use by parents affects fetal and early childhood development. It is intended to help child protective services (CPS) caseworkers understand the behaviors and problems that some children in the child welfare system may exhibit and that hold implications for their potential need for services.

The Impact on Prenatal Development

In 2006 and 2007, an average of 5.2 percent of pregnant women aged 15 to 44 years used an illicit drug during the month prior to being surveyed, and 11.6 percent had consumed alcohol. Nationwide, between 550,000 and 750,000 children are born each year after prenatal exposure to drugs or alcohol. These children often are medically fragile or born with a low birth weight. Some are born prematurely and require intensive care.

Identifying the effects of drugs and alcohol on fetuses has posed challenges for researchers. While there has been some success researching the effects of alcohol on fetal development, securing accurate information regarding the use of illicit drugs from pregnant women or women who have given birth has proven to be very difficult. In addition, women who abuse substances often have other risk factors in their lives (for example, a lack of prenatal care, poor nutrition, stress, violence, poor social support) that can contribute significantly to problematic pregnancies and births.

The information below summarizes some of what is known about the effects of substance use on prenatal development.

Pregnancy and SUDs

Women who use alcohol or illicit drugs may find it difficult or seemingly impossible to stop, even when they are pregnant. Moreover, pregnancy can be stressful and uncomfortable. For someone who commonly uses drugs and alcohol to minimize pain or stress, this practice may not only continue, but also become worse. Pregnant women can face significant stigma and prejudice when their SUDs are discovered. For these reasons, some women avoid seeking treatment or adequate prenatal care. Other pregnant women, however, do seek treatment. According to the Substance Abuse and Mental Health Services Administration, 3.9 percent of the women admitted to state licensed or certified SUD treatment programs were pregnant at the time of admission. In another study, pregnant women aged 15 to 44 years were more likely than nonpregnant women of the same age group to enter treatment for cocaine abuse.

Screening Newborns at Birth

Opinions differ about how best to respond to prenatal substance exposure. Some hospitals are reconsidering whether they should test newborns for drugs, and some courts are treating prenatal substance exposure as a public health matter, turning to CPS only if they determine the child was harmed. Decisions regarding whether and when to screen newborns for prenatal substance exposure are beyond the purview of CPS.

Child welfare legislation has provided some guidance regarding how such cases should be handled. The Keeping Children and Families Safe Act of 2003 requires that health care providers notify CPS, as appropriate, to address the needs of infants born exposed to drugs, and requires the development of a plan of safe care for any affected infants. In 2006, statutes in 15 states and the District of Columbia specified reporting procedures when there is evidence at birth that an infant was exposed prenatally to drugs, alcohol, or other controlled substances. Additionally, 13 states and the District of Columbia included prenatal substance exposure in their definitions of child abuse or neglect.

The Effects of Prenatal Exposure to Alcohol

Drinking alcohol during pregnancy can have serious effects on fetal development. Alcohol consumed by a pregnant woman is absorbed by the placenta and directly affects the fetus. A variety of birth defects to the major organs and the central nervous system, which are permanent, can occur due to alcohol use during pregnancy, though the risk of harm decreases if the pregnant woman stops drinking completely. Collectively, these defects are called fetal alcohol syndrome (FAS). FAS is one of the most commonly known birth defects related to prenatal drug exposure. Children with FAS may exhibit these characteristics:

- Growth deficiencies, both prenatally and after birth
- Problems with central nervous system functioning
- IQs in the mild to severely retarded range
- Small eye openings and poor development of the optic nerve
- A small head and brain
- Joint, limb, ear, and heart malformations

Alcohol-related neurodevelopmental disorder (ARND) and alcohol-related birth defects (ARBD) are similar to FAS. Once known as fetal alcohol effects, ARND and ARBD are terms adopted in 1996 by the National Academy of Sciences' Institute of Medicine. ARND and ARBD encompass the functional and physiological problems associated with prenatal alcohol exposure, but are less severe than FAS. Children with ARND can experience functional or mental impairments as a result of prenatal alcohol exposure, and children with ARBD can have malformations in the skeletal and major organ systems. Not all children who are exposed prenatally to alcohol develop FAS, ARND, or ARBD, but for those who do, these effects continue throughout their lives and at all the stages of development, although they are likely to present themselves differently at each developmental stage.

Childhood Behavior and Characteristics Associated with FAS, ARND, and ARBD

This information compares typical childhood behavior at each developmental stage with behaviors and characteristics associated with FAS, ARND, and ARBD.

Infants

- Typical behaviors or characteristics:
  - Develop mental and physical skills
  - Bond with caretakers
- FAS/ARND/ARBD behaviors or characteristics:
  - Problems with spatial and depth perception, muscle coordination and development, facility with speech, and processing information
  - Attention deficit disorder
  - Inability to focus
  - Possible attachment disorders

Toddlers

- Typical behaviors or characteristics:
  - Develop sense of self
  - Assert independence by saying "no"
- FAS/ARND/ARBD behaviors or characteristics:
  - Difficulty exercising self-control, which leads to self doubt and feelings of inadequacy

5–7 Year Olds

- Typical behaviors or characteristics:
  - Try new things
  - Meet or exceed academic standards
  - Learn new social skills

- FAS/ARND/ARBD behaviors or characteristics:
  - Overwhelmed with new situations and interactions with other children
  - Inability to pick up social skills by observation
  - Problems meeting academic standards

8–12 Year Olds

- Typical behaviors or characteristics:
  - Increased influence of peers
  - Games become important method of bonding and developing interpersonal skills
- FAS/ARND/ARBD behaviors or characteristics:
  - Difficulty remembering rules of games
  - Lack of remorse in breaking rules
  - Become depressed and exhibit other behavior problems

Teenagers

- Typical behaviors or characteristics:
  - Continued detachment from parents
  - Development of individual identity
  - Learn to identify with larger community
- FAS/ARND/ARBD behaviors or characteristics:
  - May lack skills to become good community members
  - Become socially isolated
  - May find their way to peer groups that engage in high risk behaviors
  - May withdraw altogether from groups

More information on FAS is available from the National Organization on Fetal Alcohol Syndrome (http://www.nofas.org) and the National Center on Birth Defects and Developmental Disabilities (http://www.cdc.gov/ncbddd/fas).

The Effects of Prenatal Exposure to Drugs

Similar to alcohol use, use of other substances can have significant effects on the developing fetus. For example, cocaine or marijuana use during pregnancy may result in premature birth, low birth weight, decreased head circumference, or miscarriage. Prenatal exposure to marijuana has been associated with difficulties in functioning of the brain. Even if there are no noticeable effects in the children at birth, the impact of prenatal substance use often can become evident later in their lives. As they get older, children who were exposed to cocaine prenatally can have difficulty focusing their attention, be more irritable, and have more behavioral problems. Difficulties surface in sorting out relevant versus irrelevant stimuli, making school participation and achievement more challenging.

The Effects of Prenatal Methamphetamine Use

Prenatal exposure to methamphetamine can cause a wide range of problems, including birth defects, fetal death, growth retardation, premature birth, low birth weight, developmental disorders, and hypersensitivity to touch in newborns. Older children who were exposed prenatally to substances may exhibit cognitive deficits, learning disabilities, and poor social adjustment.

Caseworkers should note that methamphetamine users might not be knowledgeable about the potential harm to themselves or to the fetus. Like cocaine and heroin users, methamphetamine users tend to avoid prenatal care clinics. Caseworkers also should be careful of labeling children who have been exposed prenatally to methamphetamine. For example, labeling a child as a "meth baby" can cause the child or others to have lower expectations for academic and life achievements and to ignore other causes for the physical and social problems the child may encounter.

Pregnancy as a Motivation for Treatment

Given the dangers associated with substance use during pregnancy, women who abuse substances during pregnancy should receive treatment as early as possible. Research has found that women often are more amenable to entering treatment when they are pregnant. CPS caseworkers and other professionals, therefore, should try to use the pregnancy to motivate women to change. CPS caseworkers may not have much opportunity to interact with women who have not yet given birth unless there are other children in the family who have entered the child welfare system.

Once their babies are born, significant changes can occur in the lives of women who abused alcohol or drugs during pregnancy. In the case of babies who test positive for substances at birth, the mothers may experience remorse and sadness over the actual or potential consequences of their substance use, which also can be a motivating factor to seek treatment. If CPS is involved, mothers may admit to enough drug use to explain the positive drug test, but not to an addiction, due to the fear of losing custody of their children. They may comply with treatment requirements in order to compensate for the problems their SUD may have caused their children. Nevertheless, new difficulties may begin when CPS closes the case and the pressure is off the mothers to stay clean. For instance, they may be tempted to use drugs and alcohol again.

The Impact on Childhood Development

Exposure to parental SUDs during childhood also can have dire consequences for children. Compared to children of parents who do not abuse alcohol or drugs, children of parents who do, and who also are in the child welfare system, are more likely to experience physical, intellectual, social, and emotional problems. Among the difficulties in providing services to these children is that problems affected or compounded by their parents' SUDs might not emerge until later in their lives.

The following information summarizes some of the consequences of SUDs on childhood development, including a disruption of the bonding process; emotional, academic, and developmental problems; lack of supervision; parentification; social stigma; and adolescent substance use and delinquency.

Disruption of the Bonding Process

When mothers or fathers abuse substances after delivery, their ability to bond with their child—so important during the early stages of life—may be weakened. In order for an attachment to form, it is necessary that caregivers pay attention to and notice their children's attempts to communicate. Parents who use marijuana, for example, may have difficulty picking up their babies' cues because marijuana dulls response time and alters perceptions. When parents repeatedly miss their babies' cues, the babies eventually stop providing them. The result is disengaged parents with disengaged babies. These parents and babies then have difficulty forming a healthy, appropriate relationship.

Neglected children who are unable to form secure attachments with their primary caregivers may:

- Become more mistrustful of others and may be less willing to learn from adults

- Have difficulty understanding the emotions of others, regulating their own emotions, or forming and maintaining relationships with others

- Have a limited ability to feel remorse or empathy, which may mean that they could hurt others without feeling their actions were wrong

- Demonstrate a lack of confidence or social skills that could hinder them from being successful in school, work, and relationships

- Demonstrate impaired social cognition, which is awareness of oneself in relation to others as well as of others' emotions. Impaired social cognition can lead a person to view many social interactions as stressful.

Emotional, Academic, and Developmental Problems

Children who experience either prenatal or postnatal drug exposure are at risk for a range of emotional, academic, and developmental problems. For example, they are more likely to experience symptoms of depression and anxiety, suffer from psychiatric disorders, exhibit behavior problems, score lower on school achievement tests, and demonstrate other difficulties in school.

These children may behave in ways that are challenging for biological or foster parents to manage, which can lead to inconsistent caregiving and multiple alternative care placements.

Positive social and emotional child development generally has been linked to nurturing family settings in which caregivers are predictable, daily routines are respected, and everyone recognizes clear boundaries for acceptable behaviors. Such circumstances often are missing in the homes of parents with SUDs. As a result, extra supports and interventions are needed to help children draw upon their strengths and maximize their natural potential despite their home environments. Protective factors, such as the involvement of other supportive adults (for example, extended family members, mentors, clergy, teachers, neighbors), may help mitigate the impact of parental SUDs.

Lack of Supervision

The search for drugs or alcohol, the use of scarce resources to pay for them, the time spent in illegal activities to raise money for them, or the time spent recovering from hangovers or withdrawal symptoms can leave parents with little time or energy to care properly for their children. These children frequently do not have their basic needs met and often do not receive appropriate supervision. In addition, rules about curfews and potentially dangerous activities may not be enforced or are enforced haphazardly. As a result, SUDs are often a factor in neglect cases.

Parentification

As children grow older, they may become increasingly aware that their parents cannot care for them. To compensate, the children become the caregivers of the family, often extending their caregiving behavior to their parents as well as younger siblings. This process is labeled "parentification."

Parentified children carry a great deal of anxiety and sometimes go to great lengths to control or to eliminate their parents' use of drugs or alcohol. They feel responsible for running the family. These feelings are reinforced by messages from the parents that the children cause the parents' SUDs or are at fault in some way if the family comes to the attention of authorities. Sometimes these children must contact medical personnel in the case of a parent's overdose, or they may be left supervising and caring for younger children when their parents are absent while obtaining or abusing substances.

Social Stigma

Adults with SUDS may engage in behaviors that embarrass their children and may appear disinterested in their children's activities or school performance. Children may separate themselves from their parents by not wanting to go home after school, by not bringing friends to the house, or by not asking for help with homework. These children may feel a social stigma attached to certain aspects of their parents' lives, such as unemployment, homelessness, an involvement with the criminal justice system, or SUD treatment.

Adolescent Substance Use and Delinquency

Adolescents whose parents have SUDs are more likely to develop SUDs themselves. Some adolescents mimic behaviors they see in their families, including ineffective coping behaviors such as using drugs and alcohol. Many of these children also witness or are victims of violence. It is hypothesized that substance abuse is a coping mechanism for such traumatic events. Moreover, adolescents who use substances are more likely to have poor academic performance and to be involved in criminal activities. The longer children are exposed to parental SUD, the more serious the negative consequences may be for their overall development and well-being.

Child Abuse as a Precursor to Substance Use Disorders

Many people view SUDs as a phenomenon that leads to or exacerbates the abuse or neglect of children. Research also suggests, however, that being victimized by child abuse, particularly sexual abuse, is a common precursor of SUDs. Sometimes, victims of abuse or neglect "self-medicate" (for example, drink or use drugs to escape the unresolved trauma of the maltreatment). One study found that women with a history of childhood physical or sexual abuse were nearly five times more likely to use street drugs and more than twice as likely to abuse alcohol as women who were not maltreated. In another study, childhood abuse predicted a wide range of problems, including lower self-esteem, more victimization, more depression, and chronic homelessness, and indirectly predicted drug and alcohol problems.

Chapter 37

Corporal Punishment

Chapter Contents

Section 37.1

Key Issues in the Controversy Surrounding Corporal Punishment

Excerpted from "Corporal Punishment: Key Issues," by Prue Holzer and Alister Lamont. © 2010 Commonwealth of Australia. Reprinted by permission of the Australian Institute of Family Studies, www.afis.gov.au. Although some of the information in this chapter is specific to Australia, the topics are also pertinent to people elsewhere who may be concerned about corporal punishment.

Corporal punishment is a contentious and much debated issue within the community. This text provides a brief overview of research literature on the use of corporal punishment towards children and the legal landscape regarding corporal punishment as a means of disciplining children in Australia. We examine the distinction between corporal punishment and physical abuse, and the relationship between corporal punishment and discipline. Arguments for and against changes to the law in this area are also discussed.

What is corporal punishment?

Corporal punishment is defined as the use of physical force towards a child for the purpose of control and/or correction, and as a disciplinary penalty inflicted on the body with the intention of causing some degree of pain or discomfort, however mild. Punishment of this nature is referred to in several ways, for example: hitting, smacking, spanking, and belting (Cashmore & de Haas, 1995). Although most forms of corporal punishment involve hitting children with a hand or an implement (such as a belt or wooden spoon), other forms of corporal punishment include: kicking, shaking, biting, and forcing a child to stay in uncomfortable positions (United Nations Committee on the Rights of the Child, 2006). The desired outcome of physical punishment is child compliance with adult directives (Gawlik, Henning, & Warner, 2002; Smith, Gollop, Taylor, & Marshall, 2004).

Corporal punishment or physical abuse?

The degree of physical punishment that a parent or carer can use with a child is subject to legal regulation in Australia. In most states and territories, corporal punishment by a parent or carer is lawful provided that it is carried out for the purpose of correction, control, or discipline, and that it is "reasonable" having regard to:

• the age of the child;

• the method of punishment;

• the child's capacity for reasoning (i.e., whether the child is able to comprehend correction/discipline); and

• the harm caused to the child (Bourke, 1981).

Corporal punishment that results in bruising, marking, or other injury lasting longer than a 24-hour period may be deemed to be "unreasonable" and thus classified as physical abuse. As an example, the New South Wales Crimes Act 1900 (NSW) establishes that corporal punishment is unreasonable if the force is applied to any part of the head or neck of a child or to any other part of the body of a child in such a way as to be likely to cause harm to a child that lasts for more than a short period. Corporal punishment that is unreasonable in the circumstances may lead to intervention by police and/or child protection authorities.

Are corporal punishment and discipline the same thing?

The main goal of any disciplinary strategy is to educate children about acceptable and unacceptable behavior. Corporal punishment is one disciplinary technique. However, there are many other disciplinary techniques that parents can employ, such as:

• providing appropriate supervision;

• making rules (appropriate to the child's age and stage of development);

• setting and enforcing boundaries;

• firmly saying "no";

• explaining why certain behavior is inappropriate;

• giving consequences;

- withdrawing privileges; and

- using "time out" or quiet time.

Discipline is only one part of educating children about acceptable and unacceptable behaviors. Other steps parents can take include:

- minimizing the need for discipline or punishment by planning ahead to prevent problems from occurring (e.g., avoiding grocery shopping when a toddler is tired or irritable);

- being consistent with children;

- modeling desired behaviors; and

- praising, encouraging, and rewarding children and providing them with warmth and affection (Parenting SA, 2009).

An important component in all disciplinary strategies is to maintain parental consistency. Parenting that is inconsistent can be confusing for children and lead to misbehavior. Research from the Longitudinal Study of Australian Children shows that inconsistent parenting is strongly associated with behavioral problems in children, including conduct problems, low prosocial behavior, hyperactivity, emotional difficulties and problems relating with peers (Smart, Sanson, Baxter, Edwards, & Hayes, 2008). When parents are consistent in their disciplinary strategies, children learn what to expect from their parents if they misbehave. Children are less likely to test boundaries or push limits that are firmly set when they know the consequences of poor behavior (Beltran, 2002).

Other research from the Longitudinal Study of Australian Children showed that behavioral problems were strongly linked with higher levels of parental hostility, with children being four times more likely to have conduct problems and twice as likely to have hyperactivity problems when experiencing hostile parenting (Smart et al., 2008). Evidence suggests that warmth and affection in parent-child relationships is linked with more positive outcomes for children (Smart et al., 2008). Parental warmth has been shown to increase children's self-esteem and reduce the risk of psychological and behavioral problems (Berk, 2009). In the Longitudinal Study of Australian Children, higher parental warmth was shown to reduce the risk of conduct problems, peer problems and low prosocial behavior in children 4-5 years of age (Smart et al., 2008).

For more information on discipline strategies see The Parenting Research Centre's Raising Children Network which provides helpful and practical advice about disciplining children of all ages: <http://raisingchildren.net.au/articles/discipline_introduction.html>.

What does research tell us about the use of corporal punishment towards children?

Research findings regarding the use of corporal punishment towards children point in different directions. Some reviews of the literature suggest that corporal punishment may lead to adverse child outcomes (Gershoff, 2002; Linke, 2002; Smith et al., 2004). For example, in a review of the research, Smith et al. (2004) reported a number of negative developmental consequences for children who had experienced corporal punishment, including: disruptive and anti-social behavior; poor academic achievement; poor attachment and lack of parent-child warmth; mental health problems (particularly internalizing problems such as depression); and substance and alcohol abuse.

Research has shown that corporal punishment is effective in achieving immediate child compliance. However, Gershoff (2002), Smith et al. (2004) and others have argued that the benefits associated with immediate child compliance can be offset by findings that indicate corporal punishment fails to teach a child self-control and inductive reasoning. Instead, corporal punishment teaches a child to avoid engaging in behavior that is punishable by way of force while in an adult's presence (in contrast to teaching a child not to engage in the undesirable behavior at all). In addition, Linke (2002) argued that corporal punishment teaches a child that problems can be addressed through physical aggression.

Other research suggests that the relationship between corporal punishment and adverse child outcomes is not definitive, mainly due to inconsistent definitions of corporal punishment. Baumrind, Larzelere and Cowan (2002) argued that findings such as Gershoff's may misrepresent the relationship between corporal punishment and child outcomes. They argued that the studies are often simplistic, and include in their definition of corporal punishment children who have experienced arguably more mild forms of corporal punishment such as smacking as well as children who have experienced serious physical abuse.

There is also debate in the literature regarding whether findings such as low rates of child maltreatment and child deaths can be used to illustrate the benefits of banning corporal punishment and to call for the extension of bans on all forms of corporal punishment in other jurisdictions (e.g., see Durrant (2006) and Durrant and Janson (2005) in relation to the Swedish ban on corporal punishment). Beckett (2005) argued that Sweden's low rates of child maltreatment and child deaths predate the introduction of legislation banning the use of corporal punishment, thus should not be taken as illustrative of the benefits of such legislative reform. Beckett (2005) also argued that other nations without bans on corporal punishment report lower rates of child abuse deaths than Sweden.

In brief, both Baumrind et al. (2002) and Beckett (2005) argued that we are not in a position to presuppose a clear causal link between corporal punishment (particularly parental smacking) and adverse child outcomes, and as a result, should be wary of applying the findings of correlational research to social policy decisions.

While there are no clear answers regarding the consequences of using corporal punishment as a disciplinary strategy towards children, the effects are likely to be influenced by several factors, including:

- the quality of the parent-child relationship;

- how often and how hard a child is hit;

- whether parenting is generally "hostile";

- clear boundary setting and consistency in use of discipline; and

- whether other disciplinary techniques are also used, particularly ones that are suited to a child's age, and are likely to enhance his or her learning and capacity for reasoning (Gershoff, 2002; Smart et al., 2008).

In what circumstances are children more likely to experience corporal punishment?

Research shows that children between the ages of three and five, and children who exhibit challenging behaviors and difficult temperaments are more likely than other children to be the recipients of corporal punishment (Smith et al., 2004). There are also clear gender differences, with boys more likely to experience corporal punishment than girls (Smith et al., 2004). Within the family setting, contextual factors such as family structure (e.g., number of children), economic disadvantage, and family stress increase the likelihood that parents will resort to physical punishment. In addition, Smith et al. argued that a wider social context that effectively sanctions the use of physical punishment contributes to its continuation.

The International Picture

Internationally, 23 countries have prohibited corporal punishment in all settings in legislation: Austria (1989); Bulgaria (2000); Costa Rica (2008); Croatia (1998); Cyprus (1994); Denmark (1997); Finland (1983); Germany (2000); Greece (2006); Hungary (2004); Iceland (2003); Israel (2000); Latvia (1998); Netherlands (2007); New Zealand (2007); Norway (1987); Portugal (2007); Romania (2004); Spain (2007); Sweden (1979); Ukraine (2003); Uruguay (2007); and Venezuela (2007). Corporal punishment is prohibited in Italy (1996) and Nepal (2005) by Supreme Court ruling (but not legislation) (Global Initiative to End All Corporal Punishment of Children, 2008).

Within these countries, the process of abolishing all corporal punishment typically began by legislating against the use of corporal punishment in schools. This was followed by the removal of the parental defence of "lawful correction" or "reasonable chastisement" from relevant criminal codes and finally the introduction of explicit bans on the use of corporal punishment in relevant civil codes. A number of other countries have partially abolished the use of corporal punishment in one or more settings and have expressed a commitment to enacting full prohibition (see Global Initiative to End All Corporal Punishment of Children 2008 for an overview).

Twenty-three countries have prohibited corporal punishment in all settings in legislation. Two other countries have prohibited corporal punishment by Supreme Court ruling.

Conclusion

The issue of corporal punishment is contentious. Some groups advocate for the abolition of corporal punishment arguing that it is damaging to children and a violation of children's rights. Others argue in favor of retaining the right to use corporal punishment as a form of disciplining children. While a third group—which generally takes the view that there are better or alternatives to smacking—has raised concerns that banning corporal punishment could criminalize parents and, in the process, overburden the child protection system with reports of parents who have smacked their children.

Research findings regarding the damaging effects for children of corporal punishment have been critiqued for methodological reasons. However, the research is clear that there is limited evidence to support any positive outcomes associated with corporal punishment and that there are other more preferable techniques for disciplining children.

Further Reading

For more information on the issue of corporal punishment, visit the National Child Protection Clearinghouse (http://www.aifs.gov.au/nch).

References

Baumrind, D., Larzelere, R. E., and Cowan, P. A. (2002). Ordinary physical punishment: Is it harmful? Comment of Gershoff. *Psychological Bulletin*, 128(4), 580–589.

Beckett, C. (2005). The Swedish myth: The corporal punishment ban and child death statistics. *British Journal of Social Work*, 35, 125–138.

Beltran, M. (2002). *Parenting tips: the importance of consistency*. Retrieved 6 July 2009, from <http://www.essortment.com/family/parentingtipsi_szdp.htm>.

Berk, L. E. (2009). *Child development (8th ed.)*. United States of America: Pearson Education, Inc.

Bourke, J. P. (1981). *Bourke's criminal law: Victoria*. Sydney: Butterworth's.

Cashmore, J., and de Haas, N. (1995). *Legal and social aspects of the physical punishment of children*. Canberra: Department of Human Services and Health.

Durrant, J. (2006). *Changing the landscape for children: Corporal punishment and family policy in Sweden*. Paper presented at the Australian Institute of Family Studies, Melbourne, VIC.

Durrant, J. E., and Janson, S. (2005). Law reform, corporal punishment and child abuse: The case of Sweden. *International Review of Victimology*, 12, 139–158.

Gawlik, J., Henning, T., and Warner, K. (2002). *Physical punishment of children*. Hobart, TAS: Tasmania Law Reform Institute. Retrieved 7 July 2009, from <www.law.utas.edu.au/reform/documents/PhysPunFinalReport.pdf>

Gershoff, E. T. (2002). Corporal punishment by parents and associated child behaviors and experiences: A meta-analytic and theoretical review. *Psychological Bulletin*, 124(4), 539–579.

Global Initiative to End All Corporal Punishment of Children. (2008). *Ending legalised violence against children: Global report*

2008. London, UK: Association for the Protection of All Children. Retrieved 7 July 2009, from: <http://www.endcorporalpunishment. org/pages/pdfs/reports/GlobalReport2008.pdf>.

Linke, P. (2002). Physical punishment: What does the research say? *Every Child*, 8(3), 28–29.

Milfull, C., and Schetzer, L. (2000). *Sufficient protection for Australian children's rights? Beyond the Corbett Bill: A comparative analysis of attitudes and legal responses to corporal punishment in the home*. Sydney, NSW: National Children's and Youth Law Centre.

Parenting SA. (2009). Discipline (0–12 years). *Parent Easy Guide, 2*. Retrieved 18 June 2009, from <http://www.parenting.sa.gov.au/ pegs/Peg2.pdf>

Saunders, B. J., and Goddard, C. (2003, November). *Parents' use of physical discipline: The thoughts, feelings and words of Australian children*. Paper presented at the Ninth Australasian Conference on Child Abuse and Neglect, Sydney.

Smart, D., Sanson, A., Baxter, J., Edwards, B., and Hayes, A. (2008). *Home-school transitions for financially disadvantaged children. Final Report*. Sydney: The Smith Family and Australian Institute of Family Studies. Retrieved 18 June 2009, from <http:// www.thesmithfamily.com.au/webdata/resources/files/HomeTo School_SummaryReport_WEB.pdf>

Smith, A. B., Gollop, M. M., Taylor, N. J., and Marshall, K. A. (2004). *The discipline and guidance of children: A summary of research*. Dunedin, NZ: Children's Issues Centre, University of Otago and the Office of the Children's Commissioner.

Tucci, J., Saunders, B., and Goddard, C. (2002). *Please don't hit me! Community attitudes towards the physical punishment of children* (No. 0958536376). Ringwood: Australians Against Child Abuse

United Nations Committee on the Rights of the Child. (2006). *Convention on the Rights of the Child. General comment no. 8*. Geneva: General Assembly of the United Nations. Retrieved 1 February 2009, from <http://tinyurl.com/yaqch69>.

Section 37.2

Disciplining Your Child

"Discipline for Young Children Lesson 2: Discipline and Punishment: What is the Difference?" by Valya Telep, Former Extension Specialist, Child Development, Virginia State University. © 2009 Virginia Cooperative Extension, a program of Virginia Tech and Virginia State University. Reprinted with permission.

Effective discipline helps children learn to control their behavior so that they act according to their ideas of what is right and wrong, not because they fear punishment. For example, they are honest because they think it is wrong to be dishonest, not because they are afraid of getting caught.

The purpose of punishment is to stop a child from doing what you don't want—and using a painful or unpleasant method to stop him.

There are basically four kinds of punishment:

- **Physical punishment:** Slapping, spanking, switching, paddling, and using a belt or hair brush.

- **Verbal punishment:** Shaming, ridiculing, using cruel words, saying "I don't love you."

- **Withholding rewards:** "You can't watch TV if you don't do your homework."

- **Penalties:** "You broke the window so you will have to pay for it with money from your allowance."

The first two kinds of punishment, physical and verbal, are not considered to be effective discipline methods. The other two, withholding rewards and giving penalties, can be used either as effective discipline methods or as punishment—depending on how parents administer them.

Mild or Harsh?

It is important to look at the way parents administer physical punishments.

A swat on the bottom is a mild physical punishment. While it may do no permanent physical harm, it does not help the child develop a conscience. Instead, it teaches him that physical violence is an acceptable way of dealing with problems. Parents should avoid physical punishment. If they find themselves using it, then something is wrong and their method of discipline is not working. They may as well admit that spanking is more effective in relieving the parents' frustration than in teaching the child self-control. More effective methods are needed.

Harsh physical punishment and verbal abuse can never be justified as ways to discipline children. Parents usually spank when they are angry; a parent may not realize how hard he is striking the child. Verbal abuse hurts the child's self-concept.

Why Punishment Doesn't Work

Physical punishment usually doesn't work for several reasons. First, it makes the child hate himself and others. Physical punishment makes the child think that there must be something awfully wrong with him to be treated so badly. If children think they are "bad," then they will act "bad." A vicious cycle is formed. The child who has been treated harshly has no reason to be good. Or he may be good just to keep from being punished and not learn to be good because he thinks it is the right thing to do.

Children who have been spanked feel that they have paid for their misbehavior and are free to misbehave again. In other words, spanking frees the child from feelings of remorse which are needed to prevent future misbehavior.

Parents who use physical punishment are setting an example of using violence to settle problems or solve conflicts. Children imitate their parents' behavior. When parents use physical punishment, children are more likely to use violent acts to settle their conflicts with others.

Another disadvantage of using physical punishment is that parents have to find other discipline methods when the child becomes as tall and as strong as the parent! Why not start using effective discipline methods when the child is young?

Where reward and punishment focus on the child, encouragement and reality discipline target the act. Reward and punishment teaches the child to be "good" as long as we are looking.

When rewards are our chief way of motivating children we run the risk of creating "carrot seekers": children who are always looking for and expecting a reward every time they do something good or right. If we give a child money for making his bed this week, he'll wonder where his money is next week. Instead of being self-motivated by a desire to cooperate or help other family members, we have taught the child to look to us for his source of motivation.

Effective Discipline

- Helps the child learn self-control
- Can be used with teenagers
- Builds the child's self-esteem
- Sets a good example of effective ways to solve problems

Harsh Punishment

- Teaches the child to deceive parents
- Won't work with teenagers
- Tears down self-esteem
- Teaches the child that violence is an acceptable way to solve problems.

Why Do Parents Spank?

Parents who spank their children rather than using other discipline methods usually say:

- "Nothing else works."
- "You've got to let kids know who is boss."
- "They asked for it."
- "It clears the air."
- "I was spanked and I turned out OK."

Reasons for spanking which parents seldom give are:

- They are mad at their husband or wife and take it out on the child.
- They are angry and don't stop to think of better ways to discipline.
- They don't know how to discipline more effectively.
- It relieves their feelings of frustration.
- It is easier, quicker, and requires less thinking than other discipline methods.

Some parents spank because they place a high value on obedience. Their whole aim is for the child to "mind," to do what he is told without question. There are times when a child needs to obey instantly, such as when he starts to run out in the street without looking.

When obedience is the parent's main objective, however, the child becomes passive and loses his zest for life.

The question of spanking is an emotional issue which parents feel very strongly about. They can be divided into one of three groups. They think either:

- "Spare the rod and spoil the child."

- "I can't imagine anyone laying a hand on a poor defenseless child."

- "Other kinds of discipline are more effective."

Parents who spank ask, "What's wrong with it?" It isn't a question of right or wrong, but of what is best for the child.

Perhaps parents who spank frequently should ask themselves:

- Why do I use spanking as the only way to discipline my child?

- Does spanking work?

- How did I feel when I was spanked as a child? Did it make me stop doing what I was spanked for, or Did I sneak around and try not to get caught doing it?

Often, attitudes toward physical punishment reflect religious beliefs and ideas about what children are like. Child development educators believe that the child is born neither good nor bad; they have the possibility of becoming good or bad according to how they are treated, the kind of experiences they have, and their reaction to their environment. Since these educators believe that children are not naturally bad, they think children need to be disciplined in ways which help them learn to do what is "right" rather than be punished.

Harsh discipline focuses anger on the parent. Effective discipline allows children to "hurt from the inside out" and focus on their actions.

Using Consequences as a Form of Discipline

Letting children experience the consequences of their decisions is a "hassle-free" way to discipline young people. Children learn from experiences, just like adults. We call it learning the "hard way." The child learns that every act has a consequence for which he is responsible.

Parents can declare that the consequence of not coming to the dinner table in time to eat is that the child does not eat his dinner that evening. Hunger is a natural consequence of not eating. If the child complains, mother can say, "I'm sorry you feel hungry now. It's too bad, but you'll have to wait for breakfast." The child who experiences the unpleasant consequences of his behavior will be less likely to act that way again.

Parents should tell the child, before it happens, what the consequences are for breaking a rule. If the child knows that the consequence of not getting to the dinner table in time to eat with the family is not eating, then he has a choice. He can choose to get home in time to eat, or he can choose to be late and not eat. He must understand that he has a choice and that he must accept the consequences of that choice.

The child also needs to know the reason for the consequence; for example, it is extra work to keep food warm and inconsiderate of other family members.

It is important, too, that parents be willing to accept the child's decision; that is, they must be willing to allow the child to go without dinner if he chooses to miss the meal. A general rule of thumb is: always give a couple of choices, provided they are choices the parent can live with.

Natural Consequences

Natural consequences allow children to learn from the natural order of the world. For example, if the child doesn't eat, he will get hungry. If he doesn't do his homework, he will get a low grade. The parent allows unpleasant but natural consequences to happen when a child does not act in a desirable way.

Logical Consequences

Logical consequences are arranged by parents. The consequence must logically follow the child's behavior. For example, not having clean clothes to wear is a logical consequence of not placing dirty clothes in the hamper.

Consequences Teach Responsibility

Kristin left her dirty clothes on the floor and never placed them in the dirty clothes bag as mother requested. Nagging, scolding, and threatening did no good. Kristin continued to leave her dirty clothes on the floor.

Mother decided to use logical consequences. She told Kristin, in a firm and friendly voice, that in the future she would wash only clothes that were placed in the bag. After five days, Kristin had no clean clothes to wear to school and she was very unhappy to have to wear dirty, rumpled clothes. After that, Kristin remembered to place her clothes in the bag.

Kristin's mother gave her the responsibility for placing her clothes in the proper place to be washed. If mother had relented and washed Kristin's clothes when she had not placed them in the bag, she would have deprived her of an opportunity to learn to take responsibility for herself. If parents protect children from the consequences of their behavior, they will not change their behavior.

Some parents would not be willing for their child to go to school in dirty, rumpled clothes. Only they can decide if they want to offer the child that particular consequence.

Using consequences can help a child develop a sense of accountability. It leads to warmer relationships between parents and children and to fewer conflicts. The situation itself provides the lesson to the child.

Natural Consequences Cannot Be Used in All Situations

Parents cannot use natural consequences if the health or safety of the child is involved. If a young child runs into the street without looking, it is not possible to wait until he is hit by a car—a natural consequence—to teach him not to run into the street. Instead, he should be taken into the house and told, "Since you ran into the street without looking, you cannot play outside now. You can come out when you decide to look before going into the street."

This is a logical consequence. Because running into the street can harm the child, he cannot play outside until he learns to play safely in the yard. He has a choice; he can stay out of the street or he can go inside.

He is given responsibility for his behavior and any consequences he experiences (going inside) are the result of his own behavior. You can begin giving choices as soon as the child can experience the consequence of his behavior. For example, a very young child who plays with his food instead of eating can be lovingly removed from his highchair and told, "All done!" It won't take long before he sees he has a choice: he can be up in the highchair eating and getting positive attention from the parent; or he can be hungry on the floor.

Consequences Are Learning Experiences

The purpose of using consequences is to help the child learn to make decisions and to be responsible for his own behavior. Consequences are learning experiences, not punishment. For example, if father yells angrily at his child, "Put up your toys or you can't watch TV," he is not encouraging the child to make a responsible decision. However, if he says calmly and in a friendly voice, "Stuart, feel free to watch TV as soon as your toys are picked up," he allows Stuart to make a choice. The secret of using consequences effectively is to stay calm and detached. Allow the consequences to be the "bad guy"—not you!

Parents cannot apply consequences if they are angry. They cannot conceal their anger from the child—their voices will give them away. Try to view the situation objectively—as though the child were a neighbor's child and not your own—and administer the consequences in a firm and kindly manner. Remember that giving a child a choice and allowing him to experience the consequences is one of the best ways that children learn.

Consequences work when the child is trying to get the parent's attention by misbehaving and when children fight, dawdle, and fail to do their chores. Consequences can be used to get children to school on time, to meals on time, and to take responsibility for homework. The child learns that if he doesn't pick up his toys, he can't go out and play; if he doesn't wash his hands before meals, he won't be served any food; and if he fights with his brother while in the car, the car will be stopped until calm resumes.

Using Consequences Takes Practice

It is not easy to use consequences as a way to discipline children. It is hard work to think of consequences that really are logical. And it requires lots of patience! Sometimes it takes several weeks to get results.

Parents are so used to telling children what to do that it is very difficult to sit back and let the child experience the consequences of his actions. The effort is well worth it, however, because you are sending a powerful message to the child that says, "you are capable of thinking for yourself."

Discipline vs. Punishment

The differences between consequences and punishment are:

- **Consequences:** Calm tone of voice; friendly but firm attitude; willing to accept the child's decision

- **Punishment:** Angry tone of voice; hostile attitude; unwilling to give a choice

To discipline effectively, think about these ideas:

1. Effective discipline methods work better than punishment in teaching children how to behave.

2. The more parents use effective discipline methods, the less children need punishment.

3. There is no excuse for using physical or verbal punishment to discipline a child.

4. Using consequences as a discipline method helps children learn to take responsibility for their behavior.

5. Consequences must be logically related to the misbehavior.

6. The child must see the relationship between his misbehavior and the consequences or it will not work.

7. The child must know he has a choice when consequences are used.

8. Use consequences in a firm, kind, friendly manner.

Chapter 38

Improving Parenting Skills

Chapter Contents

Section 38.1

Parenting Tips

From "Tips for Being a Nurturing Parent," U.S. Department
of Health and Human Services (http://www.childwelfare.gov), 2006.
Reviewed by David A. Cooke, MD, FACP, January 2013.

A healthy, nurturing relationship with your child is built through countless interactions over the course of time. It requires a lot of energy and work, but the rewards are well worth it. When it comes to parenting, there are few absolutes (one, of course, being that every child needs to be loved) and there is no one "right way." Different parenting techniques work for different children under different circumstances. These tips provide suggestions as you discover what works best in your family. Do not expect to be perfect; parenting is a difficult job.

Help Your Children Feel Loved and Secure

We can all take steps to strengthen our relationships with our children. Here are some examples:

- Make sure your children know you love them, even when they do something wrong.

- Encourage your children. Praise their achievements and talents. Recognize the skills they are developing.

- Spend time with your children. Do things together that you both enjoy. Listen to your children.

- Learn how to use nonphysical options for discipline. Many alternatives exist. Depending on your child's age and level of development, these may include simply redirecting your child's attention, offering choices, or using "time out."

Realize that Community Resources Add Value

Children need direct and continuing access to people with whom they can develop healthy, supportive relationships. To assist this, parents may take steps such as these:

- Take children to libraries, museums, movies, and sporting events.

- Enroll children in youth enrichment programs, such as sports or music.

- Use community services for family needs, such as parent education classes or respite care.

- Communicate regularly with childcare or school staff.

- Participate in religious or youth groups.

Seek Help If You Need It

Being a parent is difficult. No one expects you to know how to do it all. Challenges such as unemployment or a child with special needs can add to family tension. If you think stress may be affecting the way you treat your child, or if you just want the extra support that most parents need at some point, try the following:

- **Talk to someone:** Tell a friend, healthcare provider, or a leader in your faith community about what you are experiencing. Or, join a support group for parents.

- **Seek respite care when you need a break:** Everyone needs time for themselves. Respite care or crisis care provides a safe place for your children so you can take care of yourself.

- **Call a helpline:** Most states have helplines for parents. Childhelp USA offers a national 24-hour hotline (800-4-A-CHILD) for parents who need help or parenting advice.

- **Seek counseling:** Individual, couple, or family counseling can identify and reinforce healthy ways to communicate and parent.

- **Take a parenting class:** No one is born knowing how to be a good parent. It is an acquired skill. Parenting classes can give you the skills you need to raise a happy, healthy child.

- **Accept help:** You do not have to do it all. Accept offers of help from trusted family, friends, and neighbors. Do not be afraid to ask for help if you feel that you need it.

Section 38.2

Coping with Infant Crying

"What is the Period of Purple Crying?" by Marilyn Barr, Founder and Executive Director, National Center on Shaken Baby Syndrome. © National Center on Shaken Baby Syndrome, 2007, updated 2012. Reprinted with permission. For additional information, visit www.purplecrying.info or www.dontshake.org.

What Is the Period of PURPLE Crying?

The *Period of PURPLE Crying* is the phrase used to describe the time in a baby's life when they cry more than any other time. This period of increased crying is often described as colic, but there have been many misunderstandings about what "colic" really is.

The Period of PURPLE Crying is a new way to help parents understand this time in their baby's life, which is a normal part of every infant's development. It is confusing and concerning to be told your baby "has colic" because it sounds like it is an illness or a condition that is abnormal. When the baby is given medication to treat symptoms of colic, it reinforces the idea that there is something wrong with the baby, when in fact, the baby is going through a very normal developmental phase. That is why we prefer to refer to this time as the Period of PURPLE Crying. This is not because the baby turns purple while crying. The acronym is a meaningful and memorable way to describe what parents and their babies are going through.

The Period of PURPLE Crying begins at about two weeks of age and continues until about 3–4 months of age. There are other common characteristics of this phase, or period, which are better described by the acronym PURPLE. All babies go through this period. It is during this time that some babies can cry a lot and some far less, but they all go through it.

Scientists decided to look at different animal species to see if they go through this developmental stage. So far, all breast feeding animals tested do have a similar developmental stage of crying more in the first months of life as human babies do. Scientists, including developmental pediatricians, have conducted studies worldwide on early infant crying over the course of many decades.

There are other characteristics of this stage. For example, studies have shown that the crying tends to be much more common in the late afternoon and evening, just when parents are getting home from work and are the most tired. Parents try many ways to keep the baby from crying. Some of them work, some work temporarily, and some don't work at all. "I take my baby in the car and drive around the block in my PJ's," said one mom. "That worked for three nights, but on the fourth he would not stop crying. I tried several other things like warm baths, singing, swaying, and nothing worked. Then all of a sudden he would just stop, for no apparent reason. His crying was so unpredictable," she said.

When these babies are going through this period they seem to resist soothing. Nothing helps. Even though certain soothing methods may help when they are simply fussy or crying, bouts of inconsolable crying are different. Nothing seems to soothe them.

During this phase of a baby's life they can cry for hours and still be healthy and normal. Parents often think there must be something wrong or they would not be crying like this. However, even after a check-up from the doctor which shows the baby is healthy they still go home and cry for hours, night after night. "It was so discouraging," said one dad. "Our baby giggles and seems fine during the day and almost like clockwork, he starts crying around six pm. He is growing and healthy, so why does he cry like this?"

Often parents say their baby looks like he or she is in pain. They think they must be, or why would they cry so much. Babies who are going through this period can act like they are in pain even when they are not.

In my own case, I know my son was not sick. He was in the top percentile for growth, he giggled and was happy other times. Then he would start to cry, and cry, and cry. The doctor kept telling me he is just fine.

After learning all of this, we decided we needed to share this information with other parents. We had to take this information and put it into a statement that told the story about this phase in a baby's life. Dr. Ronald Barr, a developmental pediatrician who has likely done more studies on infant crying than anyone in the world, came up with the phrase the Period of PURPLE Crying. His idea was to explain this phase to parents of new babies so they would know it was normal and they would be encouraged that it would come to an end.

The acronym PURPLE is used to describe specific characteristics of an infant's crying during this phase and let parents and caregivers know that what they are experiencing is indeed normal and, although frustrating, is simply a phase in their child's development that will pass. The word *Period* is important because it tells parents that it is only temporary and will come to an end.

The letters in PURPLE stand for:

- **P**eak of crying: Your baby may cry more each week. The most at two months, then less at 3–5 months.

- **U**nexpected: Crying can come and go and you don't know why.

- **R**esists soothing: Your baby may not stop crying no matter what you try.

- **P**ain-like face: A crying baby may look like they are in pain, even when they are not.

- **L**ong lasting: Crying can last as much as five hours a day, or more.

- **E**vening: Your baby may cry more in the late afternoon and evening.

Parents, after learning about Period of PURPLE Crying have said, "Finally they have called it something that describes what we are going through. This word colic was hard to get a handle on."

Section 38.3

Parental Support Groups

Parents Need Support, Too

Parenting is a fun, exciting, rewarding, busy, and stressful job. Family life these days means being on the go and trying to do it all without enough time or enough support. If you are a parent who is feeling overwhelmed, remember that you are not alone. There are many ways to manage your stress before it becomes overwhelming. Most importantly, don't be afraid to reach out and ask for help.

Common Needs for Parents

- The need to vent
- The need to feel validated
- The need to learn
- The need to socialize
- The need to believe there is hope

When to Reach Out for Support

- Too many demands are causing you stress.
- You are frustrated because your children don't listen to you.
- You feel as though your children misbehave on purpose.
- You find yourself yelling at your children or saying hurtful things.
- You feel that your children rarely do what you expect them to do.
- You feel as though you take your frustrations out on your children.
- You feel overwhelmed and see no way out.

Tips for Dealing with Stress

- Make sure your kids are safe and then give yourself a timeout. Five minutes alone can give you time to calm down and regroup.

- Set realistic goals. Don't try to be a super-parent.

- Sometimes it's ok to take the phone off the hook, put aside the mail, use paper plates, or get pizza for dinner.

- Give yourself credit for doing a good job and try not to compare yourself to other parents. However, do share and compare your experiences with other parents because you may learn something new that works.

- Ask for help. Share your feelings with a friend, family member, or professional. Get a babysitter or ask a trusted friend or family member to watch your kids and do something for yourself.

- Take care of yourself. Get plenty of exercise, rest, and nourishment and HALT if you are Hungry, Angry, Lonely, or Tired.

If You Are the Parent of

- **A newborn:** Nap time for baby means nap time for you. Leave the housework alone. Getting the sleep you need is more important. If your baby just won't stop crying and you feel yourself becoming very frustrated, leave him safely in the crib on his back for several minutes while you leave the room to cool down.

- **A toddler:** Childproof your home so you can enjoy your baby's exploring rather than dread it. Get a babysitter to give yourself a break.

- **A preschooler:** Enroll your child in a preschool program a few days a week to give yourself a break. Check out One Tough Job's information (http://www.onetoughjob.org/) on preschoolers to enjoy the time you spend with your preschooler and make it go smooth and tantrum-free.

- **A 6–10 year old:** Find other parents you can talk to on a regular basis at activities or parent groups. Don't overwhelm yourself and your child with activities.

- **A pre-teen or teen:** You are not the meanest parent. Check out the rules with other parents and remember that this phase will pass. Enjoy your child while he/she is still a child.

Tips for Meeting Other Parents

- Get involved with child-centered activities (Boy/Girl Scouts).

- Introduce yourself to other parents at your child's school or after school activity, at the library, in your neighborhood, or at your work.

- Attend Parent Teacher Association (PTA) meetings at your child's school.

- Volunteer in your child's classroom, even just by chaperoning a field trip, at the library or other community organization, or by coaching your child's sports team or leading a youth group at your church.

- Organize a social gathering for your neighborhood or join a mothers' group or playgroup.

- Ask neighbors or parents of your child's friends for help and reciprocate with giving rides and watching each other's children.

Tips for Finding a Parent Group

- Contact a number of groups to find the one that's right for you.

- If an organization doesn't have a group that fits your needs, ask to be referred to other organizations.

- Check the phone book and internet for possible groups.

- Check places such as hospitals, health centers, childbirth education organizations, churches/synagogues, public libraries, college or university education departments, parenting newspapers or magazines, and community organizations (YMCA, YWCA, United Way).

- If you can't find a group that suits you, consider starting your own.

Tips for Starting a Support Group

There are plenty of other parents who need support. The best way to find them is to start locally. Post signs in your child's school, in a religious organization, or at the public library. Even if you can only find one other interested parent, have a meeting to talk about what each of you need and hope to get out of the group. Define the group's

521

goals, decide on a meeting place, time, and frequency, and talk about whether you want to set a size limit or other criteria for joining (such as the age of your children, just dads, etc).

Other Resources for Parent Support

- **Parents Anonymous** (http://www.parentsanonymous.org/paIndex10.html): Nationwide program that offers parents support through parent support groups and children's programs free of charge.

- **Circle of Parents** (www.circleofparents.org): Nationwide program that offers support to parents and caregivers on raising children through free, weekly support groups.

Chapter 39

Foster Care and Adoption

Chapter Contents

Section 39.1

Information for Foster Parents Considering Adoption

From: Child Welfare Information Gateway. (2012). Foster parents considering adoption. Washington, DC: U.S. Department of Health and Human Services, Children's Bureau. February 2012. The complete text of this document is available online from the Child Welfare Information Gateway at http://www.childwelfare.gov/pubs/f_fospar.cfm.

If you're a foster parent and considering adopting a child, children, or youth currently in your care, you're not alone. In fact, foster parent adoptions account for more than half the adoptions of children from foster care. According to the national Adoption and Foster Care Analysis and Reporting System (AFCARS), in fiscal year 2010, 53 percent of children adopted from foster care were adopted by their foster parents.

Foster parents who open their hearts and homes to a child in need may develop relationships as strong as those with their birth children. Adoption of children and youth by foster parents is increasingly common, and deciding whether adoption is right for you and your family can raise a lot of questions. This section is written for foster parents, like you, considering adopting a child or children in their care.

While this text does not address the specifics of how to adopt, it provides information on the differences between foster care and adoption, and it explores some of the factors you should consider before deciding to adopt.

Differences between Foster Parenting and Adopting

There are significant differences between being a foster parent and an adoptive parent.

Legal Differences

- Foster care is intended to be temporary care for children and youth unable to live with their parents because of neglect, abuse,

524

parent incarceration, or other issues. However, when reunification with birth parents or adoption by another relative isn't possible, foster parent adoption becomes a viable option. Adoption is a lifetime legal and emotional responsibility.

- Foster parents have no legal parental rights, but when you adopt, you acquire the same legal rights and responsibilities for your adopted child as parents have for their birth children. The child is no longer in the state's custody but is a full, legal member of your family.

Financial Differences

- As a foster parent, you receive a stipend or reimbursement for the care you provide. With adoption, that assistance changes.

- One of the misconceptions about adoption is that it's expensive. In reality, foster care adoption is very affordable. You aren't expected to carry the financial load alone. In many instances, federal and state assistance programs are available during and after the adoption process. Of children adopted from foster care in 2010, 90 percent received some form of adoption assistance.

- Most children and youth in foster care are covered by the federal Medicaid program. Your child also may be eligible for medical assistance from your state after adoption.

- Even if families receive adoption assistance or a subsidy, adoptive families are still responsible for everyday financial obligations such as child care and extracurricular activities.

Full Decision-Making Responsibility

- While a child is in foster care, decision-making is shared by the agency, foster parents, and perhaps the birth parents.

- When a child is adopted, the adoptive parents take full responsibility for making decisions about issues such as school enrollment, travel outside the state or country, birth family visitation, and more. While some families may choose to continue to share some decision-making and visitation with the birth family or relatives to benefit the child, the adoptive family has the ultimate decision-making responsibility after the adoption.

Attachment Issues

You likely dealt with, and perhaps continue to deal with, attachment issues after your child or youth joined your family through foster care. Attachment is formed through more than just providing food, shelter, and clothing; it's formed through consistent and predictable interaction— smiles, hugs, conversation, etc.—and it plays an important role in physical, emotional, mental, and psychological development. However, addressing attachment issues isn't a linear process. There may be new or recurring issues as your foster child or youth becomes a permanent member of your family. These may include the following:

- The idea of permanence with a foster/adoptive family and the termination of the birth parents' parental rights may trigger intense grief or a sense of loss.

- Bonds with caregivers, even abusive caregivers, are extremely strong. Additionally, past abuse or neglect may be difficult to detect as children in a temporary environment may not have felt comfortable enough to confide in others.

- Children or youth may experience conflicting feelings between love for the biological family and growing affection for and a sense of security with their foster/adoptive parents.

- Sometimes, children or youth struggle to fully commit to adoption unless they know their birth families are all right and that being adopted is acceptable. Connections and contact between foster/adoptive parents and birth parents can sometimes ease the transition.

- If your child is a regular user of social media, you may want to explore positive ways to use Facebook and other sites to maintain healthy contact between your child and his or her birth family members. Although statistics are not yet available to document the number of adopted people and birth parents who find each other through these sites, anecdotal evidence suggests that it is a growing trend.

Data on Foster Parent Adoption

- Approximately 408,000 children are in foster care in the United States, and it's estimated that 107,000 are eligible for adoption.

- In fiscal year 2010, about 53,000 children were adopted from foster care. Of those children 53 percent were adopted by foster parents, 32 percent were adopted by other relatives, and 15 percent were adopted by nonrelatives.

- Of the parents who adopt from foster care, 67 percent are married couples and 28 percent are single-parent families.

- Of the children in foster care 43 percent are white, 25 percent are African-American, and 21 percent are Hispanic.

Advantages of Foster Parent Adoption

Compared to other kinds of adoption, foster parent adoption offers the advantage of familiarity to the adopting family, the child, and the birth family. You can build on existing relationships because you may already be familiar with the child's personality, family and medical history, education plan, and other important aspects of his or her life.

Additionally, foster parents usually know about a child's background and experiences and know what behaviors to expect. If the foster parents have sufficient background information on the child, as well as some knowledge about child development and behavior, they are better able to understand and respond to the child's needs in a positive and appropriate way.

Foster parents usually have fewer fantasies and fears about the child's birth family because they often have met and know them as real people with real strengths and problems. They may have previously partnered with the birth family to work for the child's return.

Foster parents have a better understanding of their role and relationship with the agency—and hopefully a good relationship with their caseworker.

Some foster parents participate in concurrent planning in which adoption may be one of the goals. If so, some of the necessary steps toward adoption may have already been taken.

While children and youth benefit the most from foster parent adoption, this type of adoption offers a number of advantages for others as well.

- **Adoptive parents:** One of the biggest advantages of adopting your foster child or youth is seeing your child achieve permanency and complete the placement process. Foster children and youth don't always stay with one family and can't always be reunited with birth families. When you adopt your foster child, children, or youth, you and the child are granted the permanent protection of your relationship, and you both have a new, permanent family relationship—in every sense of the word.

- **Children:** Even very young infants may grieve the loss of familiar sights, sounds, smells, and touch of a family when they must move. Being adopted by foster parents means the child or youth won't have to leave familiar foster family members, friends, pets, school, and home. The biggest change for the child is the security that comes with having a permanent family and home.

- **Birth families:** Foster parent adoption also benefits birth families, including siblings and other relatives, by allowing them to know who is permanently caring for their loved one. Depending on the openness of the adoption, birth families may have ongoing contact with the child or youth and opportunities to maintain relationships and share family histories.

- **Society:** Society as a whole benefits when permanence is attained in lieu of youth aging out of foster care. Many youth transition out of foster care with few connections and little access to support, increasing the risk of negative outcomes such as jail, homelessness, substance abuse, and teen pregnancy. Research also shows that unemployment and underemployment are two common experiences among former foster youth. For instance, a study of employment by youth who aged out of foster care, youth with a history of foster care who were reunited with their parents, and youth from low-income families found that those who aged out of foster care earned less money than their peers in both the other groups, their earnings well below the poverty line. Additionally, less than two percent of former foster youth obtain a bachelor's degree compared to more than 22 percent of all young people.

What Is Concurrent Planning, and How Does It Benefit a Child?

Concurrent planning is a process of developing one permanency goal, usually reunification, while simultaneously working toward other outcomes—adoption or placement with a legal guardian (often a relative)—in order to move children and youth more quickly from out-of-home care to a permanent family. Essentially, concurrent planning is a plan with several alternative options.

The goals of concurrent planning are to promote safety of children and youth, achieve timely permanence, reduce the number of moves for children and youth, and allow for continued growth of significant relationships.

As of 2009, 42 states and the District of Columbia have statutes that address the issue of concurrent planning with language that ranges from general authorization to providing elements that must be included when developing a concurrent plan.

More information on concurrent planning can be found on Information Gateway's website: http://www.childwelfare.gov/systemwide/lawspolicies/statutes/concurrent.cfm

What Is an Open Adoption?

Open adoption, in which some kind of contact is maintained between the adoptive and birth families, may help the child adjust to being adopted. Maintaining contact with the child's relatives may help a child understand the realities of the birth family's situation and ease his or her worries about them. By acknowledging the importance of that relationship, foster/adoptive parents build the child's self-respect and help the child open up about past experiences and start to heal old wounds.

For more information about open adoption, visit the Information Gateway website: http://www.childwelfare.gov/adoption/adoptive/contacts.cfm

Strategies for Foster/Adoptive Families

What are some approaches or strategies that may contribute to a successful adoption experience? All families and children are different, but there are some things you can do to smooth the adoption process.

What the Research Shows

A 2007 report from AdoptUSKids explored characteristics of successful adoptions and barriers to adoption of children with special needs by surveying and interviewing adoptive parents, prospective adoptive parents, and adoption professionals. For the purposes of that study, the "special needs" designation referred to children who were over age eight, members of sibling groups, had specific ethnic or racial backgrounds, or children for whom agencies had difficulties finding adoptive families.

States have different definitions of "special needs." To find out about your state, read Child Welfare Information Gateway's *"Special Needs" Adoption: What Does It Mean?* at http://www.childwelfare.gov/pubs/factsheets/specialneeds

To identify characteristics of successful adoptions, 161 parents who had adopted 1–14 years earlier reported on their experiences. Parents volunteered the following factors as contributing to a successful adoption:

- They were committed to the child and the child's adoption into the family.

- They were able to fully integrate the child into the family and not treat the child differently.

- They developed and practiced good parenting skills, including patience, consistency, and flexibility.

- They sought out resources, information, and training when they needed help.

- They had a network of social support.

- They had realistic expectations of the child.

These adoptive parents also reported on postadoption services and supports. The most common were financial support, such as adoption subsidies and financial help with medical and dental care. The majority of families also noted that services such as counseling, therapy for the child or family, support groups, and training were helpful.

Conclusion

It's important to learn as much as possible about the child you want to adopt and the adoption process. Ask your caseworker or agency about resources and trainings, and make sure you are connected with other families and supports.

All children deserve loving, permanent homes. Making your family the permanent family for a child, children, or youth currently in your care is a lifetime commitment that requires careful consideration but yields a host of advantages.

Resources

Child Welfare Information Gateway offers the following resources:

- The National Foster Care and Adoption Directory, including lists of foster and adoptive support groups in each state: http://www.childwelfare.gov/nfcad

- Information on adoption assistance by state: http://www.childwelfare.gov/adoption/adopt_assistance

- Information on adoption costs: http://www.childwelfare.gov/ adoption/adoptive/expenses.cfm

- *Selecting and Working with an Adoption Therapist*, with additional information on attachment: http://www.childwelfare.gov/ pubs/f_therapist.cfm

- Information on attachment and attachment disorders: http:// www.childwelfare.gov/can/impact/development/attachment.cfm

- Adopting Children through a Public Agency (Foster Care): http:// www.childwelfare.gov/adoption/adoptive/foster_care.cfm

- After Adoption from Foster Care: http://www.childwelfare.gov/ adoption/adopt_parenting/foster

More information on the federal adoption tax credit can be found on the North American Council on Adoptable Children website: http:// www.nacac.org/taxcredit/taxcredit.html

Information on the benefits of foster care adoption can be found on the National Council for Adoption's website: https:// www.adoptioncouncil.org/images/stories/NCFA_ADOPTION_ ADVOCATE_NO35.pdf

A webinar on bridging the gap between foster and birth parents can be found on the National Resource Center for Permanency and Family Connections website: http://www.nrcpfc.org/webcasts/18.html

References

Association for Treatment and Training in the Attachment of Children. (n.d.). *What is attachment?* Retrieved from http://www .attach.org/whatisattachment.htm

Dave Thomas Foundation for Adoption. (n.d.). *Adoption costs information*. Retrieved from http://davethomasfoundation.org/ about-foster-care-adoption/myths-and-misconceptions

Fernandes, A. (2008). *Youth transitioning from foster care: Background, Federal programs, and issues for Congress*. Retrieved from the FosteringConnections website: http://www.fostering connections.org/tools/assets/files/CRS-older-youth-report.pdf

Kirk, R., and Day, A. (2010). Increasing college access for youth aging out of foster care: Evaluation of a summer camp program for foster youth transitioning from high school to college. *Children and Youth Services Review*, 33(7), 1173–1174.

McRoy, R. G. (2007). *Barriers and success factors in adoption from foster care: Perspectives of families and staff.* Retrieved from the AdoptUSKids website: http://adoptuskids.org/_assets/files/NRCRRFAP/resources/barriers-and-success-factors-family-and-staff-perspectives.pdf

Naccarato, T., Brophy, M., and Courtney, M. (2009). Employment outcomes of foster youth: The results from the Midwest evaluation of the adult functioning of foster youth. *Children and Youth Services Review*, 32(4), 551–559.

National Resource Center for Permanency and Family Connections. (n.d.). *Web-based concurrent planning toolkit.* Retrieved from http://www.nrcpfc.org/cpt/overview.htm

National Foster Parent Association and Baldino, R. (2009). *Success as a foster parent: Everything you need to know about foster care.* New York, NY: Penguin Group.

Riggs, D. (2007). *Facilitated openness can benefit children adopted from care.* Retrieved from the North American Council on Adoptable Children website: http://www.nacac.org/adoptalk/facilitated_openness.html

Sullivan, R., and Lasley, E. (2010). *Fear in love: Attachment, abuse, and the developing brain.* Retrieved from the Dana Foundation website: http://dana.org/news/cerebrum/detail.aspx?id=28926

U.S. Department of Health and Human Services. (2011). *The AF-CARS report: Preliminary FY 2010 estimates as of June 2011 (18).* Retrieved from http://www.acf.hhs.gov/programs/cb/stats_research/afcars/tar/report18.htm

Section 39.2

Helping Foster Children Transition into Adoption

From: Child Welfare Information Gateway. (2012). *Helping your foster child transition to your adopted child*. Washington, DC: U.S. Department of Health and Human Services, Children's Bureau, February 2012. The complete text of this document is available online from the Child Welfare Information Gateway at http://www.childwelfare.gov/pubs/f_transition.cfm

If you're a foster parent adopting a child, children, or youth currently in your care, you'll need to help your child make the emotional adjustment to being an adopted child. While you may appreciate the difference in the child's role within your family, children and youth may not clearly comprehend the difference between being a foster child versus being an adopted child in the same family. There are specific steps you can take to help children understand these changes.

This information was written for foster/adoptive parents, like you, who are helping their child transition from foster care to adoption.

Talking with Children about the Changes

The adoption adjustment period can be a vulnerable time as children are confronted with the reality that they will not return to their birth family. While they may have seemed fine and even happy through the foster/adoption process, children may cling to a last hope of reunification. That's why it's important to engage the child in the adoption process and listen carefully to what he or she has to say.

Children often have questions about their birth family, and you may need to address the status of your child's birth family. It is crucial to tell the truth—even when it's difficult—and to validate the child's experiences and feelings. There are several ways adoptive parents and siblings can deal with the feelings about birth families that may arise and, together, help the adopted child or youth integrate and feel secure.

- Acknowledge that adoption is important but that relationships are more important. While the names on paper might be different, the relationships already in place will remain the same.

- Encourage open discussion about any ongoing contact among birth family members, the child or youth, and members of your family.

- Create regular activities, events, or anniversaries to celebrate the adoption. Be sure to discuss the plans with your child to ensure he or she is comfortable with the attention.

- Plan regular events and activities where the focus is not on adoption but on building family memories and relationships.

- Develop relationships with other foster/adoptive children, youth, and families. Sharing common experiences, challenges, and successes will ease the feeling of being isolated or "different."

Children and youth learn best through repetition. Conversation about the differences between the foster family and the adoptive family may need to be repeated in a variety of ways. It is best if these conversations take place during activities that foster bonding and create memories.

- Help the child talk about the perceived difference in his or her own words. Ask open-ended questions, such as, "How do you think being adopted is different from being in foster care?" or "What do you think the biggest difference is, now that you're adopted?"

- Help the child draw analogies to something in his or her life. For instance, you might say, "This is like the time when ..."

There are a number of changes in status that will affect the child, and these should be discussed, depending on the child's developmental level.

- To help the child understand legal differences between foster care and adoption, you might talk about how the adoption court hearing is different from other court hearings during foster care. Some parents use marriage as an analogy for adoption and say the court hearing is like a marriage ceremony, and the adoption certificate is like the marriage certificate that makes the relationship legal and permanent. (Be prepared for questions about divorce.)

- Youth might need help in understanding the financial differences inherent in foster care and adoption. Adoption assistance payments might be compared to an allowance; older children may be able to understand the payments as costs to meet the child's needs.

- To help children understand parenting differences between foster care and adoption, you might remind the child that when in foster care, a permission slip signed by an agency caseworker was required for field trips, sleeping over at a friend's house, or traveling across state lines. After adoption, you can give permission for these activities.

Another way to explain the changes from foster care to adoption is to talk about the roles and responsibilities that different parents and agencies play in a child or youth's life.

- Birth parents give children life, gender, physical appearance, predisposition for certain diseases, intellectual potential, temperament, and talents. These aspects never change.

- State/courts/agencies provide financial responsibility, safety, and security; make major decisions; and are legally responsible for the child's actions. The court/agency plays this role while children are in foster care.

- Foster parents provide love, discipline, daily needs, transportation, life skills, values, and more. Foster parents play this role in the child welfare system.

- Adoptive parents assume the rights and responsibilities of the foster parents and the state/courts/agencies.

Helping Children Understand Their Histories and Losses

When children or youth spend extended periods of time in out-of-home care, memories of significant events and people can be lost. Children may not have a historical sense of self: who they are, where they've lived, the people they lived with, where they went to school, memories of favorite items like stuffed animals or blankets, and more. This can have negative developmental outcomes. Parents can help children review and understand their previous life experiences to clarify what happened to them in the past and help them integrate those experiences so they will have greater self-understanding.

Where Is Your Child on the Permanency Continuum?

Children's answers to the following questions will vary depending on their developmental stage, but their responses can guide you or your child's therapists or social workers in helping your child overcome past traumas and achieve feelings of permanency.

- Who am I? (question related to identity)

- What happened to me? (question related to loss and/or trauma)

- Where am I going? (question related to attachment)

- How will I get there? (question related to relationships)

- When will I know I belong? (question related to connection and safety)

For more information about helping your child deal with trauma, visit Child Welfare Information Gateway: http://www.childwelfare.gov/ systemwide/mentalhealth/common/trauma.cfm

Helpful Activities and Resources

Families can help children in answering these powerful questions and in understanding their unique history in many ways. Lifebooks, ecomaps, lifemaps, and lifepaths are tools used by foster/adoptive parents and adoption professionals to help children and youth answer questions about how they came to be separated from their birth family and where, ultimately, they belong. These tools can help children build a bridge between foster care and adoption. Working with these tools can give your child ways to experience and work through trauma and feelings of loss and grief.

Lifebook: A lifebook is an account of the child's life in words, pictures, photographs, and electronic documents. While lifebooks can take many forms, each child's lifebook is unique. You can assist in creating a lifebook by gathering information about a child and taking pictures of people and places that are—or were—meaningful. Working together on a lifebook can bring parents and children together. For free lifebook page samples, visit the Iowa Foster and Adoptive Parents Association website: http://www.ifapa.org/resources/ IFAPA_Lifebook_Pages.asp

Because a lifebook may contain personal and painful information about the child or youth's past, it is not intended to be shared outside the family. It's merely a resource to help the child cope with the transition from temporary to permanent care. For more information on lifebooks, visit the Information Gateway website: http://www.childwelfare .gov/adoption/adopt_parenting/lifebooks.cfm

Here are some suggestions for what to include in a child's lifebook:

- Pictures of the child's birth parents and/or birth relatives and information about visits

- Developmental milestones: first words, first smile, first steps, etc.

- Common childhood diseases and immunizations, injuries, illnesses, or hospitalizations

- Pictures of current or past foster family and extended family members who were/are significant to the child

- Pictures of previous foster families, their homes, and their pets

- Names of teachers and schools attended, report cards, and school activities

- Special activities such as Scouting, clubs, sports, or camping

- Faith-based activities

- What a child did when he/she was happy or excited and ways a child showed affection

- Cute things the child did, nicknames, favorite friends, activities, and toys

- Birthdays, religious celebrations, or trips taken with the foster family

W.I.S.E. UP Powerbooks: W.I.S.E. UP Powerbooks help children answer awkward or difficult questions asked by classmates or new friends. Foster care and adoption are nothing to be ashamed of, but questions like, "Why are you in foster care?" can cause added anxiety and stress for children and youth. The W.I.S.E. UP series helps children understand that they have options about how much and what kinds of information to disclose when answering these questions. The books offer example questions and responses.

- W stands for "Walk away."

- I stands for saying, "It's private."

- S stands for "Share" some information about adoption or about one's own story.

- E stands for "Educate" others about adoption with correct facts.

W.I.S.E. UP Powerbooks and similar resources can be found at the Center for Adoption Support and Education website: http://www .adoptionsupport.org/pub/index.php

Ecomap: An ecomap is a visual representation of the principal people and activities in a child or youth's life. An ecomap may have a circle in the middle of the page with a stick figure of a child in it, along with the question "Why am I here?" Lines extend from the circle like spokes to other circles representing the court, other foster families, siblings, school, or to topics such as "things I like to do" to represent what and who is important to a child and to help the child understand how he or she came to live with the foster/adoptive family.

Lifemaps and lifepaths: Lifemaps or lifepaths are visual representations to help children understand the paths their lives have taken and the decision points along the way. They may include stepping stones to represent a child's age and a statement about where and with whom they lived at that age.

Meaningful details to include in these tools that will help children understand their histories describe the child's birth, explain why and how the child entered foster care, and clarify how decisions were made about moves and new placements. If possible, include baby pictures and pictures of birth parents. If no information is available, children can draw a picture of what they might have looked like. Statements such as "There is no information about Johnny's birth father in his file" at least acknowledge the father's existence. Honesty, developmental appropriateness, and compassion are vital for children in explaining difficult and painful circumstances that brought them into foster care.

Social Media and Adoption

Social media sites like Facebook, MySpace, and Twitter have changed the face of communication today. Although statistics are not yet available to document the number of adopted people and birth parents who find each other through these sites, anecdotal evidence suggests that it is a growing trend. If your child is a regular user of social media, you may want to explore positive ways to use Facebook and other sites to maintain healthy contact between your child and his or her birth family members.

Helping Children Cope with Trauma and Losses

It may be difficult to comprehend the experience of past losses your foster child or youth encountered before adoption. Your child may still be grieving because of losses or lost connections with family members. He or she may also suffer from trauma related to those losses. There are often several stages of grief the child must experience before he or she can transfer attachment from the birth family to your family. Adoption experts acknowledge the importance of helping children integrate their previous attachments to important people in their lives in order to transition that emotional attachment to a new family. Integration is a way of helping children cope with the painful realities of the separation from their birth families.

The five-step integration process below was first described by adoption pioneer K. Donley (1988). The process is an effort to clarify permission messages children and youth receive from their birth families to be in foster care, to live with new parents, to be loved by them, and to love them back.

Five Steps to Help Your Child in the Integration Process

1. **Create an accurate reconstruction of the child's placement history:** Creating a lifebook, lifemap, or ecomap with a child helps a child to see and understand his or her own history.

2. **Identify the important attachment figures in the child's life:** Foster parents might learn who these important people are by listening to the child talk about people from previous placements. These attachment figures might be parents, but they could be siblings, former foster parents, or other family members. When adoptive families rarely talk about birth families, children or youth may feel the loss more intensely.

3. **Gain the cooperation of the most significant attachment figures available:** If possible, parents should cooperate with the birth parents, grandparents, or other relative to whom the child was attached. Even if the birth family is not happy about a child's permanency goal of adoption, there is likely one important person (a teacher, a former neighbor) who will be willing to work with you to make a child's transition easier.

4. **Clarify "the permission message":** It is necessary for children to hear and feel from people who are important to them that it is all right to love another family. The primary person in a child's life who is available to give the child that message should be sought out to do so.

5. **Communicate that permission to the child:** Whether the "permission to love your family" comes in the form of a letter from Grandma or from the birth parent during visits, it is important that children hear from that person that it is not

their fault they are in foster care and that it is all right to love another family. This "permission" will go a long way to helping a child relax and transfer his/her attachment to the new family.

During this transition phase, it's important for parents and others working with the child to use the following skills:

- Engaging the child
- Listening to the child
- Telling the truth
- Validating the child's life story
- Creating a safe space for the child
- Realizing that it is never too late to go back in time
- Acknowledging pain as part of the process

For more information on helping your child adapt to grief and loss, visit Information Gateway: http://www.childwelfare.gov/systemwide/mentalhealth/common/grief.cfm

Helping Children Transfer Attachment

While the integration process is about helping the child cope with and accept his or her past, the transfer of attachment is about moving toward the future. Attachment transfer is not an easy process but it's an important part of the transition from foster child or youth to adoptive child or youth. Children with attachment issues have missed several completions of the attachment cycle, or what is referred to as a disrupted attachment cycle, and it's critical to allow children and youth to experience the cycle with their foster/adoptive family.

The diagrams shown in Figure 39.1, adapted from Parents as Tender Healers (PATH)—a curriculum for foster parents, adoptive parents, and kinship caregivers—demonstrate the completed and disrupted attachment cycles (Jackson & Wasserman, 1997).

Relationships and Routines

Relationships and routines are key ways to fortify your child's sense of status within your family and begin the process of transferring and forming attachment to you and your family.

- Be aware of the enormous adjustment the child is making. You, too, are making a huge adjustment but have adult perceptions and skills to handle it.

- Balance structured activities with unstructured time for conversation, especially during the first few weeks. Use a prop or gimmick such as a family game or talking stick to stimulate conversation as needed.

Attachment Cycle

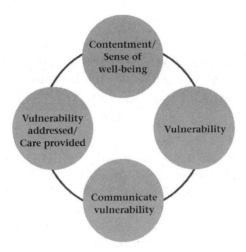

Disrupted Attachment Cycle

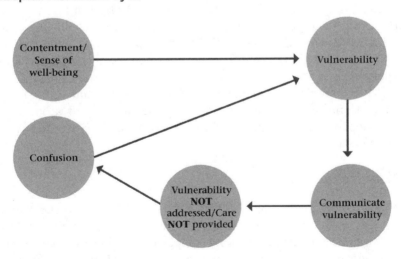

Figure 39.1. Attachment Cycle and Disrupted Attachment Cycle.

- Hold family meetings with a time set aside to evaluate "How are we doing as a family?" Encourage honesty and make adjustments as needed.

- Work together to create a written list of family rules. When everyone contributes to creating rules, everyone feels ownership of the rules. Discuss consequences for breaking the rules, procedures for modifying the rules, and family rewards for following the rules.

- As holidays or special occasions approach, encourage your child to discuss what his or her expectations are for the event.

- Incorporate elements of family traditions into your celebrations. Be sure to describe what celebrations with extended family may be like—they may seem overwhelming to your newest family members.

Conclusion

On the surface, it may seem easy for a child or youth to transition from foster care to adoption within the same family, but in reality, the internal process—both for a child and families—is much more complicated. Allowing children to "drift" into adoption without acknowledging the significant changes may lead to difficulties later.

You need to help your children consider and understand their own histories and the reasons why they cannot live with their birth families, help them adjust to this loss, and help them transfer their attachments to you and your family. In helping children, families will need to consider each child's needs as they are related to the child's age, health, personality, temperament, and cultural and racial experiences.

Other foster/adoptive parents can be a great resource for families. The National Foster Care and Adoption Directory has a list of foster and adoptive support groups in each state (http://www.childwelfare.gov/nfcad).

Resources

- "Adoption Scrapbooks Made Easy" and "Thanks for the Memories," both by Jenni Colson, published in *Adoptive Families*, offer strategies for developing adoption scrapbooks: http://www.adoptivefamilies.com/articles.php?aid=1131 and http://www.adoptivefamilies.com/articles.php?aid=1305

- "Bibliography: Lifebooks for Children and Youth in Foster Care" is a selection of resources on creating lifebooks by the Annie E. Casey Foundation and Casey Family Services: http://www.casey familyservices.org/userfiles/pdf/bib-2009-lifebooks.pdf

- "Birds, Bees, and Adoption," by Marybeth Lambe, published in *Adoptive Families*, offers tips for adoptive parents on explaining reproduction: http://www.adoptivefamilies.com/articles.php ?aid=772

- Free lifebook sample pages are available through the Iowa Foster and Adoptive Parents Association: http://www.ifapa.org/ resources/IFAPA_Lifebook_Pages.asp

- "Get Talking," published online in *Adoptive Families*, provides a number of articles on how and when adoptive parents should talk with their children about adoption: http://adoptivefamilies .com/talking

References

Adoption Resources of Wisconsin. (2009). *Moving from foster care to adoption: Changing families.* A series on adoption and foster care issues. Retrieved from http://www.wifostercareandadoption.org/ library/149/moving%20from%20foster_moving%20from%20foster.pdf

Donley, K. S. (1988). Disengagement work: Helping children make new attachments. In H. L. Craig-Oldsen (Ed.), *From foster parent to adoptive parent: A resource guide for workers.* Atlanta, GA: Child Welfare Institute.

Fahlberg, V. (1991). *A child's journey through placement.* Indianapolis, IN: Perspectives Press.

Gustavsson, N., and MacEachron, A. (2008). Creating foster care youth biographies: A role for the Internet. *Journal of Technology Services* 26(1), 45–55.

Henry, D. L. (2005). The 3-5-7 model: Preparing children for permanency. *Children and Youth Services Review*, 27(2), 197–212.

Jackson, R. P., and Wasserman, K. (1997). *PATH: Parents as tender healers. A curriculum for foster, adoptive, and kinship care parents.* Retrieved from Child Welfare Information Gateway: http://library.childwelfare.gov/cwig/ws/library/docs/gateway/ Blob/50938.pdf?w=+NATIVE%28%27recno%3D50938%27%29& upp=0&rpp=10&r=1&m=1

Keck, G., and Kupecky, R. (2002, 2009). *Parenting the hurt child.* Colorado Springs, CO: NAVPRESS. (Original work published 2002).

Laws, R. (2004). Talking to children about adoption assistance, *Adoptalk*, North American Council on Adoptable Children. Retrieved from http://www.nacac.org/adoptalk/talkingaboutaa.html

North American Council on Adoptive Children. (2009). Ambiguous loss haunts foster and adopted children. *Adoptalk*. Retrieved from http://www.nacac.org/adoptalk/ambigloss.html

Chapter 40

Parenting a Child Who Has Been Sexually Abused

You may be a foster or adoptive parent of a child who was sexually abused before coming to your home. In some cases, you will not be certain that abuse has occurred, but you may suspect it. You may even be exploring becoming a foster or adoptive parent to a child in the foster care system; many of these children have been abused or neglected—physically, emotionally, or sexually—before coming into care.

You may feel confused, frightened, and unsure of the impact the sexual abuse of a child may have on your child and family. It is important for you to understand that the term "sexual abuse" describes a wide range of experiences. Many factors—including the severity of abuse as well as others discussed later in this chapter—affect how children react to sexual abuse and how they recover. Most children who have been abused do not go on to abuse others, and many go on to live happy, healthy, successful lives. As parents, you will play an important role in your child's recovery from childhood abuse.

Although the term "parents" is used throughout this text, the information and strategies provided may be equally helpful for kinship care providers, guardians, and other caregivers.

Child Welfare Information Gateway. (2008). "Parenting a child who has been sexually abused: A guide for foster and adoptive parents," Washington, DC: U.S. Department of Health and Human Services. The complete text of this document, including references, is available online from the Child Welfare Information Gateway at www.childwelfare.gov/pubs/f_abused/index.cfm. Reviewed by David A. Cooke, MD, FACP, January 2013.

This chapter discusses how you can help children in your care by educating yourself about sexual abuse, establishing guidelines for safety and privacy in your family, and understanding when and how to seek help if you need it.

Educating Yourself

The first step to helping a child who may have been a victim of sexual abuse is to understand more about how sexual abuse is defined, behaviors that may indicate abuse has occurred, how these behaviors may differ from typical sexual behaviors in children, and how sexual abuse may affect children.

What Is Child Sexual Abuse?

Child sexual abuse is defined in federal law by the Child Abuse Prevention and Treatment Act (42 U.S.C. sec. 5106g(4)) as: "... the employment, use, persuasion, inducement, enticement, or coercion of any child to engage in, or assist any other person to engage in, any sexually explicit conduct or simulation of such conduct for the purpose of producing a visual depiction of such conduct; or the rape, and in cases of caretaker or inter-familial relationships, statutory rape, molestation, prostitution, or other form of sexual exploitation of children, or incest with children."

Within this federal guideline, each state is responsible for establishing its own legal definition of child sexual abuse. For more information, see the Child Sexual Abuse section of the Child Welfare Information Gateway website: www.childwelfare.gov/can/types/sexualabuse

For legal definitions in each state, see Information Gateway's *Definitions of Child Abuse and Neglect*: www.childwelfare.gov/ systemwide/laws_ policies/statutes/define.cfm.

Signs of Sexual Abuse

If you are a foster or adoptive parent to a child from the foster care system, you may not know whether he or she has been sexually abused. Child welfare agencies usually share all known information about your child's history with you; however, many children do not disclose past abuse until they feel safe. For this reason, foster or adoptive parents are sometimes the first to learn that sexual abuse has occurred. Even when there is no documentation of prior abuse, you may suspect abuse because of the child's behavior.

Determining whether a child has been abused requires a careful evaluation by a trained professional. While it is normal for all children to have and express sexual curiosity, children who have been sexually abused may demonstrate behaviors that are outside of the range of what might be considered normal. There is no one specific sign or behavior that can be considered proof that sexual abuse has occurred. However, many professionals and organizations agree that you might consider the possibility of sexual abuse when one or several of the following signs or behaviors are present:

- Sexual knowledge, interest, or language that is unusual for the child's age
- Sexual activities with toys or other children that seem unusual, aggressive, or unresponsive to limits or redirection
- Excessive masturbation, sometimes in public, not responsive to redirection or limits
- Pain, itching, redness, or bleeding in the genital areas
- Nightmares, trouble sleeping, or fear of the dark
- Sudden or extreme mood swings: rage, fear, anger, excessive crying, or withdrawal
- "Spacing out" at odd times
- Loss of appetite, or difficulty eating or swallowing
- Cutting, burning, or other self-mutilating behaviors as an adolescent
- Talking about a new, older friend
- Unexplained avoidance of certain people, places, or activities
- An older child behaving like a much younger child: wetting the bed or sucking a thumb, for example
- Suddenly having money

Again, these are only signs of a potential problem; they must be evaluated by a professional along with other information. The following organizations contributed to the above list and offer more information about behavioral signs of sexual abuse on their websites:

- Stop It Now! (www.stopitnow.com/warnings.html#behavioral)
- Childhelp (www.childhelp.org)

547

- National Center for Missing and Exploited Children (www.missingkids.com)

Healthy Sexual Development in Children

Children's sexual interest, curiosity, and behaviors develop gradually over time and may be influenced by many factors, including what children see and experience. Sexual behavior is not in and of itself a sign that abuse has occurred. The following lists present some of the sexual behaviors common among children of different age groups, as well as some behaviors that might be considered less common or unhealthy.

These lists are adapted from the Stop It Now! publication, "Prevent Child Sexual Abuse: Facts about Those Who Might Commit It" (2005). Additional information was provided by Eliana Gil, Ph.D., RPT-S, ATR, specialist, trainer, and consultant in working with children who have been abused and their families. See the website www.elianagil.com

Sexual Behaviors in Preschool Children (0 to 5 Years)

Common

- Sexual language relating to differences in body parts, bathroom talk, pregnancy, and birth
- Self-fondling at home and in public
- Showing and looking at private body parts

Uncommon

- Discussion of sexual acts
- Sexual contact experiences with other children
- Masturbation unresponsive to redirection or limits
- Inserting objects in genital openings

Sexual Behaviors in School Age Children (6 to 12 years)

Common

- Questions about menstruation, pregnancy, sexual behavior
- "Experimenting" with same-age children, including kissing, fondling, exhibitionism, and role-playing
- Masturbation at home or other private places

Uncommon

- Discussion of explicit sexual acts
- Asking adults or peers to participate in explicit sexual acts

Sexual Behaviors in Adolescence (13 to 16 years)

Common

- Questions about decision-making, social relationships, and sexual customs
- Masturbation in private
- Experimenting between adolescents of the same age, including open-mouth kissing, fondling, and body rubbing
- Voyeuristic behaviors
- Sexual intercourse occurs in approximately one-third of this age group
- Oral sex has been found to occur in 50 percent of teens ages 15 and older.

Uncommon

- Sexual interest in much younger children
- Aggression in touching others' genitals
- Asking adults to participate in explicit sexual acts

For a more complete list, or if you have any questions or concerns about your child's sexual behaviors, call the Stop It Now! toll-free helpline at 888-PREVENT (888-773-8368).

Factors Affecting the Impact of Sexual Abuse

If you suspect, or a professional has determined, that a child in your care has been a victim of sexual abuse, it is important to understand how children may be affected.

All children who have been sexually abused have had their physical and emotional boundaries violated and crossed. With this violation often comes a breach of the child's sense of security and trust. Abused children may come to believe that the world is not a safe place and that adults are not trustworthy.

However, children who have experienced sexual abuse are not all affected the same way. As with other types of abuse, many factors influence how children think and feel about the abuse, how the abuse affects them, and how their recovery progresses. Some factors that can affect the impact of abuse include:

- The relationship of the abuser to the child and how much the abuse caused a betrayal of trust

- The abuser's use of "friendliness" or seduction

- The abuser's use of threats of harm or violence, including threats to pets, siblings, or parents

- The abuser's use of secrecy

- How long the abuse occurred

- Gender of the abuser being the same as or different from the child

- The age (developmental level) of the child at the time of the abuse (younger children are more vulnerable)

- The child's emotional development at the time of the abuse

- The child's ability to cope with his or her emotional and physical responses to the abuse (for example, fear and arousal)

- How much responsibility the child feels for the abuse

It is very important for children to understand that they are not to blame for the abuse they experienced. Your family's immediate response to learning about the sexual abuse and ongoing acceptance of what the child has told you will play a critical role in your child's ability to recover and go back to a healthy life.

Establishing Family Guidelines for Safety and Privacy

There are things you can do to help ensure that any child visiting or living in your home experiences a structured, safe, and nurturing environment. Some sexually abused children may have a heightened sensitivity to certain situations. Making your home a comfortable place for children who have been sexually abused can mean changing some habits or patterns of family life. Incorporating some of these guidelines may also help reduce foster or adoptive parents' vulnerability to abuse allegations by children living with them. Consider whether the following tips may be helpful in your family's situation:

- Make sure every family member's comfort level with touching, hugging, and kissing is respected. Do not force touching on children who seem uncomfortable being touched. Encourage children to respect the comfort and privacy of others.

- Be cautious with playful touch, such as play fighting and tickling. These may be uncomfortable or scary reminders of sexual abuse to some children.

- Help children learn the importance of privacy. Remind children to knock before entering bathrooms and bedrooms, and encourage children to dress and bathe themselves if they are able. Teach children about privacy and respect.

- Keep adult sexuality private. Teenage siblings may need reminders about what is permitted in your home when boyfriends and girlfriends are present.

- Be aware of and limit sexual messages received through the media. Children who have experienced sexual abuse can find sexual content overstimulating or disturbing. It may be helpful to monitor music and music videos, as well as television programs, video games, and movies containing nudity, sexual activity, or sexual language. Limit access to grown-up magazines and monitor children's internet use.

If your child has touching problems (or any sexually aggressive behaviors), you may need to take additional steps to help ensure safety for your child as well as his or her peers. Consider how these tips may apply to your own situation:

- **With friends:** If your child has issues with touching other children, you may want to ensure supervision when he or she is playing with friends, whether at your home or theirs. Sleepovers may not be a good idea when children have touching problems.

- **At school:** You may wish to inform your child's school of any inappropriate sexual behavior, to ensure an appropriate level of supervision. Often this information can be kept confidential by a school counselor or other personnel.

- **In the community:** Supervision becomes critical any time children with sexual behavior problems are with groups of children, for example at day camp or after-school programs. In any case, keep the lines of communication open, so children feel more comfortable turning to you with problems and talking with you about anything—not just sexual abuse. Remember however, that sexual abuse is difficult for most children to disclose even to a trusted adult.

For more information about developing a safety plan for your family, see:

- *Create a Family Safety Plan,* Stop It Now! (www.stopitnow.org/downloads/SafetyPlan.pdf)

Seeking Help

Responding to the needs of a child who has been sexually abused may involve the whole family and will likely have an impact on all family relationships. Mental health professionals (for example, counselors, therapists, or social workers) can help you and your family cope with reactions, thoughts, and feelings about the abuse.

Impact of Sexual Abuse on the Family

Being an adoptive or foster parent to sexually abused children can be stressful to marriages and relationships. Parenting in these situations may require some couples to be more open with each other and their children about sexuality than in the past. If one parent is more involved in addressing the issue than another, the imbalance can create difficulties in the parental relationship. A couple's sexual relationship can also be affected, if sex begins to feel like a troubled area of the family's life. When these problems emerge, it is often helpful to get professional advice. For more information about sustaining a healthy marriage, visit the National Healthy Marriage Resource Center website: www.healthymarriageinfo.org

Your child's siblings (birth, foster, or adoptive) may be exposed to new or focused attention on sexuality that can be challenging for them. If one child is acting out sexually, you may need to talk with siblings about what they see, think, and feel, as well as how to respond. Children may also need to be coached on what (and how much) to say about their sibling's problems to their friends. If your children see that you are actively managing the problem, they will feel more secure and will worry less. When one child has been sexually abused, parents often become very protective of their other children. It is important to find a balance between reasonable worry and overprotectiveness. Useful strategies to prevent further abuse may include teaching children to stand up for themselves, talking with them about being in charge of their bodies, and fostering open communication with your children.

Counseling for Parents and Children

Talking with a mental health professional who specializes in child sexual abuse as soon as problems arise can help parents determine if their children's behavior is cause for concern. Specialists can also provide parents with guidance in responding to their children's difficulties and offer suggestions for how to talk with their children. A mental health professional may suggest special areas of attention in family life and offer specific suggestions for creating structured, safe, and nurturing environments.

To help a child who has been abused, many mental health professionals will begin with a thorough assessment to explore how the child functions in all areas of life. The specialist will want to know about these issues:

- Past stressors (for example, history of abuse, frequent moves and other losses)

- Current stressors (for example, a medical problem or learning disability)

- Emotional state (for example, Is the child usually happy or anxious?)

- Coping strategies (for example, Does the child withdraw or act out when angry or sad?)

- The child's friendships

- The child's strengths (for example, Is the child creative, athletic, organized?)

- The child's communication skills

- The child's attachments to adults in his or her life

After a thorough assessment, the mental health professional will decide if the child and family could benefit from therapy. Not all abused children require therapy. For those who do, the mental health professional will develop a plan tailored to the child and family's strengths and needs. This plan may include one or more of the following types of therapy:

- **Individual therapy:** The frequency and duration of therapy can vary tremendously. The style of therapy will depend on the child's age and the therapist's training. Some therapists use creative techniques (for example, art, play, and music therapy) to help children who are uncomfortable talking about their experiences. Other therapists use traditional talk therapy or a combination of approaches.

- **Group therapy:** Meeting in groups with other children who have been sexually abused can help children understand themselves; feel less alone (by interacting with others who have had similar experiences); and learn new skills through role plays, discussion, games, and play.

- **Family therapy:** Many therapists will see children and parents together to support positive parent-child communication and to guide parents in learning new skills that will help their children feel better and behave appropriately.

Whether or not family therapy is advised, it is vital for parents to stay involved in their child's therapy or other kinds of treatment. Skilled mental health professionals will always seek to involve the parents by asking for and sharing information.

Your Child Welfare Agency

If you are a foster parent or seeking to adopt a child, you may wish to talk with your social worker about what you discover about your child's history and any behaviors that worry you. Sharing your concerns will help your social worker help you and your family. If your child exhibits problematic sexual behaviors, be aware that you may also be required to report these to child protective services in order to comply with mandated reporting laws in your jurisdiction. See Information Gateway's *Mandatory Reporters of Child Abuse and Neglect* at www.childwelfare.gov/systemwide/laws_policies/statutes/manda.cfm.

Many adoptive parents also call their local child welfare agency to seek advice if their child shows troubling behaviors. Child welfare workers are often good sources of information, can offer advice, and are familiar with community resources. Adoption agencies may also be able to provide additional postadoption services or support to adoptive parents who find out about their child's history of sexual abuse after the adoption is finalized. For more information about postadoption services, see the Information Gateway web section: www.childwelfare. gov/adoption/postadoption

What to Look for in a Mental Health Professional

The following information is adapted from the National Center for Missing and Exploited Children's *Parental Guidelines in Case Your*

Child Might Someday Be the Victim of Sexual Exploitation: www .missingkids.com.

Finding a knowledgeable and experienced mental health professional is key to getting the help your family needs. Some communities have special programs for treating children who have been sexually abused, such as child protection teams and child advocacy centers. You may also find qualified specialists in your community through the organizations noted below.

- Child advocacy centers

- Rape crisis or sexual assault centers

- Local psychological or psychiatric association referral services

- Child abuse hotlines (see the Information Gateway publication, Child Abuse Reporting Numbers: www.childwelfare.gov/pubs/ reslist/rl_dsp.cfm?rs_id=5&rate_chno=11-11172)

- Child protective services (CPS) agencies

- Nonprofit service providers serving families of missing or exploited children

- University departments of social work, psychology, or psychiatry

- Crime victim assistance programs in the law enforcement agency, prosecutor's, or district attorney's office

- Family court services, including court appointed special advocate (CASA) groups or guardians *ad litem*

Therapy for children who have been sexually abused is specialized work. When selecting a mental health professional, look for the following:

- An advanced degree in a recognized mental health specialty such as psychiatry (M.D.), psychology (Ph.D. or Psy.D.), social work (M.S.W.), counseling (L.P.C.), or psychiatric nursing (R.N.)

- Licensure to practice as a mental health professional in your state. (Some mental health services are provided by students under the supervision of licensed professionals.)

- Special training in child sexual abuse, including the dynamics of abuse, how it affects children and adults, and the use of goal-oriented treatment plans

- Knowledge about the legal issues involved in child sexual abuse, especially the laws about reporting child sexual victimization, procedures used by law enforcement and protective services, evidence collection, and expert testimony in your state

Conclusion

Many people want to help children who have been sexually abused, but many struggle with feelings of anger and disgust as they learn more about the abuse. You may need help to resolve these struggles and to move toward acceptance of your child's background.

If you were (or suspect you may have been) sexually abused as a child, dealing with your own child's difficulties may be particularly challenging, and reading this information may have brought up difficult thoughts and feelings. Your courage in facing these issues and tackling a personally difficult and painful subject can actually be helpful to your children by demonstrating to them that sexual abuse experiences can be managed and overcome.

Creating a structured, safe, and nurturing home is the greatest gift that you can give to all of your children. Seek help when you need it, share your successes with your social worker, and remember that a healthy relationship with your children allows them to begin the recovery process. It is in the parent-child relationship that your child learns trust and respect, two important building blocks of your children's safety and well-being.

Part Seven

Additional Help and Information

Chapter 41

Glossary of Terms Related to Child Abuse

abandonment: A situation in which the child has been left by the parent(s), the parent's identity or whereabouts are unknown, the child suffers serious harm, or the parent has failed to maintain contact with the child or to provide reasonable support for a specified period of time.[a]

adoption: The social, emotional, and legal process through which children who will not be raised by their birth parents become full and permanent legal members of another family while maintaining genetic and psychological connections to their birth family.[a]

adoption services: Services or activities provided to assist in bringing about the adoption of a child.[b]

adoptive parent: A person with the legal relation of parent to a child not related by birth, with the same mutual rights and obligations that exist between children and their birth parents.[b]

alcohol abuse: Compulsive use of alcohol that is not of a temporary nature. Applies to infants addicted at birth, or who are victims of fetal alcohol syndrome, or who may suffer other disabilities due to the use of alcohol during pregnancy.[b]

This chapter includes terms marked [a] excerpted from "Glossary," Child Welfare Information Gateway, DHHS, available online at www.childwelfare.gov/admin/glossary/index.cfm; accessed September 27, 2012; and terms marked [b] from "National Child Abuse and Neglect Data System (NCANDSSS) Glossary," Administration for Children and Families, U.S. Department of Health and Human Services (http://www.acf.hhs.gov), March 2000.

alcohol-related birth defects: Physical or cognitive deficits in a child that result from maternal alcohol consumption during pregnancy. This includes but is not limited to fetal alcohol syndrome.[a]

alleged perpetrator report source: An individual who reports an alleged incident of child abuse or neglect in which he/she caused or knowingly allowed the maltreatment of a child.[b]

alleged victim: Child about whom a report regarding maltreatment has been made to a child protective services (CPS) agency.[b]

alleged victim report sources: A child who alleges to have been a victim of child maltreatment and who makes a report of the allegation.[b]

anonymous or unknown report source: An individual who reports a suspected incident of child maltreatment without identifying himself or herself; or the type of reporter is unknown.[b]

assessment: The ongoing practice of informing decision-making by identifying, considering, and weighing factors that impact children, youth, and their families. Assessment occurs from the time children and families come to the attention of the child welfare system and continues until case closure.[a]

behavior problem: Behavior of the child in the school and/or community that adversely affects socialization, learning, growth, and moral development. May include adjudicated or non-adjudicated behavior problems. Includes running away from home or a placement.[b]

biological parent: The birth mother or father of the child rather than the adoptive or foster parent or the stepparent.[b]

birth mother: An individual's biological mother, after an adoption has occurred. Prior to an adoption decision and legal adoption, birth mother is referred to as a pregnant woman, or expectant mother.[a]

birth parent: An individual's biological mother or father, after an adoption has occurred. Prior to an adoption decision and legal adoption, birth parents are referred to as a child's parents or expectant parents.[a]

bonding: The process of developing lasting emotional ties with one's immediate caregivers; seen as the first and primary developmental achievement of a human being and central to a person's ability to relate to others throughout life.[a]

caregiver: One who provides for the physical, emotional, and social needs of a dependent person. The term most often applies to parents or parent surrogates, child care and nursery workers, health-care specialists, and relatives caring for children, elderly, or ill family members.[a]

case management: Coordination and monitoring of services on behalf of a client. In general, the role of the case manager does not involve the provision of direct services but the monitoring of services to assure that they are relevant to the client, delivered in a useful way, and effective in meeting the goals of the case plan. A key element of case management in child welfare is the ongoing assessment of the client's needs and progress in services.[a]

child: A person less than 18 years of age or considered to be a minor under state law.[b]

child abuse and neglect: Defined by the Child Abuse Prevention and Treatment Act (CAPTA) as any recent act or failure to act on the part of a parent or caretaker that results in death, serious physical or emotional harm, sexual abuse, or exploitation, or an act or failure to act that presents an imminent risk of serious harm. Child abuse and neglect are defined by federal and state laws. CAPTA is the federal legislation that provides minimum standards that states must incorporate in their statutory definitions of child abuse and neglect.[a]

child protective services (CPS): The social services agency designated (in most states) to receive reports, conduct investigations and assessments, and provide intervention and treatment services to children and families in which child maltreatment has occurred. Frequently, this agency is located within larger public social service agencies, such as departments of social services.[a]

child victim: A child for whom an incident of abuse or neglect has been substantiated or indicated by an investigation or assessment. A state may include some children with other dispositions as victims.[b]

closed without a finding: Disposition that does not conclude with a specific finding because the investigation could not be completed for such reasons as: the family moved out of the jurisdiction; the family could not be located; or necessary diagnostic or other reports were not received within required time limits.[b]

corporal punishment: Inflicting physical pain for the purpose of punishment in an effort to discipline a child.[a]

counseling services: Beneficial activities that apply the therapeutic processes to personal, family, situational or occupational problems in order to bring about a positive resolution of the problem or improved individual or family functioning or circumstances.[b]

court action: Legal action initiated by a representative of the CPS agency on behalf of the child. This includes, for instance, authorization to place the child, filing for temporary custody, dependency, or termination of parental rights. It does not include criminal proceedings against a perpetrator.[b]

court-appointed special advocate (CASA): A person, usually a volunteer appointed by the court, who serves to ensure that the needs and interests of a child in child protection judicial proceedings are fully protected.[a]

court-appointed representative: A person required to be appointed by the court to represent a child in a neglect or abuse proceeding. May be an attorney or a court-appointed special advocate (or both) and is often referred to as a guardian ad litem. Makes recommendations to the court concerning the best interests of the child.[b]

custody: Refers to the legal right to make decisions about children, including where they live. Parents have legal custody of their children unless they voluntarily give custody to someone else or a court takes this right away and gives it to someone else. For instance, a court may give legal custody to a relative or to a child welfare agency. Whoever has legal custody can enroll the children in school, give permission for medical care, and give other legal consents.[a]

cycle of abuse: A generational pattern of abusive behavior that can occur when children who have either experienced maltreatment or witnessed violence between their parents or caregivers learn violent behavior and learn to consider it appropriate.[a]

discipline: Training that develops self-control, self-sufficiency, and orderly conduct. Discipline is based on respect for an individual's capability and is not to be confused with punishment.[a]

domestic/family violence: A pattern of assaultive and/or coercive behaviors, including physical, sexual, and psychological attacks, as well as economic coercion, that adults or adolescents use against their intimate partners. Intimate partners include spouses, sexual partners, parents, children, siblings, extended family members, and dating relationships.[a]

drug abuse: Compulsive use of drugs that is not of a temporary nature. Applies to infants addicted at birth.[b]

educational neglect: Failure to ensure that a child's educational needs are met. Such neglect may involve permitting chronic truancy, failure to enroll a child in school, or inattention to special education needs.[a]

emotional neglect: Failure to provide adequate nurturing and affection or the refusal/delay in ensuring that a child receives needed treatment for emotional or behavioral problems. Emotional neglect may also involve exposure to chronic or extreme domestic violence.[a]

family: A group of two or more persons related by birth, marriage, adoption, or emotional ties.[b]

family preservation services: Short-term, family-focused, and community-based services designed to help families cope with significant stresses or problems that interfere with their ability to nurture their children. The goal of family preservation services (FPS) is to maintain children with their families or to reunify the family, whenever it can be done safely. These services are applicable to families at risk of disruption/out-of-home placement across systems and may be provided to different types of families—birth or biological families, kinship families, foster families, and adoptive families—to help them address major challenges, stabilize the family, and enhance family functioning.[a]

family support services: Community-based preventative activities designed to alleviate stress and promote parental competencies and behaviors that will increase the ability of families to successfully nurture their children, enable families to use other resources and opportunities available in the community, and create supportive networks to enhance childrearing abilities of parents.[b]

fetal alcohol spectrum disorders (FASDs): A group of conditions that can occur in a person whose mother drank alcohol during pregnancy. These effects can include physical problems and problems with behavior and learning. Often, a person with an FASD has a mix of these problems.[a]

foster care: Twenty-four-hour substitute care for children placed away from their parents or guardians and for whom the state agency has placement and care responsibility. This includes, but is not limited to, family foster homes, foster homes of relatives, group homes, emergency shelters, residential facilities, child care institutions, and pre-adoptive homes regardless of whether the facility is licensed and whether payments are made by the state or local agency for the care of the child, or whether there is federal matching of any payments made.[b]

foster child: Child who has been placed in the state's or county's legal custody because the child's custodial parents/guardians are unable to provide a safe family home due to abuse, neglect, or an inability to care for the child.[a]

foster parent: Individual licensed to provide a home for orphaned, abused, neglected, delinquent or disabled children, usually with the approval of the government or a social service agency. May be a relative or a non-relative.[b]

group home: Residence intended to meet the needs of children who are unable to live in a family setting and do not need a more intensive residential service. Homes normally house 4–12 children in a setting that offers the potential for the full use of community resources, including employment, health care, education, and recreational opportunities. Desired outcomes of group home programs include full incorporation of the child into the community, return of the child to his or her family or other permanent family, and/or acquisition by the child of the skills necessary for independent living.[a]

guardian ad litem (GAL): A lawyer or layperson who represents a child in juvenile or family court. Usually this person considers the best interest of the child and may perform a variety of roles, including those of independent investigator, advocate, advisor, and guardian for the child. A layperson who serves in this role is sometimes known as a court-appointed special advocate (CASA).[a]

guardianship: The transfer of parental responsibility and legal authority for a minor child to an adult caregiver who intends to provide permanent care for the child. This can be done without terminating the parental rights of the child's parents. Transferring legal responsibility removes the child from the child welfare system, allows the caregiver to make important decisions on the child's behalf, and establishes a long-term caregiver for the child. In subsidized guardianship, the guardian is provided with a monthly subsidy for the care and support of the child.[a]

inadequate housing: A risk factor related to substandard, over-crowded, or unsafe housing conditions, including homelessness.[b]

incest: Sexual intercourse between persons who are closely related by blood. In the United States, incest is prohibited by many state laws as well as cultural tradition.[a]

investigation: The gathering and assessment of objective information to determine if a child has been or is at risk of being maltreated. Generally includes face-to-face contact with the victim and results in a disposition as to whether the alleged report is substantiated or not.[b]

juvenile and family court: Court that specializes in areas such as child maltreatment, domestic violence, juvenile delinquency, divorce, child custody, and child support. These courts were established in most states to resolve conflict and to otherwise intervene in the lives of families in a manner that promotes the best interest of children.[a]

kinship care: Kinship care is the full time care, nurturing, and protection of a child by relatives, members of their tribe or clan, godparents, stepparents, or any adult who has a kinship bond with the child. This definition is designed to be inclusive and respectful of cultural values and ties of affection. It allows a child to grow to adulthood in a family environment.[a]

learning disability: A disorder in basic psychological processes involved in understanding or using language, spoken or written, that may manifest itself in an imperfect ability to listen, think, speak, read, write, spell or use mathematical calculations. The term includes conditions such as perceptual disability, brain injury, minimal brain dysfunction, dyslexia, and developmental aphasia.[b]

maltreatment: An act or failure to act by a parent, caretaker, or other person as defined under state law which results in physical abuse, neglect, medical neglect, sexual abuse, emotional abuse, or an act or failure to act which presents an imminent risk of serious harm to a child.[b]

mandated reporter: Individuals required by state statutes to report suspected child abuse and neglect to the proper authorities (usually child protective services or law enforcement agencies). Mandated reporters typically include educators and other school personnel, health-care and mental health professionals, social workers, child care providers, and law enforcement officers or others who have frequent contact with children and families. Some states identify all citizens as mandated reporters.[a]

medical neglect: A type of maltreatment caused by failure by the caretaker to provide for the appropriate health care of the child although financially able to do so, or offered financial or other means to do so.[b]

mental health services: Beneficial activities which aim to overcome issues involving emotional disturbance or maladaptive behavior adversely affecting socialization, learning, or development. Usually provided by public or private mental health agencies and includes both residential and non-residential activities.[b]

not substantiated: See unsubstantiated.

other planned permanent living arrangement (OPPLA): A permanency option in which the child welfare agency maintains care and custody responsibilities for and supervision of the child, and places the child in a setting in which the child is expected to remain until adulthood. This might be with foster parents or relative caregivers who have made a commitment to care for the child permanently, or in a long-term care facility (for children with developmental disabilities who require long-term residential care, for example). This term was created when the Adoption and Safe Families Act struck the term "long-term foster care" from statute. OPPLA (or APPLA) is selected only when reunification, adoption, legal guardianship, and relative placements have been determined to be inappropriate.[a]

parens patriae: A legal term referring to the state's power to act for or on behalf of children who cannot act on their own behalf, in their best interest.[a]

parent: The birth mother/father, adoptive mother/father, or step mother/father of the child.[b]

parental rights: The legal rights and corresponding legal obligations that go along with being the parent of a child.[a]

paternity: Legal or biological fatherhood. Paternity establishment is the legal procedure to determine if a man is the biological father of a particular child and to establish his rights and responsibilities in regard to that child.[a]

perpetrator: The person who has been determined to have caused or knowingly allowed the maltreatment of the child.[b]

physical abuse: Child abuse that results in physical injury to a child. This may include, burning, hitting, punching, shaking, kicking, beating, or otherwise harming a child. Although an injury resulting from physical abuse is not accidental, the parent or caregiver may not have intended to hurt the child. The injury may have resulted from severe discipline, including injurious spanking, or physical punishment that is inappropriate to the child's age or condition. The injury may be the result of a single episode or of repeated episodes and can range in severity from minor marks and bruising to death.[a]

physical neglect: Failure to provide for a child's basic survival needs, such as nutrition, clothing, shelter, hygiene, and medical care. Physical neglect may also involve inadequate supervision of a child and other forms of reckless disregard of the child's safety and welfare.[a]

post-investigation services: Beneficial activities provided or arranged by the child protective services agency, social services agency, and/or the child welfare agency for the child/family as a result of needs discovered during the course of the investigation. Include such services as Family Preservation, Family Support, and foster care provided as a result of the report of alleged child maltreatment, or offered prior to the report and continued after the disposition of the investigation. Post-investigation services are delivered within the first 90 days after the disposition of the report.[b]

prenatal substance exposure: Fetal exposure to maternal drug and alcohol use that can significantly increase the risk for developmental and neurological disabilities in the child. The effects can cause severe neurological damage and growth retardation in the substance-exposed newborn.[a]

preventive services: Beneficial activities aimed at preventing child abuse and neglect. Such activities may be directed at specific populations identified as being at increased risk of becoming abusive and may be designed to increase the strength and stability of families, to increase parents' confidence and competence in their parenting abilities, and to afford children a stable and supportive environment. [b]

prior victim: A child victim with previous substantiated or indicated incidents of maltreatment.[b]

protective custody: A form of custody required to remove a child from his or her home and place in out-of-home care. Law enforcement may place a child in protective custody based on an independent determination that the child's health, safety, and welfare is jeopardized. A child can also be placed in protective custody via court order.[a]

protective/promotive factor: Strengths and resources that appear to mediate or serve as a buffer against risk factors that contribute to maltreatment. These factors may strengthen the parent-child relationships, ability to cope with stress, and capacity to provide for children. Protective factors include nurturing and attachment, knowledge of parenting and of child and youth development, parental resilience, social connections, and concrete supports for parents.[a]

psychological or emotional maltreatment: Type of maltreatment that refers to acts or omissions, other than physical abuse or sexual abuse, that caused, or could have caused, conduct, cognitive, affective, or other mental disorders. Includes emotional neglect, psychological abuse, mental injury, etc. Frequently occurs as verbal abuse or excessive demands on a child's performance and may cause the child to have a negative self-image and disturbed behavior.[b]

relinquishment: Voluntary termination or release of all parental rights and duties that legally frees a child to be adopted. This is sometimes referred to as a surrender or as making an adoption plan for one's child.[a]

resilience: The ability to adapt well to adversity, trauma, tragedy, threats, or even significant sources of stress. Parental resilience is considered a protective factor in child abuse and neglect prevention. Resilience in children enables them to thrive, mature, and increase competence in the midst of adverse circumstances. Resilience can be fostered and developed in children as it involves behaviors, thoughts, and actions that can be learned over time and is impacted by positive and healthy relationships with parents, caregivers, and other adults.[a]

respite care: Child care offered for designated periods of time to allow a caregiver to tend to other family members; alleviate a work, job, health, or housing crisis; or take a break from the stress of caring for a seriously ill child. Respite for foster and adoptive parents is a preventive measure that enhances quality of care for the child, gives the caregiver a deserved and necessary break, and ensures healthy and stable placements for children.[a]

risk: In child welfare, the likelihood that a child will be maltreated in the future. A risk assessment is a measure of the likelihood that a child will be maltreated in the future, frequently through the use of checklists, matrices, scales, and other methods of measurement.[a]

risk factor: Behaviors and conditions present in the child, parent, or family that will likely contribute to child maltreatment occurring in the future. Major risk factors include substance abuse, domestic/family violence, and mental health problems.[a]

safe haven: When applied to legislation, refers to the policy in which a parent can relinquish a child, usually a newborn, to lawfully designated places such as a hospital. When a child is surrendered in this way, the parent is protected from criminal prosecution. The scope and specifications of the rule vary widely across the states.[a]

safety plan: A casework document developed when it is determined that a child is in imminent or potential risk of serious harm. In the safety plan, the caseworker targets the factors that are causing or contributing to the risk of imminent serious harm to the child and identifies, along with the family, the interventions that will control the safety factors and assure the child's protection.[a]

sexual abuse: According to the Child Abuse Prevention and Treatment Act (CAPTA), the employment, use, persuasion, inducement, enticement, or coercion of any child to engage in, or assist any other person to engage in, any sexually explicit conduct or simulation of such conduct for the purpose of producing a visual depiction of such conduct; or the rape, and in cases of caretaker or interfamilial relationships, statutory rape, molestation, prostitution, or other form of sexual exploitation of children, or incest with children.[a]

shaken baby syndrome: The collection of signs and symptoms resulting from the violent shaking of an infant or small child. The consequences of less severe cases may not be brought to the attention of medical professionals and may never be diagnosed. In severe cases that usually result in death or severe neurological consequences, the child usually becomes immediately unconscious and suffers rapidly escalating, life-threatening central nervous system dysfunction.[a]

sibling abuse: The physical, emotional, or sexual maltreatment of a child by a brother or sister.[a]

stepparent: The husband or wife, by a subsequent marriage, of the child victim's mother or father.[b]

substance abuse services: Beneficial activities designed to deter, reduce, or eliminate substance abuse or chemical dependency.[b]

substantiated: An investigation disposition concluding that the allegation of child maltreatment or risk of maltreatment was supported or founded by state law or state policy. A child protective services determination means that credible evidence exists that child abuse or neglect has occurred.[a]

Temporary Assistance for Needy Families (TANF): A program that provides assistance and work opportunities to needy families by granting states the federal funds and wide flexibility to develop and implement their own welfare programs. The focus of the program is to help move recipients into work and to turn welfare into a program of temporary assistance.[a]

termination of parental rights (TPR): Voluntary or involuntary legal severance of the rights of a parent to the care, custody, and control of a child and to any benefits that, by law, would flow to the parent from the child, such as inheritance.[a]

therapeutic foster care: Intensive care provided by foster parents who have received special training to care for a wide variety of children and adolescents, usually those with significant emotional, behavioral, or social problems or medical needs. Therapeutic foster parents typically receive additional supports and services.[a]

unsubstantiated: Not substantiated. An investigation disposition that determines that there is not sufficient evidence under state law or policy to conclude that a child has been maltreated or is at risk of maltreatment. A child protective services determination means that credible evidence does not exist that child abuse or neglect has occurred.[a]

well-being: The result of meeting a child's educational, emotional, and physical and mental health needs. Well-being is achieved when families have the capacity to provide for the needs of their children or when families are receiving the support and services needed to adequately meet the needs of their children.[a]

youth permanency: The opportunity for a continuous, lifetime relationship with a nurturing parent, caregiver, or other adult. Includes unconditional commitment by a caring adult, lifelong support, involvement of the youth as a participant, a legal arrangement, where possible, and the opportunity to maintain contacts with important people, including birth family members and siblings.[a]

Chapter 42

Where to Report Child Abuse

The chapter includes a list of state contact numbers for specific agencies designated to receive and investigate reports of suspected child abuse and neglect.

Alabama
Phone: 334-242-9500
Website: http://dhr.alabama.gov/services/Child_Protective_Services/Abuse_Neglect_Reporting.aspx
Additional information: Visit the website above for information on reporting or call Childhelp (800-422-4453) for assistance.

Alaska
Toll-Free: 800-478-4444
Website: http://www.hss.state.ak.us/ocs/default.htm

Arizona
Toll-Free: 888-SOS-CHILD (888-767-2445)
Website: https://www.azdes.gov/dcyf/cps/reporting.asp

Arkansas
Toll-Free: 800-482-5964
Website: http://www.arkansas.gov/reportARchildabuse

Reprinted from "State Child Abuse Reporting Numbers," U.S. Department of Health and Human Services, January 5, 2012. All contact information was verified and updated in July 2012.

California
Website: http://www.dss.cahwnet.gov/cdssweb/PG20.htm
Additional information: Visit the website above for information on reporting or call Childhelp (800-422-4453) for assistance.

Colorado
Phone: 303-866-5932
Website: http://www.cdhs.state.co.us/childwelfare/FAQ.htm
Additional information: Visit the website above for information on reporting or call Childhelp (800-422-4453) for assistance.

Connecticut
Toll-Free: 800-842-2288
Toll-Free TDD: 800-624-5518
Website: http://www.state.ct.us/dcf/HOTLINE.htm

Delaware
Toll-Free: 800-292-9582
Website: http://kids.delaware.gov/services/crisis.shtml

District of Columbia
Phone: 202-671-SAFE (202-671-7233)
Website: http://cfsa.dc.gov/DC/CFSA/Support+the+Safety+Net/Report+Child+Abuse+and+Neglect

Florida
Toll-Free: 800-96-ABUSE (800-962-2873)
Website: http://www.dcf.state.fl.us/abuse

Georgia
Website: http://dfcs.dhs.georgia.gov
Additional information: Visit the website above for information on reporting or call Childhelp (800-422-4453) for assistance.

Hawaii
Phone: 808-832-5300
Website: http://www.hawaii.gov/dhs/protection/social_services/child_welfare

Idaho
Toll-Free: 800-926-2588
TDD: 208-332-7205

Website: http://healthandwelfare.idaho.gov/
Children/AbuseNeglect/ChildProtectionContactPhone
Numbers/tabid/475/Default.aspx

Illinois
Toll-Free: 800-25-ABUSE (800-252-2873)
Phone: 217-785-4020
Website: http://www.state.il.us/dcfs/child/index.shtml

Indiana
Toll-Free: 800-800-5556
Website: http://www.in.gov/dcs/protection/dfcchi.html

Iowa
Toll-Free: 800-362-2178
Website: http://www.dhs.state.ia.us/dhs2005/dhs_homepage/
children_family/abuse_reporting/child_abuse.html

Kansas
Toll-Free: 800-922-5330
Website: http://www.dcf.ks.gov/Pages/Default.aspx

Kentucky
Toll-Free: 877-KYSAFE1 (877-597-2331)
Website: http://chfs.ky.gov/dcbs/dpp/childsafety.htm

Louisiana
Toll-Free: 855-4LA-KIDS (855-452-5437)
Website: http://dss.louisiana.gov/index.cfm?md=
pagebuilder&tmp=home&pid=109

Maine
Toll-Free: 800-452-1999
Toll-Free TTY: 800-963-9490
Website: http://www.maine.gov/dhhs/ocfs/hotlines.htm

Maryland
Website: http://www.dhr.state.md.us/cps/report.htm
Additional information: Visit the website above
for information on reporting or call Childhelp
(800-422-4453) for assistance.

Massachusetts

Toll-Free: 800-792-5200
Website: http://www.mass.gov/eohhs/consumer/
family-services/child-abuse-neglect

Michigan

Toll-Free: 855-444-3911
Website: http://www.michigan.gov/dhs/0,1607,7-124-5452
_7119---,00.html

Minnesota

Website: http://www.dhs.state.mn.us/main/idcplg?IdcService
=GET_DYNAMIC_CONVERSION&RevisionSelectionMethod
=LatestReleased&dDocName=id_000152
Additional information: Visit the website above for information
on reporting or call Childhelp (800-422-4453) for assistance.

Mississippi

Toll-Free: 800-222-8000
Phone: 601-432-4570
Website: http://www.mdhs.state.ms.us/fcs_prot.html

Missouri

Toll-Free: 800-392-3738
Phone: 573-751-3448
Website: http://www.dss.mo.gov/cd/rptcan.htm

Montana

Toll-Free: 866-820-5437
Website: http://www.dphhs.mt.gov/cfsd/index.shtml

Nebraska

Toll-Free: 800-652-1999
Website: http://dhhs.ne.gov/children_family_services/
Pages/children_family_services.aspx

Nevada

Toll-Free: 800-992-5757
Phone: 702-399-0081
Website: http://dcfs.state.nv.us/DCFS
_ReportSuspectedChildAbuse.htm

New Hampshire
Toll-Free: 800-894-5533
Toll-Free TDD: 800-735-2964
Phone: 603-271-6556
Fax: 603-271-6565 (Report Child Abuse Fax)
Website: http://www.dhhs.state.nh.us/dcyf/cps/contact.htm

New Jersey
Toll-Free: 877-NJ ABUSE (877-652-2873)
Toll-Free TDD/TTY: 800-835-5510
Website: http://www.state.nj.us/dcf/abuse/how

New Mexico
Toll-Free: 855-333-SAFE (855-333-7233)
Website: http://www.cyfd.org/content/reporting-abuse-or-neglect

New York
Toll-Free: 800-342-3720
Toll-Free TDD/TTY: 800-638-5163
Phone: 518-473-7793
Website: http://www.ocfs.state.ny.us/main/cps

North Carolina
Website: http://www.dhhs.state.nc.us/dss/cps/index.htm
Additional information: Visit the website above for information
on reporting or call Childhelp (800-422-4453) for assistance.

North Dakota
Website: http://www.nd.gov/dhs/services/childfamily/cps/#reporting
Additional information: Visit the website above for information on
reporting or call Childhelp (800-422-4453) for assistance.

Ohio
Website: http://jfs.ohio.gov/County/County_Directory.pdf
Additional information: Contact the county Public Children
Services Agency or call Childhelp (800-422-4453) for assistance.

Oklahoma
Toll-Free: 800-522-3511
Website: http://www.okdhs.org/
programsandservices/cps/default.htm

Oregon
Website: http://www.oregon.gov/DHS/children/
abuse/cps/report.shtml
Additional information: Visit the website above for information
on reporting or call Childhelp (800-422-4453) for assistance.

Pennsylvania
Toll-Free: 800-932-0313
Toll-Free TDD: 866-872-1677
Website: http://www.dpw.state.pa.us/forchildren/
childwelfareservices/calltoreportchildabuse!/index.htm

Puerto Rico
Toll-Free: 800-981-8333
Phone: 787-749-1333
Website (Spanish): http://www.gobierno.pr/GPRPortal/
StandAlone/AgencyInformation.aspx?Filter=177

Rhode Island
Toll-Free: 800-RI-CHILD (800-742-4453)
Website: http://www.dcyf.ri.gov/child_welfare/index.php

South Carolina
Phone: 803-898-7318
Website: http://dss.sc.gov/content/customers/protection/cps/
index.aspx
Additional information: Visit the website above for information on
reporting or call Childhelp (800-422-4453) for assistance.

South Dakota
Website: http://dss.sd.gov/cps/protective/reporting.asp
Additional information: Visit the website above for information on
reporting or call Childhelp (800-422-4453) for assistance.

Tennessee
Toll-Free: 877-237-0004 or 877-54ABUSE (877-542-2873)
Website: https://reportabuse.state.tn.us

Texas
Department of Family and Protective Services
Toll-Free: 800-252-5400

Toll-Free TTY: 800-735-2989
Website: https://www.dfps.state.tx.us/Child_Protection/
About_Child_Protective_Services/reportChildAbuse.asp
Spanish: http://www.dfps.state.tx.us/default-sp.asp

Utah
Toll-Free: 855-323-3237
Website: http://www.hsdcfs.utah.gov

Vermont
After hours: 800-649-5285
Website: http://www.dcf.state.vt.us/fsd/reporting_child_abuse

Virginia
Toll-Free: 800-552-7096
Phone: 804-786-8536
Website: http://www.dss.virginia.gov/family/cps/index.html

Washington
Toll-Free: 800-562-5624 or 866-END-HARM (866-363-4276)
Toll-Free TTY: 800-624-6186
Website: http://www1.dshs.wa.gov/ca/safety/abuseReport.asp?2

West Virginia
Toll-Free: 800-352-6513
Website: http://www.wvdhhr.org/bcf/children_adult/cps/report.asp

Wisconsin
Website: http://dcf.wisconsin.gov/children/CPS/cpswimap.htm
Additional information: Visit the website above for information on reporting or call Childhelp (800-422-4453) for assistance.

Wyoming
Website: http://dfsweb.state.wy.us/protective-services/cps/index.html
Additional information: Visit the website above for information on reporting or call Childhelp (800-422-4453) for assistance.

Chapter 43

A Directory of Organizations Dedicated to Promoting Healthy Families

Adult Survivors of Child Abuse
The Morris Center
P.O. Box 14477
San Francisco, CA 94114
Website: http://www.ascasupport.org

Adult Survivors of Child Abuse is a support group program for adults who experienced child abuse. The program began in San Francisco, and groups now exist in several other states and in other parts of the world.

Advocates for Youth
2000 M Street NW, Suite 750
Washington, DC 20036
Phone: 202-419-3420
Fax: 202-419-1448
Website: http://www.advocatesforyouth.org

Information in this chapter was compiled from resources listed in "Child Abuse and Neglect Prevention: Related Organizations Lists," Child Welfare Information Gateway (www.childwelfare.gov-and other sources deemed reliable. To search Child Welfare Information Gateway for child-welfare related national organizations by topic, use the Related Organizations Search at http://www.childwelfare.gov/organizations/search.cfm. Inclusion does not constitute endorsement, and there is no implication associated with omission. All contact information was verified in December 2012.

Advocates for Youth provides resources, technical assistance and training to help ensure that young people receive accurate and complete information about sexual health and that they are treated with respect.

American Academy of Pediatrics
141 Northwest Point Boulevard
Elk Grove Village, IL 60007-1098
Toll-Free: 800-433-9016
Phone: 847-434-4000
Fax: 847-434-8000
Website: http://aap.org
Parent Information Website: http://www.healthychildren.org

The American Academy of Pediatrics is a professional organization of healthcare providers who provide services to patients from birth through age 21. Through a special website for parents, it offers information about wide-variety of issues related to child development, healthy living, and family life.

American Humane Association
1400 16th Street NW, Suite 360
Washington, DC 20036
Toll-Free: 800-227-4645
Phone: 303-792-9900
Fax: 303-792-5333
Website: http://www.americanhumane.org
E-mail: info@americanhumane.org

The mission of the American Humane Association (AHA) is to prevent cruelty, abuse, neglect, and the exploitation of children and animals. AHA offers education and resources to professionals, conducts conferences, roundtables and training, and provides consultation and technical assistance to state and county child welfare and community agencies. In addition, AHA conducts research and evaluation, disseminates knowledge on child welfare, and advocates for social service systems that promote the best interest of children, youth, and families. AHA also offers membership subscriptions.

AHA promotes collaboration across systems, including its recent focus on the juvenile justice system and the restorative justice approach for youth justice. AHA is also known for its work on the human-animal bond which includes programs that strengthen families and their connection to animals. AHA is actively involved in child welfare legislation and public policy at both the state and federal levels.

American Professional Society on the Abuse of Children
350 Poplar Avenue
Elmhurst, IL 60126
Toll-Free: 877-402-7722
Phone: 630-941-1235
Fax: 630-359-4274
Website: http://www.apsac.org
E-mail: apsac@apsac.org

The American Professional Society on the Abuse of Children (AP-SAC) addresses all facets of the professional response to child maltreatment: prevention, assessment, intervention, and treatment. APSAC is committed to preventing and eliminating the recurrence of child maltreatment, promoting research and guidelines to inform professional practice, connecting professionals from the many disciplines to promote the best response to child maltreatment, and educating the public about child abuse and neglect.

Association for Play Therapy
3198 Willow Avenue, Suite 110
Clovis, CA 93612
Phone: 559-294-2128
Fax: 559-294-2129
Website: http://www.a4pt.org
E-mail: info@a4pt.org

The Association for Play Therapy is a professional society for therapists who use a systematic approach that employs play to help children who may not have the verbal ability to participate in other forms of psychotherapy.

Association for the Treatment of Sexual Abusers
4900 SW Griffith Drive, Suite 274
Beaverton, OR 97005
Phone: 503-643-1023
Fax: 503-643-5084
Website: http://www.atsa.com
E-mail: atsa@atsa.com

The Association for the Treatment of Sexual Abusers is a professional organization that seeks to enhance community safety through the prevention of sexual abuse. It supports research and education for the purpose of effectively assessing, treating, and managing people who have sexually abused others or who are considered to be at risk for becoming abusers.

Australian Institute of Family Studies
Level 20 South Tower
485 La Trobe Street
Melbourne, Victoria 3000
Australia
Phone: +61 3 9214 7888
Fax: +61 3 9214 7839
Website: http://www.aifs.gov.au

The Australian Institute of Family Studies is an agency of the Australian government. It conducts research and provides information on matters that impact family health, including childhood development and sexual assault.

AVANCE, Inc.
National Headquarters
118 North Medina
San Antonio, TX 78207
Phone: 210-270-4630
Fax: 210-270-4636
Website: http://www.avance.org

AVANCE's mission is to provide support and education services that will strengthen low-income families. AVANCE's focus is on community-based intervention that is family-centered, preventive, comprehensive, and continuous through the integration and collaboration of services. The AVANCE Family Support and Education Program is an example of one of AVANCE's programs: Targeted primarily at Hispanic at-risk parents with young children, the program aims to strengthen parent-child relationships and the parental role of advocate for the child. To find local contact information, see the drop-down box, "Our Chapters," on the homepage of the organization's website.

Center for Effective Discipline
327 Groveport Pike
Canal Winchester, OH 43110
Phone: 614- 834-7946
Fax: 614- 321-6308
Website: http://www.stophitting.org
E-mail: Info@StopHitting.org

The Center for Effective Discipline (CED) provides educational information to the public on the effects of corporal punishment of children and alternatives to its use. CED is the headquarters for and the coordinator of both the National Coalition to Abolish Corporal Punishment in Schools (NCACPS) and End Physical Punishment of Children (EPOCH-USA).

Center for Violence and Injury Prevention
Washington University in St. Louis
CB 1007
700 Rosedale Avenue
St. Louis, MO 63112
Phone: 314-935-8129
Website: http://cvip.wustl.edu/Pages/Home.aspx
E-mail: bcvip@wustl.edu

The Center for Violence and Injury Prevention (CVIP) promotes healthy young families and healthy young adults by advancing evidence-based violence prevention through a range of education, research, and training activities on topics that include child abuse and neglect and sexual violence. CVIP's partners and collaborators include multiple universities and community-based agencies serving the most vulnerable populations.

Chadwick Center for Children and Families
3020 Children's Way, MC 5017
San Diego, CA 92123
Phone: 858-966-5814
Fax: 858-966-8535
Website: http://www.ChadwickCenter.org
E-mail: chadwickcenter@rchsd.org

The Chadwick Center's mission is to protect children and strengthen families through prevention, treatment, education, public policy, advocacy, and research in the areas of child maltreatment and family violence. The Center uses a multidisciplinary, family-centered approach. The Chadwick Center offers accredited professional education to those involved in fields of prevention, investigation, diagnosis, treatment, and prosecution of child abuse and family violence.

Chapel Hill Training-Outreach Project, Inc.
800 Eastowne Drive, Suite 105
Chapel Hill, NC 27514
Phone: 919-490-5577
TDD: 919-490-5577
Fax: 919-490-4905
Website: http://chtop.org

The mission of the Chapel Hill Training-Outreach Project, Inc. (CHTOP) is to develop and deliver programs and strategies that will enhance the lives of children, youth and families. Of principal concern are families in poverty, families caring for the elderly, children with disabilities or chronic illness, and children at risk of abuse and neglect.

Child Abuse Prevention Network
Website: http://www.child-abuse.com

The Child Abuse Prevention Network, originally launched as an outreach effort of the Family Life Development Center at Cornell University, is sponsored by LifeNET, Inc. Child maltreatment, physical abuse, psychological maltreatment, neglect, sexual abuse, and emotional abuse and neglect are key areas of concern. Through internet linkages, the Network provides professionals with online tools and support for the identification, investigation, treatment, adjudication, and prevention of child abuse and neglect.

Child AbuseWatch.NET
One Child International, Inc.
590 SW 9th Terrace, Suite 2
Pompano Beach, FL 33069
Website (English): http://www.abusewatch.net
Website (Spanish): http://www.abusewatch.net/CAN_esp.php
E-mail: info@abusewatch.net

Child AbuseWatch.NET is a resource center operated by One Child International, Inc. It provides information and resources about child abuse, child abuse awareness, and child abuse education for professionals as well as other community members involved in child abuse prevention activities.

Child Lures Prevention
5166 Shelburne Road
Shelburne, VT 05482
Toll-Free: 800-552-2197
Phone: 802-985-8458
Fax: 802-985-8418
Website: http://www.childluresprevention.com
E-mail: info@childluresprevention.com

The primary goals of Child Lures Prevention are to raise public awareness concerning the prevalence of childhood sexual exploitation and related crimes against children and to make prevention of these crimes a national priority.

Child Molestation Research and Prevention Institute
2515 Santa Clara Avenue, Suite 208
Alameda, CA 94501
Phone: 510-740-1410
Website: http://www.childmolestationprevention.org
E-mail: contact@childmolestationprevention.org

The Child Molestation Research and Prevention Institute is a national, science-based nonprofit organization dedicated to preventing child sexual abuse through research, education, and family support. Its focus is on providing information to professionals and to families about the early warning signs of a problem, as well as the availability of early diagnosis and effective treatment.

Child Safe
St. Vincent's Center/Catholic Charities
2600 Pot Spring Road
Timonium, MD 21093
Phone: 410-252-4000
Website: http://www.childsafeeducation.com
E-mail: childsafe@catholiccharities-md.org

The Child Safe program is a national outreach and educational program aimed at preventing and reducing the negative impact of abuse on children, with a special emphasis on sexual abuse. The Child Safe program offers workshops, educational materials, and online training programs for primary caregivers, professionals, volunteers and children around the topics of sexual abuse awareness, prevention, and intervention.

Child Welfare Information Gateway
Children's Bureau/ACYF
1250 Maryland Avenue SW, Eighth Floor
Washington, DC 20024
Toll-Free: 800-394-3366
Fax: 703-225-2357
Website: http://www.childwelfare.gov
E-mail: info@childwelfare.gov

Child Welfare Information Gateway connects professionals and the general public to information and resources targeted to the safety, permanency, and well-being of children and families. A service of the Children's Bureau, Administration for Children and Families, U.S. Department of Health and Human Services, Child Welfare Information

Gateway provides access to programs, research, laws and policies, training resources, statistics, and much more.

Child Welfare League of America

1726 M Street NW, Suite 500
Washington, DC 20036
Phone: 202-688-4200
Fax: 202-833-1689
Website: http://www.cwla.org

The Child Welfare League of America (CWLA) is the oldest national organization serving vulnerable children, youth, and their families. CWLA provides training, consultation, and technical assistance to child welfare professionals and agencies while also educating the public on emerging issues that affect abused, neglected, and at-risk children. Through its publications, conferences, and teleconferences, CWLA shares information on emerging trends, specific topics in child welfare practice (family foster care, kinship care, adoption, positive youth development), and federal and state policies.

Childhelp USA

15757 North 78th Street, Suite B
Scottsdale, AZ 85260
Toll-Free: 800-4-A-CHILD (800-422-4453)
Toll-Free TDD: 800-2-A-CHILD (800-222-4453)
Phone: 480-922-8212
Fax: 480-922-7061
Website: http://www.childhelp.org

Childhelp is dedicated to helping victims of child abuse and neglect. Childhelp's approach focuses on prevention, intervention and treatment. The Childhelp National Child Abuse Hotline, 800-4-A-CHILD, operates 24 hours a day, seven days a week, and receives calls from throughout the United States, Canada, the U.S. Virgin Islands, Puerto Rico and Guam. Childhelp's programs and services also include residential treatment services; children's advocacy centers; therapeutic foster care; group homes; child abuse prevention, education and training; and the National Day of Hope, part of National Child Abuse Prevention Month every April.

Children Without a Voice USA

P.O. Box 4351
Alpharetta, GA 30023
Website: http://www.childrenwithoutavoiceusa.org
E-mail: email@childrenwithoutavoiceusa.org

The mission of Children Without a Voice USA is to raise awareness and to prevent crimes against children and child abuse and neglect through advocacy and education.

Circle of Parents
2100 South Marshall Boulevard, Suite 305
Chicago, IL 60623
Phone: 773-257-0111
Fax: 773-277-0715
Website: http://www.circleofparents.org

The mission of the Circle of Parents is to prevent child abuse and neglect and to strengthen families through friendly, supportive, mutual self-help parent support groups and children's programs. Currently the Circle of Parents national network represents a partnership of parent leaders and 26 statewide organizations in 25 states and Puerto Rico. The organization was formed after a successful collaborative project of Prevent Child Abuse America and the National Family Support Roundtable, which was made possible by the Children's Bureau, Administration on Children, Youth and Families, U.S. Department of Health and Human Services. The Circle of Parents website provides links to information about the program model, its state network member organizations, training and technical assistance to its membership, parenting resources, and more.

Committee for Children
2815 Second Avenue, Suite 400
Seattle, WA 98121
Toll-Free: 800-634-4449
Fax: 206-438-6765
Website: http://www.cfchildren.org
E-mail: clientsupport@cfchildren.org

Committee for Children creates research-based learning materials that focus on social and emotional learning. Their curricula address such topics as skills for learning, violence prevention, bullying, child abuse, and personal safety.

Cooperative Extension System
United States Department of Agriculture
National Institute of Food and Agriculture
1400 Independence Avenue SW, Stop 2201
Washington, DC 20250-2201
Phone: 202-720-4423

Website: http://www.csrees.usda.gov/Extension
E-mail: webcomments@csrees.usda.gov

The Cooperative Extension System is a nationwide educational collaboration of federal, state, and local governments and state land-grant universities. The mission of the Cooperative Extension System is to disseminate research-based information on topics as varied as family and child development, health, nutrition, agriculture, horticulture, small business and personal finance. Each state Extension serves its residents through a network of local or regional offices staffed by educators in their field.

Court Appointed Special Advocates for Children
100 West Harrison Street, North Tower, Suite 500
Seattle, WA 98119
Toll-Free: 800-628-3233
Website: http://www.casaforchildren.org

Court Appointed Special Advocates (CASA) for Children is a network of programs in which volunteers monitor child abuse and neglect cases as they move through the legal and social services systems. The goal is to ensure that cases are resolved efficiently and that children find permanent homes.

Crime Victims' Institute
College of Criminal Justice
Sam Houston State University
P.O. Box 2180
Huntsville, TX 77341-2180
Phone: 936-294-3100
Fax: 936-294-4296
Website: http://www.crimevictimsinstitute.org
E-mail: crimevictims@shsu.edu

A Texas-based organization, the Crime Victims' Institute seeks to assist victims of criminal activity, conduct research, and inform policymakers.

Darkness to Light
7 Radcliffe Street, Suite 200
Charleston, SC 29403
Toll-Free: 866-FOR-LIGHT (866-367-5444)
Phone: 843-965-5444
Fax: 843-965-5449
Website: http://www.darkness2light.org

Darkness to Light is a primary prevention program whose mission is to engage adults in the prevention of child sexual abuse; to reduce the incidence of child sexual abuse nationally through education and public awareness aimed at adults; and to provide adults with information to recognize and react responsibly to child sexual abuse.

Doris Duke Charitable Foundation
650 Fifth Avenue, 19th Floor
New York, NY 10019
Phone: 212-974-7000
Fax: 212-974-7590
Website: http://www.ddcf.org
E-mail: webmaster@ddcf.org

The mission of the Doris Duke Charitable Foundation's Child Abuse Prevention Program is to protect children from abuse and neglect in order to promote their healthy development. The program awards grants to organizations to improve parent-child interactions and to increase parents' access to information and services that help prevent child maltreatment before it occurs.

Every Child Matters Education Fund
1023 15th Street NW, Suite 401
Washington, DC 20005
Phone: 202-223-8177
Fax: 202-223-8499
Website: http://www.everychildmatters.org
E-mail: info@everychildmatters.org

By employing systematic public education campaigns, the Every Child Matters Education Fund provides opportunities for focusing public attention on children's issues including the prevention of child abuse and neglect. The Every Child Matters Education Fund works with children's organizations and volunteers to conduct campaigns of public opinion polling, press outreach, and community and voter outreach.

FaithTrust Institute
2900 Eastlake Avenue East, Suite 200
Seattle, WA 98102
Toll-Free: 877-860-2255
Phone: 206-634-1903
Fax: 206-634-0115
Website: http://www.faithtrustinstitute.org
E-mail: info@faithtrustinstitute.org

The FaithTrust Institute is an interreligious educational resource that addresses issues of sexual and domestic violence. The Institute's goals are to engage religious leaders in the task of ending abuse, and to serve as a bridge between the religious and secular communities.

Family Life Development Center
Cornell University
Beebe Hall
Ithaca, NY 14853-4401
Phone: 607-255-7794
Fax: 607-255-8562
Website: http://www.human.cornell.edu/fldc
E-mail: fldc@cornell.edu

The mission of the Family Life Development Center is to improve professional and public efforts to understand and act upon risk and protective factors in the lives of children, youth, families, and communities that affect family strengths, child well-being, and youth development. The FLDC accomplishes its mission through research, training, outreach, education, and program development and implementation. Current areas of special interest include childhood violence prevention and evaluation of programs designed to prevent abuse and neglect. The FLDC operates the National Data Archive on Child Abuse and Neglect (NDACAN), which promotes scholarly exchange among researchers and makes original data available for secondary analysis.

Fight Crime: Invest in Kids
1212 New York Ave NW, Suite 300
Washington, DC 20005
Phone: 202-776-0027
Fax: 202-776-0110
Website: http://www.fightcrime.org
E-mail: info@fightcrime.org

Fight Crime: Invest in Kids is dedicated to reviewing research about what really works and what does not work to keep children from becoming criminals. The organization strives to educate policymakers, the mass media, and the public through briefings about effective crime prevention programs while also serving as an information clearinghouse for journalists, policymakers, and the public. Major topics of interest include child abuse and neglect prevention, prevention programs for prekindergartners, bullying prevention, and more.

Freddie Mac Foundation
8250 Jones Branch Drive
Mailstop A40
McLean, VA 22102-3110
Phone: 703-918-8888
Fax: 703-918-8895
Website: http://www.freddiemacfoundation.org
E-mail: freddiemac_foundation@freddiemac.com

The Freddie Mac Foundation provides funds for various nonprofit organizations that work on behalf of children, youth, and families. The Foundation focuses on children and prevention-oriented programs. Typically, grants are awarded to programs that build strong families, prevent child abuse and neglect, and recruit foster and adoptive parents. Among the Foundation's major programs are Healthy Families America and Wednesday's Child USA, a campaign to promote adoptions.

Future of Children
267 Wallace Hall
Princeton University
Princeton, NJ 08544
Phone: 609-258-5894
Website: http://www.princeton.edu/futureofchildren
E-mail: foc@princeton.edu

The Future of Children, part of the Center for Research on Child Wellbeing at the Princeton University's Woodrow Wilson School, conducts research to help provide information to policymakers, the media, and others about issues that impact children.

General Federation of Women's Clubs
1734 N Street NW
Washington, DC 20036-2990
Toll-Free: 800-443-4392
Phone: 202-347-3168
Fax: 202-835-0246
Website: http://www.gfwc.org
E-mail: gfwc@gfwc.org

The General Federation of Women's Clubs is the world's largest and oldest women's volunteer organization. GFWC's members include business owners, teachers, elected officials, homemakers, corporate executives, college students, and retirees. The organization's members

591

are united by dedication to community improvement through volunteer service. GFWC advocates for conservation, quality education, health, civic awareness, safety, and crime prevention. The Federation's Advocates for Children Program is a referral and networking resource for Club members interested in assisting children. The program focuses on advocacy on behalf of children, prevention, and on improving public awareness of the importance of early intervention.

Generation Five
P.O Box 1715
Oakland, CA 94604
Website: http://generationfive.org
E-mail: info@generationFIVE.org

The mission of Generation Five is to end the sexual abuse of children within five generations. Through survivor leadership, community organizing, and public action, Generation Five works to interrupt and mend the impact of child sexual abuse on individuals, families, and communities. Generation Five offers training and consulting on child sexual abuse to professionals and community organizations. This training helps people to develop child sexual abuse programs and pilot projects or to incorporate child sexual abuse issues into their existing programs.

Healthy Families America
200 South Wabash, 10th Floor
Chicago, IL 60604
Phone: 312-663-3520
Fax: 312-939-8962
Website: http://healthyfamiliesamerica.org

Healthy Families America, a program of Prevent Child Abuse America, promotes child health and development and positive parenting through voluntary home visits by trained staff.

International Center for Assault Prevention (ICAP)
107 Gilbreth Parkway, Suite 200
Mullica Hill, NJ 08062
Toll-Free: 800-258-3189
Phone: 856-582-7000
Fax: 856-582-3588
Website: http://www.internationalcap.org
E-mail: childassaultprevention@gmail.com

The International Center for Assault Prevention (ICAP) is an international prevention program that works with individuals, groups, and communities who desire to advocate and protect children by starting a CAP project in their town. Training programs for various age groups, from preschool through the teens years, as well as training for adults, is available.

International Initiative to End Child Labor
1016 South Wayne Street, Suite 702
Arlington, VA 22204
Phone/Fax: 703-920-0435
Website: http://www.endchildlabor.org
E-mail: IIECL@endchildlabor.org

The International Initiative to End Child Labor was founded in 1998 to help eliminate child slavery, human trafficking in children, hazardous child labor, and the use of child labor in prostitution, soldiering, and illegal activities.

International Society for Prevention of Child Abuse and Neglect
13123 East 16th Avenue, B390
Aurora, CO 80045-7106
Phone: 303-864-5220
Fax: 303-864-5222
Website: http://www.ispcan.org
E-mail: ispcan@ispcan.org

The International Society for the Prevention of Child Abuse and Neglect (ISPCAN) is the only multidisciplinary international organization that brings together a global cross-section of committed professionals to work towards the prevention and treatment of child abuse, neglect, and exploitation. ISPCAN's mission is to prevent cruelty to children in every nation, in every form: physical abuse, sexual abuse, neglect, street children, child fatalities, child prostitution, children of war, emotional abuse, and child labor.

Jacob Wetterling Resource Center
2324 University Avenue W, Suite 105
St. Paul, MN 55114
Toll-Free: 800-325-HOPE (800-325-4673)
Phone: 651-714-4673
Fax: 651-714-9098
Website: http://www.jwrc.org

With a vision that every child grows up in a healthy, safe world free from exploitation and/or abduction, the Jacob Wetterling Resource Center (JWRC) focuses on educating families and communities to prevent the exploitation of children.

Kempe Foundation for the Prevention and Treatment of Child Abuse and Neglect
Anschutz Medical Campus, Gary Pavilion
13123 East 16th Avenue, B390
Aurora, CO 80045
Phone: 303-864-5250
Website (English): http://www.kempe.org
Website (Spanish): http://www.kempe.org/index.php?s=10667
E-mail: questions@kempe.org

The Kempe Children's Center is a clinically based resource providing training, consultation, program development and evaluation, and research in child abuse and neglect. The Center is committed to multidisciplinary approaches to the prevention, identification, and treatment of all forms of abuse and neglect. Kempe provides advanced training for front-line professionals who will subsequently become child abuse and neglect experts in their communities.

Kidpower Teenpower Fullpower International
P.O. Box 1212
Santa Cruz, CA 95061
Toll-Free: 800-467-6997
Website: http://www.kidpower.org
E-mail: safety@kidpower.org

Kidpower Teenpower Fullpower International (Kidpower works to create cultures of caring, respect, and safety for all. Its mission is to teach people of all ages and abilities, especially children in need, to use their power to stay safe, act wisely, and believe in themselves. Kidpower provides information, resources, and training on bullying prevention, child abuse prevention, stranger awareness, and personal safety for children, teens, and adults, including those with special needs.

Liberty House
2685 4th Street NE
Salem, OR 97301
Phone: 503-540-0288
Website: http://libertyhousecenter.org

Liberty House is a child abuse assessment center, offering services to children and families in Marion and Polk Counties (Oregon).

Massachusetts Children's Trust Fund
55 Court Street, 4th Floor
Boston, MA 02108
Toll-Free: 888-775-4KID (800-775-4543; Massachusetts only)
Phone: 617-727-8957
Fax: 617-727-8997
Website (English): http://www.onetoughjob.org
Website (Spanish): http://espanol.onetoughjob.org
E-mail: info@mctf.org

The Massachusetts Children's Trust Fund provides an online resource for parents through OneThoughJob.org. The website includes information about positive parenting, child development, family issues, and other common areas of concern.

Maternal Infant Health Outreach Worker Program
Center for Community Health Solutions
Vanderbilt University, Station 17
Nashville, TN 37232-8180
Phone: 615-322-4184
Fax: 615-343-0325
Website: http://www.mc.vanderbilt.edu/root/vumc.php?site=MIHOW

The Maternal Infant Health Outreach Worker Program, a partnership between Vanderbilt University and community-based organizations, seeks to identify disadvantaged families and provide parent-to-parent support through home visits and parenting groups.

National Alliance of Children's Trust and Prevention Funds
P.O. Box 15206
Seattle, WA 98115
Phone: 206-526-1221
Fax: 206-526-0220
Website: http://www.ctfalliance.org
E-mail: info@ctfalliance.org

The National Alliance of Children's Trust and Prevention Funds initiates and engages in national efforts that assist state Children's Trust and Prevention Funds in strengthening families to prevent child abuse and neglect. This includes promoting and supporting a system of services, laws, practices, and attitudes that supports families by enabling them to provide their children with a safe, healthy, and nurturing childhood.

National Association of State Mental Health Program Directors
66 Canal Center Plaza, Suite 302
Alexandria, VA 22314
Phone: 703-739-9333
Fax: 703-548-9517
Website: http://www.nasmhpd.org

The National Association of State Mental Health Program Directors is a national organization that provides advocacy for mental health agencies within the United States. Its goals include the delivery of person-centered and family-centered mental health services.

National Center for Mental Health Promotion and Youth Violence Prevention
Education Development Center, Inc.
43 Foundry Avenue
Waltham, MA 02453
Toll-Free: 877-217-3595
Fax: 617-969-5951
Website: http://www.promoteprevent.org
E-mail: info@promoteprevent.org

The National Center for Mental Health Promotion and Youth Violence Prevention offers assistance to school districts and communities to help foster mental wellbeing and prevent violence and behavior disorders among young people.

National Center for Missing and Exploited Children
Charles B. Wang International Children's Building
699 Prince Street
Alexandria, VA 22314-3175
Toll-Free: 800-THE-LOST (800-843-5678)
Phone: 703-224-2150
Fax: 703- 224-2122
Website: http://www.missingkids.com

The National Center for Missing and Exploited Children provides assistance to parents, children, law enforcement, schools, and the community in recovering missing children and raising public awareness about ways to help prevent child abduction, molestation, and sexual exploitation. The Center sponsors the CyberTipLine for online reporting of the sexual exploitation or molesting of children. One special program offered by the Center is the NetSmartz Workshops, for teaching internet safety.

National Center on Shaken Baby Syndrome
1433 North Highway 89, Suite 110
Farmington, UT 84025
Phone: 801-447-9360
Fax: 801-447-9364
Website: http://www.dontshake.org
E-mail: mail@dontshake.org

The National Center on Shaken Baby Syndrome offers information on shaken baby syndrome, shaken baby syndrome prevention programs, and training for professionals and parents nationwide. The Online Training Center contains three training modules: the Period of PURPLE Crying program overview, Basic Shaken Baby Syndrome (SBS/AHT) education, and Intermediate Shaken Baby Syndrome (SBS/AHT) education.

National Child Protection Training Center
Winona State University Campus
Maxwell Hall, 2nd Floor
Winona, MN 55987
Phone: 507-457-2890
Fax: 507-457-2899
Website: http://www.ncptc.org
E-mail: trainings@ncptc-jwrc.org

The National Child Protection Training Center strives to reduce and seek an end to child abuse, neglect, and all other forms of child maltreatment through education, training, awareness, prevention, and advocacy. The Center promotes reformation of current training practices by providing an educational curriculum to current and future front-line child protection professionals around the nation so that they will be prepared to recognize and report the abuse of a child.

National Children's Advocacy Center
210 Pratt Avenue
Huntsville, AL 35801
Phone: 256-533-KIDS (256-533-5437)

Fax: 256-534-6883
Website: http://www.nationalcac.org
E-mail: intervention@nationalcac.org

The National Children's Advocacy Center (NCAC) provides prevention, intervention, and treatment services to physically and sexually abused children and their families with a child-focused team approach. NCAC also operates the Southern Regional Children's Advocacy Center, which provides education and training to support the development of Children's Advocacy Centers nationwide. The NCAC is one of the providers of training for professionals working with abused children and their families. These trainings are both multidisciplinary and discipline-specific.

National Children's Alliance
516 C Street NE
Washington, DC 20002
Toll-Free: 800-239-9950
Phone: 202-548-0090
Fax: 202-548-0099
Website: http://www.nationalchildrensalliance.org

The National Children's Alliance, a professional membership organization, works to help communities and local child advocacy centers in their efforts to respond to, investigate, and prosecute cases of child abuse.

National Coalition to Prevent Child Sexual Abuse and Exploitation
Website: http://www.preventtogether.org
E-mail: PreventTogether@gmail.com

The mission of the National Coalition to Prevent Child Sexual Abuse and Exploitation is to promote the healthy development of children and youth, and prevent and end their sexual abuse and exploitation.

National Council on Child Abuse and Family Violence
1025 Connecticut Avenue NW, Suite 1000
Washington, DC 20036
Phone: 202-429-6695
Fax: 202-521-3479
Website: http://www.nccafv.org
E-mail: info@nccafv.org

The National Council on Child Abuse and Family Violence is a non-profit organization serving as a private sector response to the problems of child, spousal, and elderly abuse. The Council's primary purpose is to strengthen, professionally and practically, community child abuse and family violence prevention and treatment programs nationwide. A broad range of activities is included in the Council's three major program areas: public awareness and education, professional development, and organizational development.

National Indian Child Welfare Association
5100 SW Macadam Avenue, Suite 300
Portland, OR 97239
Phone: 503-222-4044
Fax: 503-222-4007
Website: http://www.nicwa.org
E-mail: info@nicwa.org

The National Indian Child Welfare Association (NICWA) functions as the only Native American organization focused specifically on issues of child abuse and neglect and tribal capacity to prevent and respond effectively to these problems. NICWA provides workshops and training programs, using culturally appropriate resources, including training materials, curricula, and books. NICWA also offers technical assistance and training on child care, family preservation, and substance abuse.

National Parent Helpline
Parents Anonymous, Inc.
981 Corporate Center Drive, Suite 100
Pomona, CA 91768
Toll-Free: 855-4-A-PARENT (855-427-2736)
Phone: 909-621-6184
Website: http://www.nationalparenthelpline.org
E-mail: info@nationalparenthelpline.org

The National Parent Helpline, operated by Parents Anonymous Inc., is a new resource for parents and caregivers of children all across America. When parents reach out and call the National Parent Helpline, a trained Helpline Advocate will provide them with emotional support and link them to a wide range of services, if necessary.

NetSafeKids
Computer Science and Telecommunications Board
The National Academies
500 Fifth Street NW
Washington, DC 20001

Phone: 202-334-2605
Fax: 202-334-2318
Website: http://www.nap.edu/netsafekids
E-mail: cstb@nas.edu

NetSafeKids, sponsored by the National Academy of Sciences, is a resource for concerned parents regarding child safety and the internet. It provides practical information and tips on types and sources of sexually explicit content, ways that inappropriate material can reach children and teens, the threat of cyberstalking, the pros and cons of filtering and monitoring tools, and other issues involving internet safety.

Office for Victims of Crime

U.S. Department of Justice
810 Seventh Street NW, Eighth Floor
Washington, DC 20531
Phone: 202-307-5983
Fax: 202-514-6383
Website: http://www.ovc.gov

The Office for Victims of Crime, a component of the Office of Justice Programs of the U.S. Department of Justice, offers information and services to crime victims, including a Directory of Crime Victim Services, which can be downloaded through a link available at ovc.ncjrs .gov/findvictimservices.

Parents Anonymous, Inc.

981 Corporate Center Drive, Suite 100
Pomona, CA 91768
Phone: 909-236-5757
Fax: 909-236-5758
Website: http://www.parentsanonymous.org
National Parent Helpline: http://www.nationalparenthelpline.org
E-mail: Parentsanonymous@parentsanonymous.org

Parents Anonymous Inc. is a family strengthening organization dedicated to the prevention of child abuse and neglect. Parents Anonymous Inc. operates numerous programs and initiatives, including an international Network of accredited organizations that implement Parents Anonymous groups and complementary children and youth programs based on a mutual support-shared leadership model. In addition, Parents Anonymous provides many services, including specialized trainings, customized technical assistance, public awareness and outreach strategies, and evaluation services to states, counties, and community-based organizations on a wide range of topics related to children and families.

Parents for Megan's Law and the Crime Victims Center
Toll-Free: 888-ASK-PFML (888-275-7365)
Phone: 631-689-2672
Website (English): http://www.parentsformeganslaw.org/welcome.jsp
Website (Spanish): http://www.parentsformeganslaw.org/public/
paraEspanoleOprime.html
E-mail: pfmeganslaw@aol.com

Parents for Megan's Law and the Crime Victims Center (PFML/CVC) provide national Helpline community support and assistance on issues related to Megan's Law, sex offender management, and sexual assault prevention. PFML/CVC is funded by the U.S. Justice Department to staff the National Megan's Law Helpline to support the community when sex offender notifications are implemented and to provide appropriate law enforcement referrals when registrants are failing to comply with registration requirements or are in positions of trust which may pose a risk to public safety.

Prevent Child Abuse America
228 South Wabash Avenue, 10th Floor
Chicago, IL 60604
Phone: 312-663-3520
Fax: 312-939-8962
Website: http://www.preventchildabuse.org
E-mail: mailbox@preventchildabuse.org

Prevent Child Abuse America (PCAA) is committed to promoting legislation, policies, and programs that help prevent child abuse and neglect, support healthy childhood development, and strengthen families. Working with state chapters, PCCA provides leadership to promote and implement prevention efforts at the national and local levels.

Rape, Abuse and Incest National Network (RAINN)
2000 L Street NW, Suite 406
Washington, DC 20036
Toll-Free: 800-656-HOPE (800-656-4673)
Phone: 202-544-3064
Fax: 202-544-3556
Website: http://www.rainn.org
E-mail: info@rainn.org

Rape, Abuse and Incest National Network (RAINN) provides help to people who have experienced sexual assault. Services include the National Sexual Assault Hotline (800-656-HOPE) and the National Sexual Assault Online Hotline (http://online.rainn.org). In addition, RAINN provides resources and educational materials to media, policymakers, law enforcement personnel, and others.

Safe4Athletes

P.O. Box 650
Santa Monica, CA 90406
Phone: 855-SAFE-4-AA (855-723-3422)
Website: http://safe4athletes.org
E-mail: info@safe4athletes.org

Safe4Athletes works to help ensure that sports organizations provide programs that are free of inappropriate behaviors including sexual misconduct, bullying, and harassment.

Safe Child Program

Coalition for Children, Inc.
P.O. Box 6304
Denver, CO 80206
Phone: 303-320-6328
Fax: 303-809-6328
Website: http://www.safechild.org
E-mail: info@safechild.org

The Safe Child Program is a curriculum which teaches prevention of sexual, emotional, and physical abuse by people known to the child; prevention of abuse and abduction by strangers; and safety in self-care. Presented in a preschool through third grade series, it teaches a broad base of life skills.

Safer Society Foundation, Inc.

P.O. Box 340
Brandon, VT 05733-0340
Phone: 802-247-3132
Fax: 802-247-4233
Website: http://www.safersociety.org

The Safer Society Foundation, Inc., a nonprofit agency, is a national research, advocacy, and referral center on the prevention and treatment of sexual abuse. The Foundation provides training and consultation, research, sex offender treatment referrals, a computerized program network, and a resource library. It also publishes materials for the prevention and treatment of sexual abuse. The Safer Society will help individuals, agencies, states, and organizations develop specialized training institutes on current and emerging topics related to sexual abuse prevention and treatment.

Sexuality Information and Education Council of the United States (SIECUS)
90 John Street, Suite 402
New York, NY 10038
Phone: 212-819-9770
Fax: 212-819-9776
Website: http://www.siecus.org

The Sexuality Information and Education Council of the United States (SIECUS) was founded during the 1960s in response to a concern that young people and adults lacked accurate information about sexuality. It works to provide fact-based information about healthy sexuality to teens, families, educators, and policymakers.

Stop It Now!
351 Pleasant Street, Suite B-319
Northampton, MA 01060
Toll-Free: 888-PREVENT (888-773-8368)
Phone: 413-587-3500
Fax: 413-587-3505
Website: http://www.StopItNow.org
E-mail: info@stopitnow.org

Stop It Now! prevents the sexual abuse of children by mobilizing adults, families, and communities to take action before a child is harmed. Stop It Now! provides support, information and resources for adults to take responsibility for creating safer communities.

Stop The Silence, Inc.
P.O. Box 127
Glenn Dale, MD 20769
Phone: 301-464-4791
Website: http://www.stopcsa.org

The mission of Stop the Silence is to increase awareness about and conduct programming to address the prevention and treatment of child sexual abuse, and to address the relationships between this issue and the broader issues of overall family and community violence.

Substance Abuse and Mental Health Services Administration
SAMHSA's Health Information Network
P.O. Box 2345
Rockville, MD 20847-2345
Toll-Free: 877-SAMHSA-7 (877-726-4727)
Toll-Free TTY: 800-487-4889
Phone: 240-221-4036
Fax: 240-221-4292
Website: http://store.samhsa.gov
E-mail: SAMHSAInfo@samhsa.hhs.gov

The Substance Abuse and Mental Health Services Administration's (SAMHSA) mission is to reduce the impact of substance abuse and mental illness on America's communities. The Center for Mental Health Services focuses on the prevention and treatment of mental disorders. The Center for Behavioral Health Statistics and Quality has primary responsibility for the collection, analysis and dissemination of behavioral health data. Other Centers seek to prevent and reduce substance abuse and to support effective treatment and recovery services.

Survivors of Incest Anonymous
World Service Office
P.O. Box 190
Benson, MD 21018-9998
Phone: 410-893-3322
Website: http://www.siawso.org

Survivors of Incest Anonymous provides referrals to self-help groups and other information to adults who experienced sexual abuse during childhood.

Wind and Fire Missions Base
(Formerly Center to Restore Trafficked and Exploited Children)
P.O. Box 126
Hiawatha, IA 52233
Phone: 319-294-5307
Fax: 319-892-0203
Website: http://wfmmissionsbase.org/
E-mail: info@windandfire.org

The vision of Wind and Fire Missions Base is to provide a safe environment for trafficked children to heal and be restored so that they have every opportunity to live as healthy children in a safe community.

This vision will be accomplished through the efforts of staff and community service providers advocating on behalf of trafficked children and utilizing human trafficking prevention and intervention tools and resources to heal and restore children and families.

Witness Justice
P.O. Box 2516
Rockville, MD 20847-2516
Phone: 301-846-9110
Website: http://witnessjustice.org
E-mail: info@witnessjustice.org

Witness Justice is a nationwide, nonprofit organization that works to help victims of violence find sources of information and support.

Index

Index

Page numbers followed by 'n' indicate a footnote. Page numbers in *italics* indicate a table or illustration.

family preservation
  services, defined 563
family support services,
  defined 563
family therapy
  described 433
  sexual behavior problems 554
family violence, defined 562
Federal Family Educational
  Rights and Privacy Act
  (FERPA; 1974) 413
Federal Trade Commission
  (FTC), online protection
  publication 287n
fetal alcohol spectrum
  disorders (FASD)
  childhood behavior 488–89
  defined 563
  parental substance abuse 480
Fight Crime: Invest in Kids,
  contact information 590
filicide
  versus homicide 41–44
  overview 39–41
financial considerations
  adoption 525
  child abuse 125
  emotional abuse 265–66
  sexual abuse 158
  truancy reduction 259–60
"Finding Care and Support"
  (ASCA) 445n
Finkelhor, David 57n
first responders, child abuse
  identification 135–39
Florida
  child abuse reporting
    contact information 572
  clergy mandatory
    reporting *399*, 400
  reporting
    requirements 390, 391, 397
  sexual age of consent *176*
  statutory rape legislation 182, *191*
foster care
  child maltreatment 56
  defined 563
  described 427–28
  see also therapeutic foster care

foster children
  adoption transition 533–44
  defined 563
foster parents
  adoption 524–32
  defined 564
"Foster parents considering
  adoption" (Child Welfare
  Information Gateway) 524n
Freddie Mac Foundation,
  contact information 591
friends, sexual behavior
  problems 551
FTC *see* Federal Trade
  Commission
Future of Children, contact
  information 591

G

gender factor
  child maltreatment 46
  domestic violence 460
General Federation
  of Women's Clubs,
  contact information 591
Generation Five,
  contact information 592
Georgia
  child abuse reporting
    contact information 572
  clergy mandatory
    reporting *399*, 400
  reporting requirements 396
  sexual age of consent *176*
  statutory rape legislation 181,
    186–89
global neglect, described 116–17
"Glossary" (Child Welfare
  Information Gateway) 559n
group homes
  defined 564
  foster care 427
group therapy, sexual
  behavior problems 554
Guam, clergy mandatory
  reporting *399*
guardian ad litem (GAL),
  defined 564
guardianship, defined 564

Y, Z